FAMILIAL BRAIN TUMOURS

A Commented Register

DEVELOPMENTS IN ONCOLOGY 9

Other titles in this series:

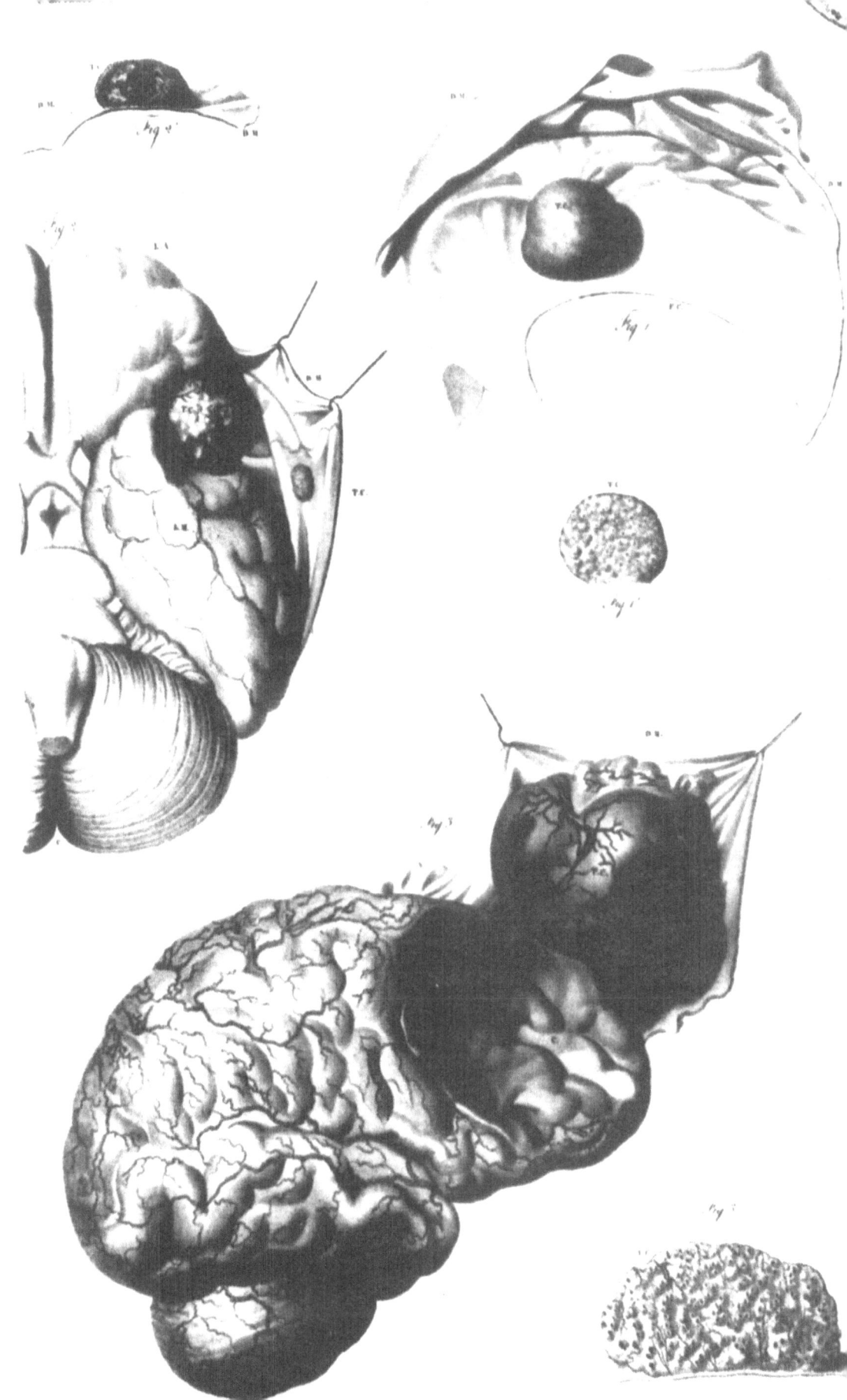

The frontispiece is a reproduction of the coloured lithograph
illustrating fascicle 8 of Jean Cruveilhier's famous atlas
Anatomie pathologique du corps humain (J.B. Baillière, Paris,
1835-1842). Figure 3 clearly represents a meningioma.

(Courtesy of the Bibliothèque Charcot,
Paris)

Authors' note:

Examples of other early representations of tumours such as
pontine glioma and pontine angle tumour are found in Charles
Bell's The nervous system of the human body (Longmans, London,
1830). Possibly the earliest drawing of an (unspecified) brain
tumour ever published may be found in V. Chiarugi's Della pazzia
in genere (L. Carlieri, Firenze, 1794).

FAMILIAL BRAIN TUMOURS
A Commented Register

Cornelis C. Tijssen, M.D.
Department of Neurology
Municipal Hospitals / The Hague, The Netherlands

Michael R. Halprin, M.D.
Psychiatric Hospital Rosenburg
The Hague, The Netherlands

Lambertus J. Endtz, M.D.
Department of Neurology
Municipal Hospitals / The Hague, The Netherlands

with an introductory chapter by

F.J. Cleton, M.D.
Professor of Medical Oncology
University of Leyden / Leyden, The Netherlands

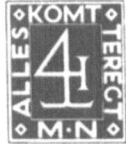

1982

Martinus Nijhoff Publishers
The Hague / Boston / London

VI

Distributors:

for the United States and Canada

Kluwer Boston, Inc.
190 Old Derby Street
Hingham, MA 02043
USA

for all other countries

Kluwer Academic Publishers Group
Distribution Center
P.O. Box 322
3300 AH Dordrecht
The Netherlands

Library of Congress Cataloging in Publication Data   CIP

```
Tijssen, Cornelis C.
   Familial brain tumours.

   (Developments in oncology ; v. 9)
   1. Brain--Tumors--Genetic aspects.  2. Familial
diseases.  I. Halprin, Michael R.  II. Endtz,
Lambertus J.  III. Title.  IV. Series.
[DNLM: 1. Brain neoplasms--Familial and genetic
--Case studies.  2. Registries.  Wl DE998N v. 9 /
WL 358 T568f]
RC280.B7T54  1982      616.99'481042      82-14149
ISBN-13: 978-94-009-7602-3    e-ISBN-13: 978-94-009-7600-9
DOI: 10.1007/978-94-009-7600-9
```

TABLE OF CONTENTS

Preface

Heredity, environment, the role of infectious agents, and other influences
have been cited within a multiplicity of factors of possible relevance to the
problem of neoplasm etiology. In some cases, such as that of retinoblastoma
the influence of hereditary factors has been clearly established. The influence
of genetic factors in cerebral tumour development has been under discussion
since as early as 1896 when Besold reported two sisters suffering from brain
tumours. Although much more is now known about the classification, prognosis,
and treatment of these tumours, and a number of familial cases have been
reported, the present data are insufficient to permit conclusions regarding
the influence of hereditary factors in the etiology of most types of cerebral
neoplasms, and research in this area is urgently required.

Research on familial brain tumours must still be largely based upon the
cumulative case histories which have been reported. Although a number of papers
contain historical reviews, some in tabulated form, the actual data have not
been readily available to the researcher, each investigator being obliged to
compile anew all reports published on the subject over an 80 year period.

This book represents an attempt by the present authors to assemble the
pertinent data on individual cases of familial brain tumours published since
1896. For this purpose the essential information from the original articles
in German, French, Dutch, Spanish, Italian, Polish, and Czechoslovakian have
been translated into English. Exact quotations from reports in the English
language have been presented here in italics to facilitate the flow of reading
of the material. Relevant material relating to the original reports, i.e.
reproductions of anatomical specimens, pedigrees, et cetera have been repro-
duced where possible. The surname of the first author, the author's location,
and the year of publication have been used as a reference heading for each
case report. If not specified, the nationality of the patient has been assumed
to be in conformity with that of the country of publication. Special attention
has been given to the presence or absence of data providing validation of the
diagnosis in each case. This, as well as the available information concerning
hereditary influence and other aspects of relevance, has been noted in the
case comments. In the description of the case reports and the tables the
diagnoses are presented as stated by the authors; in the discussions on

familial aspects they have been adapted, when relevant, to the present classification of the World Health Organization.

Where possible, an attempt has been made to supplement existing information
by requesting authors of publications to submit additional data (see standard
request form as addendum). In this manner a number of new familial cases have
been collected from The Netherlands and are published here as personal communi-
cations.

Six groups of brain tumours have been examined: medulloblastoma, meningioma,
choroid plexus papilloma, cerebral fibrosarcoma, pinealoma, and glioma. The
reports on familial occurrence have been subdivided into brain tumours occurring
in twins, siblings, and more than one generation. The reports were designated as
concordant when the brain tumours in relatives were verified histologically or
at autopsy. Cases not meeting these criteria were regarded as discordant. In
each chapter a short summary of the general aspects of the involved tumour group
has been given, without pretence of being complete, intended for the more generally interested reader in the fields of neurology, neurosurgery, oncology, and
genetics. An introductory chapter on general hereditary factors in oncology has
been provided by Professor F.J. Cleton.

This book does not lead to definite conclusions as to the validity of a
genetic basis for the occurrence of brain tumours. Its main purpose has been to
constitute a body of actual knowledge concerning cases in which familial occurrence was noted and therefore it must be essentially regarded as a working tool
for research. The present data do seem to indicate promising results for future
studies of genetic influence in the etiology of glioma. Compilation of further
reports will be required before a sufficient amount of information is available
to support evaluative attempts in regard to these or other neoplasms. For this
reason a permanent International Register of Familial Brain Tumours (IRFBT) is
to be established in the Comprehensive Cancer Centre in Leyden[*]. The IRFBT will
be engaged in the active search for newly published cases of familial brain
tumours and will invite clinicians worldwide to submit cases to this register.
Care will be taken to update the register at appropriate times.

The project executor for this book was C.C. Tijssen, M.D., with the assistance of M.R. Halprin, M.D., who also wrote the chapters on cerebral fibrosarcoma
and pinealoma and was responsible for the English language supervision, and
L.J. Endtz, M.D., responsible for general supervision and editing.

---

[*] Address Comprehensive Cancer Centre: Vondellaan 47,
2332 AA Leyden, The Netherlands

Acknowledgements

The authors would like to express their gratitude to a number of persons for their invaluable assistance and contributions:

Professor F.J. Cleton, M.D., medical oncologist at the University of Leyden, for writing an introductory chapter on general aspects of hereditary factors in oncology;

Professor G.T.A.M. Bots, M.D., neuropathologist at the University of Leyden, for permission to use his photographs of macroscopic and microscopic preparations;

R.E.M. Hekster, M.D., neuroradiologist at the Municipal Hospitals of The Hague, for selecting and providing the computerized tomography (made with a General Electric CT/T 8800 scanner);

J. te Velde, M.D., pathologist at the Municipal Hospitals of The Hague, for his critical reading of the general aspects;

C. Fortgens, medical physicist, for assisting in the statistical evaluation.

We are indebted to our colleagues of the neurological department for the cooperation that made the realization of this book possible.

Some of the case reports have been illustrated by use of the original material. We thank the authors concerned for their permission in the use of these photographs.

Technical assistance was given by C.Th. Ruygrock and C.A. van Beek in the preparation of the photographs, and by C.H. Bootsma and A.R. Rensen in the drawing of the pedigrees.

Our special thanks to Mrs. A.M. Henkus. The preparation of this book would not have been possible without her efficient and conscientious secretarial assistance. Mrs. J.E.M. Mol assisted in typing the references.

We would also like to express our gratitude to the staff of Martinus Nijhoff Publishers for their patient and supportive literary collaboration.

This work was supported by a grant from the Queen Wilhelmina Cancer Foundation.

Chapter I

GENERAL ASPECTS OF HEREDITARY FACTORS IN ONCOLOGY

by F.J. Cleton, M.D.

Professor of Medical Oncology,
University of Leyden, The Netherlands

The exact cause of cancer is not known, but considerable evidence has been accumulated in favour of the somatic mutation hypothesis. This means that a genetic change in somatic cells is thought to be the initiating event in the origin of cancer. Both environmental and constitutional factors are involved in the origin of cancer. It has been estimated that 80 percent of human cancer is determined by the environment via ionizing radiation, ultraviolet light, chemical carcinogens and dietary factors. This hypothesis is supported by the finding of large geographic differences in the frequency of certain tumour types. The convenient term for the sum of these factors is 'life style'.

The first lesion in the multiple step process that leads to the malignant transformation of a cell is probably located in the DNA molecule. When this change is not repaired, the change in the genetic information will be transmitted to daughter cells (somatic mutation).

Most known carcinogens are indeed mutagenic substances. In a similar manner oncogenic viruses can introduce changes in DNA by the insertion of new nuclear acids into the genome. Most carcinogens can induce the initiation step towards malignant transformation. Different substances (promotors) are needed to cause proliferation of the initiated cells. Examples are phorbolesters (tar), hormones, effect of viral infection and repeated mechanical trauma.

The proliferating initiated cells show a loss of differentiation and after many divisions more defects can be the result of the first trauma. Some of these effects may be epigenetic and not be directly caused by the somatic mutation. In most carcinogenic processes multiple steps are necessary to produce a full carcinogenic effect, involving many stimulating and permitting factors. This process may take many years, as is well demonstrated by the late effects of radiation.

Our interest is also directed to the target of this carcinogenic action, the cell. The genetic background of the cells can interfere with the mutation process. Differences in DNA repair mechanisms, metabolic activation of carcinogenic substances and immune-resistance all play a role in the origin of a tumour. There is evidence from cytogenetic studies that somatic mutations can occur at specific sites. The first known example is the Philadelphia chromosome (Ph[1]), which results from a translocation between chromosome 22 and usually chromosome 9. Less consistent changes have been described for several lymphomas including Burkitt's lymphoma, acute leukaemias and renal carcinoma. If such lesions are associated with the appearance of a neoplastic clone of cells and if these lesions are specific for any type of human cancer, there may be more than a hundred cancer genes.

Knudson (1) has stated that virtually every human cancer exists in a dominantly heritable form as well as in a non-hereditary form. The two most well-known examples are retinoblastoma (40% hereditary) and carcinoma of the colon. The latter tumour may originate from polyposis coli, a dominantly hereditary disease with a high penetrance, from familial colon polyps or occur as a non-hereditary condition. More than one gene may be involved in the carcinogenic event. In familial pheochromocytoma, two varieties can be recognized, one associated with medullary thyroid cancer and one which is not. The hypothesis put forward by Knudson is that cancer results from mutation at 100 - 200 human cancer genes. In the hereditary forms of cancer the first mutation occurs in a germinal cell and somatic mutations later occur at the same site. In non-hereditary cancer multiple mutations of somatic cells are needed for malignant transformation. In clinical studies of members of pedigrees of families with a hereditary form of cancer, developmental defects have been found in the target tissues in constitutional heterozygotes. This could mean that the alleles of the so-called cancer genes are important in tissue differentiation. Hyperplasia of undifferentiated cells may be pre-neoplastic lesions, susceptible for carcinogenic (mutagenic) agents.

More than a thousand proved single gene traits are listed in the catalogue 'Mendelian inheritance in man' (2); about 9% of these conditions are associated with cancer (3). Only a few cancers show a clear-cut pattern of inheritance. Most of these tumours show an autosomal dominant inheritance pattern (polyposis coli, retinoblastoma, Sipple's syndrome); some show autosomal recessive inheritance (xeroderma pigmentosa, Bloom's syndrome, ataxia telangiectasia) and a few a sex-linked recessive inheritance. The majority of cancers occur as sporadic cases. The risk of individuals belonging to a retinoblastoma family may be increased over the risk of the normal population by a factor of 100,000.
In the so-called sporadic cases of cancer the relative risk for first-degree relatives is usually in the order of 2 - 3 times that of the normal population.

It has been argued by Peto (4) that the ratio of the risk in susceptible individuals to that in non-susceptibles may be more than 10 times greater.

Such differences do not appear in the classical studies of siblings or even in twin partners of cancer patients. The study of cancer in twins has provided little evidence for inherited differences in susceptibility for cancer. These studies will have to be repeated with the modern tools that are now available for linkage studies.

The classical epidemiological studies of familial cancer are often difficult to interpret. In most studies genetic factors have not been taken into account and the genetic studies are influenced by environmental variations. In studies of common tumours, such as breast cancer, a familial aggregation may easily occur by chance. It is therefore necessary to carry out detailed genetic investigations such as analysis of linkage with known genetic markers. This is the only conclusive evidence for the presence of a major gene. Presently this type of analysis has yielded little information for gene mapping. Recent advances in recombinant DNA technology may give us the solution to this problem using DNA polymorphisms obtained with restriction enzymes (5).

The tumours of the central nervous system are of particular interest with regard to genetics for several reasons. It has already been mentioned that many tumours with a dominant pattern of heredity are often associated with changes in the differentiation of tissues. There is a long list of congenital malformations associated with CNS tumours, including medulloblastoma with gastrointestinal and genitourinary system anomalies and glioblastoma with arteriovenous malformations. CNS tumours are also frequently associated with genetic disorders such as the phacomatoses (tuberous sclerosis, Von Hippel-Lindau's disease, Sturge-Weber disease and multiple basal cell naevus syndrome) and Von Recklinghausen's disease. A different type of association may relate to immunological susceptibility to cancer. In this respect two disorders of genetic origin, the Wiskott Aldrich syndrome (recurrent bacterial infections, thrombocytopenia and eczema) a defect in both humoral and cellular immunity exists. Primary malignant lymphoma of the brain has been reported several times in this rare syndrome. Patients with ataxia telangiectasia may present with medulloblastoma of the cerebellum or glioma. Apart from these associations several families with multiple cases of CNS tumours have been described. The important question of increased genetic susceptibility versus increased exposure to environmental carcinogenic factors should again be raised and the possibility of transplacental carcinogenesis should be entertained.

The application of modern techniques in cytogenetics of human tumours has revealed that many tumours are characterized by specific non random abnormal chromosome patterns. In meningiomas, about one third of the tumours with aberrations show a loss of one chromosome in addition to the characteristic monosomy or deletion of one chromosome 22. The biological importance of such chromosome changes in tumour formation is not yet known.

The genetic basis of human cancer is still not clear. There are several well defined dominant types of cancer, but the gene or genes involved in the origin of these tumours have not yet been defined or located. There is ample evidence that most forms of cancer can occur in a hereditary form. The risk of family members of cancer patients is usually increased above that of the normal population. This risk may be severely underestimated for the susceptible individuals in the family. It may be important to recognize these susceptible persons. In some dominant forms of cancer, like polyposis coli, preventive colon surgery has been successful in eliminating the tumours. Studies of familial cancer including modern linkage analysis techniques may locate certain cancer susceptibility genes and enable us to detect the susceptible individuals. The present register may encourage clinical investigators to undertake such studies.

REFERENCES

1.   KNUDSON AG, STRONG LC, ANDERSON DE   1973
        Heredity and cancer in man.
        Prog Med Genet 9:113-158
2.   McKUSICK VA   1974
        Mendelian inheritance in man.
        The John Hopkins Press, Baltimore
3.   MULVIHILL JJ   1977
        Genetic repertory of human neoplasia.
        In: Mulvihill JJ, Fraumeni JF (eds) Genetics of Human Cancer.
        Raven Press, New York
4.   PETO J   1980
        Genetic predisposition to cancer.
        In: Banbury report 4. Cancer incidence in defined populations.
        Cold Spring Harbor Laboratory
5.   WHITE R   1980
        In search of DNA polymorphism in humans.
        In: Banbury report 4. Cancer incidence in defined populations.
        Cold Spring Harbor Laboratory

Chapter II

FAMILIAL MEDULLOBLASTOMA

CASE REPORTS

CLASSIFICATION

A. *TWINS*

    1. Monozygotic twins with concordant tumour

    2. Monozygotic twins with discordant tumour

    3. Monozygotic twins, one demonstrating medulloblastoma

    4. Dizygotic twins

B. *SIBLINGS*

    1. Siblings with concordant tumour

    2. Siblings with discordant tumour

C. *OTHER GENERATIONS AND DISTANT RELATIVES*

    1. Other generations and distant relatives with concordant tumour

    2. Other generations and distant relatives with discordant tumour

TABLES

II.A.   *TWINS*

II.A.1.   MONOZYGOTIC TWINS WITH CONCORDANT TUMOUR

II.A.1.1. Griepentrog and Pauly 1957 - Berlin, Germany (31)

Monozygotic twins. Female. German.

Case 1

History: The patient was born in breech presentation with a birthweight of
4000 g. At birth there was an irregular tumour in the left supra- and infra-
clavicular region, which lead to a hypotone paresis of the left arm 10 days
before death. At the age of 8 weeks the patient was taken to hospital because
of the sudden occurrence of high fever. A few hours later she died unexpectedly.
There were no cerebral symptoms. X-thorax showed an unhomogeneous process in
the upper part of the lung.

Autopsy: In the left clavicular region a tumour was found which had grown
into the left plexus brachialis and into the upper part of the left lung.
Metastases were present in the left lymph nodules of the neck, in the right
kidney and in the left adrenal gland.
A brain tumour the size of a walnut was also found. It was located in the
fourth ventricle and was growing into the right cerebellar hemisphere. There
was serious oedema of the brain.

Microscopic study: The brain tumour was composed of undifferentiated cells
with oval or round nuclei and weak protoplasm forming a sort of network. The
cells were lying close to each other, in groups or in series. Several small
areas of necrosis of tumour tissue were seen. There was growth into the brain
tissue in several areas. A diagnosis of medulloblastoma was made.
Histology of the breast tumour revealed a large teratoid tumour with parts of
medulloblastoma tissue.

Diagnosis: Cerebellar medulloblastoma. Teratoid tumour with medulloblastoma
tissue in the left clavicular region.

Case 2

History: At birth a left-sided facial nerve paralysis existed. In the last
weeks before death there was a rapid increase of head circumference from 32 to
40 cm. The patient died at 11 weeks of age.
An unusual haematological differentiation was noted with 22% eosinophils.

<u>Autopsy</u>: A brain tumour was found the size of a walnut, partly necrotic, partly haemorrhagic in the fourth ventricle with infiltration into the cerebellum. Occlusion of the mesencephalic aqueduct by fresh bleeding from the tumour existed with a serious internal hydrocephalus.

<u>Microscopic study</u>: Histologically this tumour had the same appearance as the tumour of case 1. It was composed of undifferentiated cells with oval to round nuclei, varying little in size, and weak protoplasm formed as a network.

<u>Diagnosis</u>: Cerebellar medulloblastoma.

<u>Family</u>:

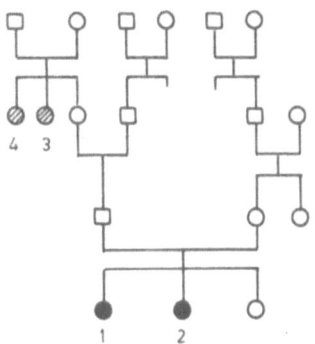

1 = case 1

2 = case 2

3 = grand-aunt, she was a dwarf of 1 m length and died at 16 years of age from a kidney disease

4 = grand-aunt, she died suddenly as a baby of unknown cause

<u>COMMENT</u>

Unfortunately microscopic studies of the right kidney and left adrenal were not performed. The question as to the metastatic character of the medulloblastoma remained open. The assumption seemed more probable that these tumour elements were primary extracranial tumours, or primary components of the teratoid.

These twins are the same as those reported by Zülch (95) in his 'Handbuch der Neurochirurgie' on page 120.

II.A.1.2. Waldbaur et al. 1976 - Erlangen, Germany (88)

Monozygotic twins. Female. German.
Identical bloodtypes. Normal pregnancy.

Case 1

History: The patient was born in cephalic presentation with the use of a vacuum extractor. The apgar score was 10. Her birthweight was 2490 g and length 44 cm. She had a normal growth.

At the age of 4 1/2 months the patient was taken to hospital because of paleness and vomiting. Her physical condition had declined and she was dehydrated. On examination the patient was soporific. The pupils showed isocoria with normal reaction. She had hypotonic muscles and tendon reflexes were absent. There was a hip-joint dysplasia on both sides. Ophthalmological investigations were normal until a few days before death, when retinal bleedings were seen. Radiographs of the skull were normal, but the EEG showed slow waves over the left hemisphere, and echography a displacement of the median structures 1 to 2 mm to the right. A brain scan was suspect for higher activity on the left side. Cerebrospinal fluid showed a pleiocytosis with an elevated protein content and a low pressure.

During her stay in the hospital the patient continued vomiting. She had generalized convulsions and respiration difficulties. Artificial respiration was necessary. She died at 5 months of age.

Autopsy: There was serious general brain oedema, but no herniation. The ventricle system was normal. In the left cerebellar hemisphere a tumour the size of a cherry was found. It consisted of dark brown friable material. There was a connection between the tumour and the fourth ventricle, where also dark brown, friable tissue parts were found.

Microscopic study: A cell-rich tumour was seen, consisting of little cells often without a nucleus and several others with round, oval or bean-shaped nuclei full of chromatin. Many mitoses were present. Now and then cells were shaped as pseudo-rosettes. The central part of the tumour was necrotic. Diffuse infiltration of the subarachnoid space with tumour cells existed.

Diagnosis: Medulloblastoma of the cerebellum. Metastasis in the subarachnoid space.

Case 2

History: The patient was born in transverse presentation by manual extraction. Her birthweight was 2190 g, length 44 cm and apgar score 8. She had a normal

growth. At 7 weeks she demonstrated anaemia, which was treated with iron
injections. At the age of 5 months a hip-joint dysplasia on both sides was
discovered and treated with a pelvic plaster. At the age of 16 months the
patient was taken to hospital because of vomiting.

On examination the patient was mentally and physically retarded. There was a
progressive decline of consciousness. She had extensor-spasms. Later she lost
consciousness, was hypotonic and showed a low reaction to pain stimuli.
Ophthalmological examination revealed bilateral signs of papilloedema. The EEG
was diffusely abnormal and the echo showed serious ventricle enlargement. At
ventriculography in the pinealis region a tumour mass in the dorsal, upper part
of the third ventricle was seen. There was compression of the mesencephalic
aqueduct by the tumour.

The tumour was inoperable and palliative cerebrospinal fluid drainage was
applied. Nevertheless there was no improvement in her clinical state. Artificial respiration was necessary. The patient died at the age of 16 months.

Autopsy: Slight general signs of brain oedema were present. A tumour the
size of a plum was found in the epiphysis with some bleeding and necrosis. The
front half was lying in the third ventricle. There was compression of the
mesencephalic aqueduct. The lateral ventricles were moderately enlarged.

Microscopic study: A cell-rich tumour was seen, most cells without nucleus,
lying in an irregular structure close to each other. In some areas tumour cells
formed pseudo-rosettes. The nuclei were round, oval or bean-shaped, and full of
chromatin. Many mitoses were present. The central parts of the tumour were
necrotic. There was infiltration of the thalamus and hypothalamus.

Diagnosis: Pineoblastoma or undifferentiated pinealis tumour with medulloblastoma character.

Family: The family history revealed no nervous system disorders. There was
no consanguinity. The parents were healthy. The twins had two brothers and one
sister, all healthy. The mother had had four abortions.

1   = case 1
2   = case 2
3 - 6 = abortions

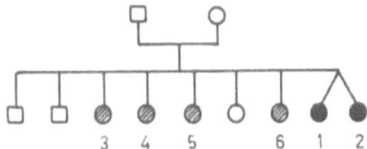

COMMENT

In the article it is stressed that the tumours were perhaps not concordant in regard to localization but, according to the authors, concordant as regards histological examination. Generally there is little difference between the histological features of pineoblastoma and medulloblastoma. For this reason we have classified this report among the concordant tumours.

II.A.2.   MONOZYGOTIC TWINS WITH DISCORDANT TUMOUR

II.A.2.1. <u>Leavitt 1928 - Philadelphia, U.S.A.</u> (44)

Identical twins. Male. American.
Normal birth, growth and development. Birthweight 2.4 kg each.

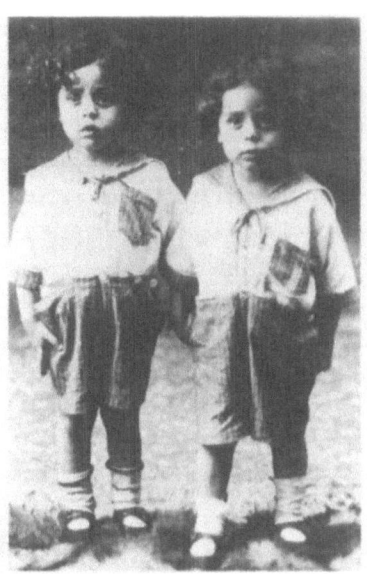

Fig. 1.
Photograph of case 1
(the smaller) and
case 2, showing the
striking similarity
in appearance.
(Leavitt FH (44),
Copyright 1928,
American Medical Association)

Case 1
    History: The patient was taken ill at the age of 6 years and 4 months
demonstrating headache, gradually increasing in severity and frequency, followed
by projectile vomiting and disturbance in walking. One month later he was taken
to hospital because of several generalized convulsions.
*Ophthalmologic examination ... revealed bilateral choked disk with an elevation
of from 3 to 4 diopters above the retinal level.* No extraocular palsies were
present and a lumbar puncture did not reveal any abnormalities.
The patient died in the hospital one month later at the age of 6 1/2 years.
    Autopsy: A tumour was found in the vermis of the cerebellum. The tumour
measured approximately 5 cm in diameter. *It was of spongy consistency, not
definitely infiltrating in character and apparently arose from the region of
the roof of the fourth ventricle.* Other tissues of the brain were found to be
normal. *The meninges were not involved.*

Microscopic study: *The types of cells present vary, but for the most part they fit in with what has been described ... as 'medullo-blastomas', but other glial type cells are present as is common in this type of tumour. Neuroblasts and spongioblasts are present to a small degree. The connective tissue stroma, which has a tendency to divide the tumour up into small islets, is a little more abundant than in the usual blastoma.*

Diagnosis: Cerebellar medulloblastoma.

Case 2

History: The patient became ill at the age of 5 years with increasing head-ache, projectile vomiting and disturbance in walking, symptoms comparative to those of his twin brother. *He soon developed a distinctively cerebellar gait and became constipated.* A few months later he had a series of generalized convulsions, lasting several hours. *Subsequently, he became totally blind in the right eye, and the vision of the left eye was limited to perception of light. He developed skew deviation of the eyeballs and bilateral deafness.* Ophthalmological examination showed 4 diopters of choking in the right and 3 diopters in the left disks, with marked blurring of each.
The patient died at home at 8 1/2 years of age.

Autopsy: Was not permitted by the parents.

Diagnosis: A clinical diagnosis of cerebellar tumour was made.

COMMENT

Unfortunately autopsy of the second twin was not permitted, so the exact location and histopathologic type of tumour for this twin is not known. We have therefore registered this report among the discordant occurrences. The identical symptomatology and age of occurrence suggest a cerebellar tumour, i.c. a medulloblastoma.

II.A.2.2. Sugita 1960 - Japan
            (personal communication in Metzel 1963) (54)

Female twins. Japanese.

These female twins were reported by Metzel (1963) as a personal communication
from Sugita. The report concerns twins of similar appearance for whom the mono-
zygocity had not been ascertained. One twin died at the age of 8 years of a
clinically diagnosed tumour of the posterior fossa. The other twin had been
operated upon because of a brain tumour which was reported as a *Kleinhirn-
astrocytom*.
Discussing these twins the author states that a medulloblastoma was probably
present. For this reason these cases have been registered here. Concordancy,
however, might be suspected if one considers the age of occurrence and the
localization of the tumours.

II.A.3.   MONOZYGOTIC TWINS, ONE DEMONSTRATING MEDULLOBLASTOMA

II.A.3.1. Cushing 1930 - Boston, U.S.A. (20)

Female twin. American.

   History: The patient had primary symptoms at the age of 13 years: morning
vomiting, listlessness, blindness.
A suboccipital exploration revealed metastases over the cerebellum. The tumour
presented between herniated tonsils. A laminectomy of the atlas was performed.
The patient died 9 months after operation.
   Microscopic study: Medulloblastoma.
   Diagnosis: Cerebellar medulloblastoma.

The twin sister died soon after birth.

COMMENT
It is not noted in the article whether the twins were mono- or dizygotic.
This twin-pair was tabulated as a concordant occurrence of medulloblastoma in
the review by Metzel (54). No further information, however, is given concerning
the twin sister in the original article.

II.A.3.2. Cushing 1930 - Boston, U.S.A. (20)

Female monozygotic twin. American.

   History: Primary symptoms started at the age of 7 years with vomiting. There
was a slight internal squint of the left eye from early childhood.
A suboccipital exploration revealed a large midline tumour. A radical extirpa-
tion of the tumour was performed and the fourth ventricle widely opened.
Postoperatively the patient received radiotherapy of the cerebellum and spine.
She was still alive 22 months later and in good condition.
   Microscopic study: Medulloblastoma
   Diagnosis: Cerebellar medulloblastoma.

The twin sister had a less noticeable internal squint of the right eye.

II.A.3.3. <u>Macklin 1941 - Ontario, Canada</u> (50)

Male monozygotic twin. Canadian.

    The patient, a boy aged 14 years, had a medulloblastoma of the cerebellum removed which had been histologically verified.
Radiation was given and the patient was still alive and well 5 years later.

The twin brother had a sarcoma of the left scapula at the age of 14 years. The diagnosis was confirmed by a biopsy specimen. The tumour was treated by radiation and the boy was still alive and well 5 years later.

20

II.A.3.4. Ende 1955 - Texas, U.S.A. (24)

Female monozygotic twin. American.

  History: The mother was a 24-year-old white woman, gravida 1, para 0. In the 34th week of gestation she had a spontaneous rupture of her membranes, and regular uterine contractions followed. *Roentgenographic examination on admission to the hospital revealed a twin pregnancy, with both fetuses in the cephalic presentation and with the first twin having a hydrocephalus. The first baby was a stillborn girl that weighed 5 lb., 9 3/4 oz.; the other twin, delivered immediately afterward, was an apparently normal, viable, premature girl who weighed 2 lb., 15 oz.*
On examination there appeared to be one placenta, one chorion and two amnions.

  Autopsy: The still-born baby *was found to be entirely normal except for the hydrocephalic head. ... the cerebral hemispheres were seen to be enlarged. The surface of the entire left hemisphere had a yellow discoloration. On cut sections, the left hemisphere was found to be almost completely replaced by gray-white neoplastic tissue showing areas of hemorrhage and soft yellow areas of necrosis. The right hemisphere had a markedly thin cortex and there was blood in the right ventricle. The third and fourth ventricles ... appeared to be normal and not dilated.*

  Microscopic study: *The neoplastic tissue was very vascular and there were scattered areas of hemosiderin pigment. The cell pattern was variable. In general the cells were arranged in nests and cords. In some areas the tumor cells were arranged concentrically around necrotic areas. Most of the cells were elongated and variably staining, with an ovoid vesicular nucleus and a moderate amount of pink cytoplasm. Mitotic figures were infrequent.*

  Diagnosis: Medulloblastoma (or ependymoma) in the left hemisphere.

The twin sister suffered from anaemia for approximately four months and received several blood transfusions. In a follow-up period of one year she had a normal growth and development. She had no serious illness and appeared normal in all respects at 13 months of age.

COMMENT

The tumour has been examined microscopically by various investigators. The diagnoses of medulloblastoma and ependymoma have been made.

II.A.3.5. <u>Norris and Jackson 1970 - California, U.S.A.</u> (59)

The authors studied 52 childhood cancer deaths in a California twin-birth cohort. Among them were seven cases of medulloblastoma in one of twins. The other twins were healthy with the exception of one case in which the co-twin died at 14 years of age because of accidental drowning, probably associated with epileptic seizure. One of the medulloblastomas was located in the cervical cord. In four of the seven cases the twins were of different sex and therefore dizygotic. The other three twins (A-C) were of the same sex, but the authors do not mention whether they were mono- or dizygotic (table 3).

II.A.3.6. <u>Bodor et al. 1974 - Lund, Sweden</u> (10)

Male monozygotic twin. Swedish.

<u>History</u>: The patient was the first-born, his weight at birth was 3050 g and his length 49 cm. At the age of 5 years he was admitted to hospital.
On examination *choked discs of 1 to 1.5 D, nystagmus bilaterally of cerebellar type, and slight ocular motor paresis to the right and general ataxia* were found. He was operated upon. *Between the ruptured tonsils a large, bluish-red tumour bulged forth. This proved to be an off-shoot of a tumour, at least the size of a hen's egg, which occupied the dilated fourth ventricle, extended into the vermis, and especially into the medial part of the right cerebellar hemisphere.* The main part of the tumour was removed.
Postoperatively the patient received a course of radiotherapy to the head and spinal canal. Thirteen years later the patient was still alive and in good condition.
<u>Microscopic study</u>: Medulloblastoma.
<u>Diagnosis</u>: Cerebellar medulloblastoma.

The twin brother was healthy at 18 years of age.

II.A.4.   DIZYGOTIC TWINS

No publications of dizygotic twins with concordant tumour (medulloblastoma) are available in the literature.

There are several publications of dizygotic twins, one twin having a medullo-blastoma.

The first is from Geyer and Pedersen (28). They describe a dizygotic male twin having a tumour of the posterior fossa with obstructive internal hydrocephalus, and papilloedema on both sides. He died at the age of 4 years. No operation or microscopic investigation was conducted. A medulloblastoma is suspected by the authors. The twin brother was healthy.

Another publication by Hauge and Harvald (39) reports on male dizygotic twins. One of the twins had a medulloblastoma which was operated upon when the patient was 10 years of age. He died at the age of 10. His twin brother was alive and well at the age of 20 years.

Macklin (49) describes one of male twins with a medulloblastoma at the age of 11 months. The healthy twin was alive and well at the age of six years with no cerebral symptoms.

Four other cases of medulloblastoma in one of dizygotic twins are described by Norris and Jackson (59) in their study on childhood cancer deaths in twins (II.A.3.5).

II.B.   *SIBLINGS*

II.B.1.   SIBLINGS WITH CONCORDANT TUMOUR

II.B.1.1. <u>Bennet 1946 - Army Institute of Pathology, U.S.A.</u> (5)

Two brothers. American.

This article describes the study of primary intracranial neoplasms in a
selected group, namely in Army personnel during the second world war. The
patients were all between the ages of 18 and 38 years.
The material was sent to the Army Institute of Pathology from hospitals all
over the world. Material from 84,615 cases was received at the institute.
Included were 543 intracranial tumours. Forty-five intracranial neoplasms
were diagnosed as medulloblastomas. *One history recorded the fact that the*
patient's brother had died of a medulloblastoma.
No further data are given in the article.

II.B.1.2. Kjellin et al. 1960 - Stockholm, Sweden (43)

A half-brother and half-sister. Swedish.

Case 1

History: The patient was admitted to hospital at the age of 10 years. His complaints were *diplopia, impaired vision, poor balance, vomiting and increasing headaches for 2 months.*

Examination revealed *neck rigidity, paresis of the left superior rectus muscle, bilateral papilledema, nystagmus, and impairment of gait with a tendency to fall towards the right side.*

At operation a *soft, friable, poorly defined tumor was found originating in the vermis of the cerebellum and occupying the posterior part of the fourth ventricle. It was partially removed. The patient died 3 days after operation, approximately 2 months after the onset of the disease* (at age 10).

Autopsy: *showed a large hydrocephalus with great distortion of the third ventricle. The fourth ventricle was filled with tumor mass and old blood.*

Microscopic study (of the biopsy): *showed a very cellular tumor with occasional mitoses. The cells had rounded or elongated dark-staining nuclei and were frequently arranged in bands, whirls, or pseudorosettes. Several pale round cell areas were encountered.*

Diagnosis: Cerebellar medulloblastoma.

Case 2

History: The patient was admitted to hospital at the age of 11 years. Her complaints were *paroxysms of headache and vomiting for 2 years.*

On examination *incipient papilledema on the left side* was found.

At operation a *tumor in the cerebellum was removed. It was soft, greyish-red, and poorly defined, and had apparently originated in the vermis.*

The patient died 9 months after the operation, approximately 2 years and 9 months after the onset of the disease.

Autopsy: Was not performed.

Microscopic study (of the biopsy): *showed a very cellular tumor with occasional mitoses. The cells had rounded, elongated, or carrot-shaped dark-staining nuclei surrounded by sparse cytoplasm, and were occasionally arranged in pseudorosettes. Some rounded, light-staining areas were seen. There was a moderate number of thin-walled blood vessels.*

Diagnosis: Cerebellar medulloblastoma.

<u>Family</u>: The medulloblastoma occurred in a half-brother and a half-sister in a family of 4 children. No additional information concerning the family is given.

II.B.1.3. Bickerstaff et al. 1967 - Smethwick, England (7)

Two brothers. English.

Case 1

History: At the age of 2 years and 4 months the patient began to hold his head slightly to the left. *The following month he had measles, from which he failed to recover his former good health, being much less active than previously, tending to sit and stare. Three months later it was noticed that he could not walk more than a few steps without falling forward. Just before admission he became progressively more unsteady and fell to the left ... He complained of pains in the front and back of the head mainly in the evenings and during the night lasting for 15-45 min.*

On examination *he was found to have bilateral papilloedema and sixth nerve palsies. There were no cerebellar signs.* At walking *he appeared to stagger to the right and held head and neck extended.* Radiographs of the skull showed sutural diastasis. A ventriculogram *showed a large mid-line posterior fossa space-occupying lesion with an associated upward herniation through the tentorium.* ... C.S.F. *contained 10 mgm protein per 100 ml.*

A suboccipital craniectomy was performed 2 days after admission as a matter of urgency. A soft grey very vascular tumour was found in the lower part of the vermis at a depth of 1-2 cm. The patient collapsed because of profuse bleeding from the tumour and died during operation.

Autopsy: Cerebellar tonsils extended 1 cm into the spinal canal. *The posterior and inferior surfaces of the vermis and lateral lobes of the cerebellum showed a greyish white material infiltrating along the vessels and away from them in the subarachnoid space. Patches of a similar infiltration were present over the dorsal aspect of the spinal cord. On sagittal section in the midline a large well defined area of uniform greyish pink tissue was seen to occupy the centre of the vermis and almost the whole of the roof of the fourth ventricle.*

Microscopic study: *A large section of the tumour was predominantly necrotic but viable portions were composed of circular or polyhedral cells with round nuclei with a high chromatin content. The cell bodies were mostly circular (hydropic) with bulky basophilic cytoplasm.*

Diagnosis: Medulloblastoma of the cerebellum.

Case 2

History: The patient had fallen out of bed and bumped his head. Five days later *he was slightly sleepy and unsteady on his feet*, so he was admitted to hospital. In the hospital the patient began to vomit *and became increasingly drowsy with slowing of the pulse*. Radiographs of the skull showed a fracture over the left parietal region. The patient then developed neck stiffness. *He rapidly became more drowsy. There was a slight right facial weakness. The abdominal reflexes were slightly less brisk on the left and he was not moving the right arm and leg*. On suspicion of a left subdural haematoma exploratory burr holes were made, but no haematoma was found. The patient remained drowsy and unsteady on his feet, and occasionally vomited. *Bilateral carotid angiograms showed a hydrocephalus*. Ventriculography *showed a left sided posterior fossa tumour, displacing the fourth ventricle forward and to the right*.
Posterior fossa craniectomy showed high tension in the posterior fossa. Both cerebellar tonsils were displaced downwards into the spinal canal. A grey tumour was found, growing from the anterior surface of the vermis and roof of the fourth ventricle and completely filling the lower two-thirds of the ventricle.
Ten days after operation the patient developed ptosis of the left eyelid. He received deep X-ray therapy. A few months later *he was found to have a secondary deposit in the left orbit and thereafter deteriorated rapidly and was discharged home*.

Microscopic study: A partly necrotic tumour was seen. The surviving part *was very cellular without any division into stroma and parenchyma. The nuclei were mostly oval or more elongated with a moderate chromatin content and mitoses were very numerous*.

Diagnosis: Medulloblastoma of the cerebellum.

Family:

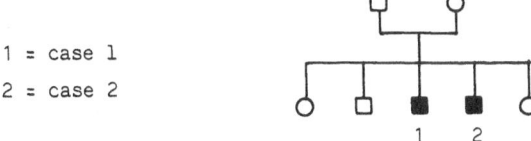

1 = case 1
2 = case 2

There were three other siblings, two sisters and one brother. No further data concerning the family are mentioned in the article.

II.B.1.4. <u>Belamaric and Chau 1969</u> - Hong Kong, B.C.C. (4)

Two sisters. Chinese family from Hong Kong.

Case 1

<u>History</u>: The patient was the sixth child in the family. *She was born at full term of a normal pregnancy, but her weight at birth was only 2,400 gm. No abnormalities were detected until the 15th day when progressive expansion of the skull was noted* ... The patient was admitted to hospital when she was 33 days old.

On examination the patient *was conscious, active, and appeared well-nourished. The head was abnormally large, measuring 36 cm. in greatest circumference. The cranial sutures were excessively separated, and the anterior fontanelle was bulging. There was slight rigidity in the legs. Tendon reflexes were brisk but not abnormal. Cranial nerve dysfunction was not observed.* Cerebrospinal fluid was turbid and contained 60 mg of protein and 51 mg of glucose per 100 cc. There were 300 cells per cu mm; 80% had irregular nuclei, and the rest were lymphocytes. One week after admission the hydrocephalus became complicated by meningitis. A pneumoventriculogram (at the age of 65 days) *showed dilated lateral and third ventricles.*

The patient developed bronchopneumonia and died at the age of 68 days.

<u>Autopsy</u>: *The fronto-occipital circumference measured 42 cm. The cranial sutures were wide. The cerebral hemispheres were markedly enlarged, the convolutions wide and flat, and the sulci narrow. The third ventricle also was markedly dilated. A layer of granular, friable, pale greyish-brown tumor tissue averaging 0.5 cm in thickness covered and, in places, replaced the substance of the superior vermis and the superior surface of both cerebellar hemispheres.* Infiltration of the dorsal surface of the midbrain with compression of the cerebellar aqueduct occurred. *Caudally, it extended into the cerebello-medullary cistern and the 4th ventricle.*

<u>Microscopic study</u>: *A highly cellular tumor growing in sheets. The bulk of it was composed of small, sometimes "carrot-shaped", cells with scant, ill-defined, generally wispy cytoplasm. Most nuclei were round or oval but some tended to be wedge-shaped or irregular. Foci of necrosis and hemosiderin deposition were seen within the tumor.*

<u>Diagnosis</u>: Cerebellar medulloblastoma complicated by obstructive hydrocephalus and purulent meningitis.

Case 2

History: The patient *was the seventh child in the family. She was born at*
the end of an uneventful 36 1/2-week gestation period. Delivery was uncompli-
cated. *The weight at birth was 2,440 gm. Immediately after delivery the patient*
had a single episode of cyanosis promptly relieved by oxygen administration.
She had obvious hydrocephalus at birth. The skull was abnormally expanded,
measuring 37 cm in circumference; the cranial sutures and the anterior
fontanelle were broad. Reflexes were normal. *The liver was palpable 4 cm below*
the right costal margin. Cerebrospinal fluid was clear, yellowish and *containing*
240 mg of protein, less than 10 mg of glucose and 660 mg of chloride per 100 cc.
There were 121 cells per cu mm. Many of these were described as being larger
than lymphocytes and having a single nucleus. In some cells the nucleus was
hyperchromatic.
At the age of 6 days the patient developed meningitis and she died at the age
of 12 days.

Autopsy: The fronto-occipital circumference measured 39 cm. *The cranial*
sutures and the fontanelles were broad. Greenish fibrinopurulent exudate
covered the leptomeninges. The third and lateral ventricles were markedly
dilated ... An irregular, solid, friable, grayish-white tumor infiltrated the
vermis and both cerebellar hemispheres. From there ... it involved and exten-
sively damaged the medulla oblongata, pons, 4th ventricle, midbrain, and the
undersurface of both occipital lobes. The cerebral aqueduct and foramina of
Magendie and Lushka were completely obliterated. There were many firm, whitish
tumor nodules up to 0.5 cm in diameter scattered over the spinal cord and the
brain surface.

Microscopic study: The microscopic features were *strikingly similar* to those
described in case 1, *except for the presence of slightly larger and paler nuclei,*
the finding of a single rosette, and involvement of the spinal cord meninges ...

Diagnosis: Congenital cerebellar medulloblastoma complicated by obstructive
hydrocephalus and purulent meningitis.

Family:

1 = case 1
2 = case 2
3 = eldest sister

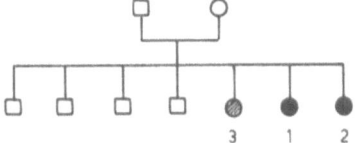

The four brothers were healthy. The eldest sister (3) *developed progressive hydrocephalus of undetermined etiology some time after birth and died at the age of 4 months. Unfortunately, post-mortem examination was not performed and detailed hospital records are not available. It might be justifiable to speculate that in this child cerebellar medulloblastoma may also have been the underlying cause of hydrocephalus.*

COMMENT

In case 1 the inception of the neoplastic growth began either before birth or at least only a short time afterwards. In case 2 the tumour must have originated during intrauterine life, external environmental factors having only a limited influence.

This is the only report in literature in which possibly three siblings of one family have a medulloblastoma. It is remarkable that only females were affected, four other male siblings being healthy.

II.B.1.5. <u>Chen et al. 1970 - Rochester, Minn., U.S.A.</u> (14)

Two sisters and two brothers. Guamanian.

<u>History</u>: The authors investigated the clinical and genetic patterns of
neurological diseases on Guam. They discovered a family demonstrating 4
patients (2 male and 2 female) with brain tumours and 2 with acute myelogenous leukaemia in a sibship of 14. The brain tumours were diagnosed from
material collected at autopsy and included 2 medulloblastomas, 1 glioblastoma
and 1 paraventricular haemangioma. The two patients with medulloblastomas were
sisters who died at the ages of 7 and 13 years. One sister had black naevi on
the back and hypoplasia of the corpus callosum, the other had several café-
au-lait spots and haemangiomata on the right leg and also in the spleen. One
brother had a glioblastoma in the left hemisphere and died at the age of 5
years. He also had café-au-lait spots on the back. The other brother having
a paraventricular haemangioma, who died at the age of 5 years of a rupture,
also had a haemangioma in the right hemisphere.

<u>Family</u>:

1 = case 1
2 = case 2
3 = case 3
4 = case 4
5 = acute myelogenous leukaemia
6 = acute myelogenous leukaemia
7 = hepatoma
8 = hepatoma
9 = laryngeal cancer

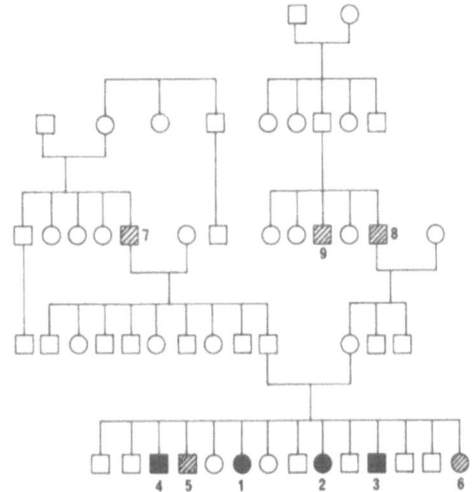

Both paternal (7) and maternal (8) grandfathers died of a primary hepatoma,
and a maternal great-uncle died of laryngeal cancer (9). Amyotrophic lateral
sclerosis had been diagnosed in a great-uncle of the patients and in his son.
Other members of the sibship had clinical features associated with the phacomatosis complex, such as café-au-lait spots and black naevi. *There was no*

roentgenographic evidence of jaw cyst or forking ribs.

COMMENT

The association of the brain tumours with stigmata of phacomatosis, such as café-au-lait spots and black naevi (neurofibromatosis), and haemangiomata (Hippel-Lindau) makes a relationship very likely. Considering the occurrence of leukaemia and other forms of cancer (hepatoma, laryngeal cancer), a manifestation of the family cancer syndrome (SBLA syndrome) also cannot be excluded.

II.B.1.6. <u>Yamashita et al. 1975 - Kyoto, Japan</u> (92)

Two brothers. Japanese.

Case 1

<u>History</u>: The patient was born 50 days earlier than expected, weighing 2000 g at birth. His development appeared normal. At the age of 2 1/2 years he was admitted to hospital because of a month long *disturbance of gait, associated with headache and vomiting.*

On examination the patient *was drowsy and irritable. Babinski sign was equivocal bilaterally. There was no other focal neurological abnormality. Plain X-ray films of the skull showed diastasis of the coronal suture and enlargement of the posterior cranial fossa.* A ventriculogram *suggested the presence of a midcerebellar tumor.*

At operation one week after admission (suboccipital craniectomy) *there were tumor infiltrations over both cerebellar hemispheres and the vermis. The main portion of the tumor was in the fourth ventricle. The tumor appeared bluish gray, friable and hemorrhagic.* A biopsy was taken.

Postoperatively the patient received a ventriculoperitoneal shunt. In spite of radiotherapy there was no marked improvement in his condition. He died 7 months after operation.

<u>Autopsy</u>: Was not performed.

<u>Microscopic study</u>: *A highly cellular tumor packed with small cells in which the cytoplasm was scanty and poorly defined, and the nuclei round or oval, variable in size and abundant in chromatin.*

<u>Diagnosis</u>: Cerebellar medulloblastoma.

Case 2

<u>History</u>: The patient was born at full term with a body weight of 2950 g. His development was normal and he had been able to walk normally prior to his illness. At the age of 1 1/2 years he was admitted to hospital because of a *disturbance of gait for one and half months and of headache and vomiting for one week.*

On examination the patient was drowsy. *The major fontanelle was open and bulging. There was nuchal stiffness. The optic fundi showed bilateral choked discs. Deep reflexes were bilaterally hyperactive.* Babinski sign was positive on both sides. *Plain X-ray films of the skull showed diastasis of all cranial sutures and enlargement of the posterior cranial fossa. A right carotid angiogram revealed a symmetrical hydrocephalus.* A left retrograde brachial angiogram showed a mid-cerebellar process.

At operation 18 days after admission (suboccipital craniectomy) *there were
tumor infiltrations over both cerebellar hemispheres and vermis. The tumor
was soft, friable, hemorrhagic, grayish pink and moderately demarcated. Some
of it was taken for biopsy.*

Postoperatively the patient had an irregular respiration. He died on the
seventh postoperative day.

Autopsy: Was not performed.

Microscopic study: *A highly cellular tumor with occasional mitoses. The
cells had round or elongated nuclei and scanty cytoplasm. In some places there
were cord-like arrangements.*

Diagnosis: Cerebellar medulloblastoma.

Family:

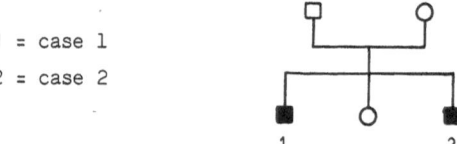

1 = case 1

2 = case 2

The parents were healthy without consanguinity. The only sister was also
healthy.

II.B.1.7. <u>Wakai et al. 1980 - Tokyo/Chiba, Japan</u> (87a)

Two brothers. Japanese.

In their article *Teratoma in the pineal region in two brothers* the authors also report in their discussion the occurrence of medulloblastoma in two brothers. ... *one was 11 years old and the other 10 years old at the onset of symptoms*.
No further information is given about these cases.

II.B.2. SIBLINGS WITH DISCORDANT TUMOUR

II.B.2.1. Turcot et al. 1959 - Quebec, Canada (87)

A brother and sister. Canadian.

Case 1

    History: This 17-year-old boy had to be hospitalized as an emergency because
of acute myelitis. He died two months later.
The patient was known to have polyposis of the colon since 15 years of age.
He had been operated upon several times for this disease. From the specimens
removed at these operations two malignant tumours were reported, both adeno-
carcinomas, in sigmoid and rectum.
    Autopsy: *It was discovered that he had a complete destruction of the spinal
cord by a malignant tumor diagnosed as a medulloblastoma invading the medulla
spinalis. The brain was not examined.*
    Microscopic study: No additional information given.
    Diagnosis: Medulloblastoma of the spinal cord. Polyposis of the colon with
adenocarcinoma of rectum and sygmoid.

Case 2

    History: At the age of 21 years the patient was admitted to hospital because
of *two or three episodes of headache during which she became unconscious.*
Examinations indicated that she had a cerebral tumour. Before treatment could
be administered, the patient died suddenly.
The patient was known to have polyposis of the colon since 13 years of age. She
was operated upon several times for this condition.
    Autopsy: *A large tumor of the posterior zone of the left frontal lobe was
discovered.* The diameter was 5.5 cm.
    Microscopic study: Glioblastoma. *There was also a small chromophobe adenoma
(3 mm. in diameter) of the hypophysis.*
    Diagnosis: Glioblastoma of the left frontal lobe. Chromophobe adenoma of the
hypophysis. Polyposis of the colon.

    Family: The family history of two generations failed to disclose any other
occurrences of significant disorders.

COMMENT

In this family there is an association of polyposis of the colon with tumours of the central nervous system. This association is known as the glioma-polyposis or Turcot syndrome, which has a probably autosomal recessive mode of inheritance. The authors of this article conclude that the two cases *support the theory that hereditary transmission of familial polyposis as a dominant characteristic can be associated with other potentialities residing in the same gene.*

II.B.2.2. <u>Thomas et al. 1977 - Glasgow, Scotland</u> (83)

Two sisters. Scottish.

Case 1

<u>History</u>: Normal birth and development. At the age of 5 years the patient was *admitted to hospital with a four day history of headache, vomiting and intermittent drowsiness.*
On examination no abnormal neurological signs were found apart from mild hypotonia. *Lumbar CSF was clear and contained 2 mononuclear cells per ml., protein 0.5 g/l, and 4.2 mmol/l (76 mg/dl) of sugar.* Four days later the patient was discharged home without symptoms. *Over the next few days, however, her symptoms recurred and worsened, and she developed anorexia and enuresis.*
She was readmitted to hospital.
Examination then revealed *truncal ataxia with a tendency to stagger to the left, hypotonic limbs, and papilloedema.* A ventriculogram *confirmed the clinical impression of a left cerebellar tumour.*
At operation a *well-circumscribed tumour high up in the left cerebellar hemisphere and attached to the dura mater* was excised.
Postoperatively the patient *received a course of radiotherapy to the neuraxis. She remained apathetic ..., slept more and frequently refused food.*
She died some six months after the onset of her illness.
<u>Autopsy</u>: Permission was not obtained.
<u>Microscopic study</u>:

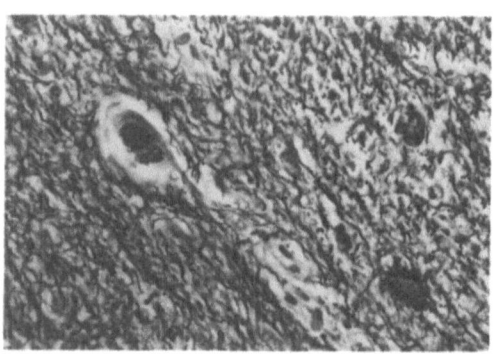

Fig. 1.
Ganglioneuromatous part
of tumour of case 1.
Palmgren.
(Thomas M, Adams JH,
Doyle D 1977 (83))

... showed two distinct types of tissue. Part ... was of low cellularity and contained many large cells, some of which were binucleate or multinucleate. The nuclei were large and vesicular and contained prominent nucleoli. Within

39

*the cytoplasm of most of these cells Nissl granules and neurofibrils were
identifiable .... Among these cells, which were clearly ganglionic in type,
there was a dense plexus of axis cylinders. There was also a scanty fibrovascular stroma.*

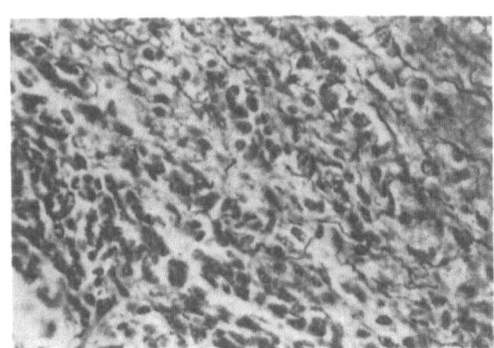

Fig. 2.
Neuroblastomatous part
of tumour of case 1.
Palmgren.
(Thomas M, Adams JH,
Doyle D 1977 (83))

There was a fairly sharp transition to the second type of tissue: a *densely
cellular tumour which was similar in appearance to all of the other pieces of
tissue submitted. The cells were small, round or oval, and had scanty cytoplasm.
The nuclei had well-developed nuclear membranes and contained many small
chromatin dots .... Mitotic figures were frequent. Among these cells there were
numerous delicate axons, ... and there was only scanty collagen and reticulin
in relation to vessels. Because of the network of axons in the highly cellular
part of the tumour, mixed ganglioneuroma and neuroblastoma seemed to be the
most appropriate diagnosis.*

Diagnosis: Mixed ganglioneuroma and neuroblastoma in the left cerebellar
hemisphere.

Case 2

History: Normal birth. *Early development was normal apart from delayed and
unsteady walking, and she was never able to walk more than a few steps on her
own. Speech, however, developed normally.* At the age of 2 years and 2 months
the patient *had a right sided clonic seizure after which she was unable to
walk by herself at all. One month later she had a further seizure and was
admitted to hospital ....*
On examination *truncal and symmetrical limb ataxia, hypotonia and brisk tendon
reflexes were noted. Radiographs of the skull showed starting of the sutures.*
A ventriculogram revealed a midline tumour of the posterior fossa.

40

Operation *revealed a midline cerebellar tumour with extensive subpial infiltration over both hemispheres. Subtotal removal was undertaken.*
Postoperatively *a course of radiotherapy to the neuraxis was given.*
The condition of the patient, however, deteriorated progressively and she
died seven months after the onset of her illness.

Autopsy: Permission was not obtained.

Microscopic study (biopsy):

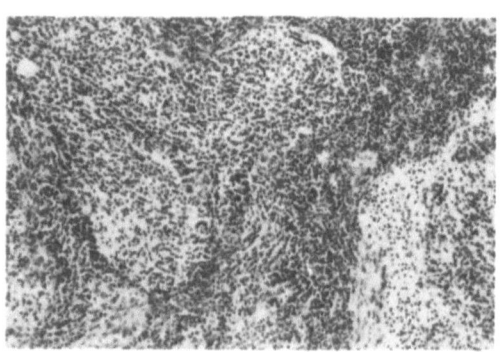

Fig. 3.
Microscopic appearance
of tumour of case 2.
HE.
(Thomas M, Adams JH,
Doyle D 1977 (83))

*A highly cellular tumour composed partly of sheets of small cells with hyper-
chromatic, slightly elongated nuclei, distinct 'pale islands' of slightly
larger cells ... and narrow cords of tumour cells running in parallel lines.
Mitotic figures were numerous.* Abundant collagen and reticulin throughout the
highly cellular areas.

Diagnosis: Midline cerebellar desmoplastic medulloblastoma.

COMMENT

In medulloblastoma varying degrees of differentiation along several distinct
neuroepithelial cell lines can occur. However, according to the authors, the
tumours of the two cases must be regarded as discordant. We have also registered
them among the discordant tumours. The opinion expressed here remains open to
discussion.

II.B.2.3. Blattner et al. 1979 - Miami, U.S.A. (9)

Two brothers. American.

Case 1

History: This male was hospitalized at the age of 37 years. His early development had been normal, *although the left testicle did not descend into the*
scrotal sac until age 13 years. At the age of 33 years he *experienced psycho-*
motor seizures ..., which increased in frequency in the years preceding
admission.
An EEG showed a right temporal lobe focus, and computerized tomography *disclosed*
a right temporal lobe lesion ..., for which the patient was operated upon.
Microscopic study: Low-grade astrocytoma.
Diagnosis: Right temporal low-grade astrocytoma.

Case 2

History: This 2-year-old male was admitted to hospital as he had *experienced*
a stiff back, anorexia, weight loss, drowsiness, and projectile vomiting during
a two-month period ....
A clinical diagnosis of tuberculous meningitis was made, but autopsy showed a
tumour *originating in the wall of the fourth ventricle.*
Microscopic study: Medulloblastoma.
Diagnosis: Medulloblastoma of the fourth ventricle.

Family: A sister had a single grand mal seizure at the age of 27 years, but
cerebral CAT was normal. A distant relative was hospitalized at 27 years of age
with headache, visual problems, vertigo, mental confusion and vomiting. *A mid-*
line cerebellar tumor was excised. It was a highly cellular papillary, rosette-
forming tumor possibly of choroid epithelial origin; it may have been metastatic,
but no other primary tumor was found. A comprehensive family study showed a
constellation of tumours in the family - a total of 16 cases of cancer -
including bony and soft tissue sarcomas, neural tumours, brain tumours, leukaemia
and breast carcinoma.

COMMENT

The tumours in this family are a manifestation of the so-called SBLA cancer
syndrome, a dominantly inherited predisposition to certain kinds of cancer.

II.C.   *OTHER GENERATIONS AND DISTANT RELATIVES*

II.C.1.   OTHER GENERATIONS AND DISTANT RELATIVES WITH CONCORDANT TUMOUR

Reports of concordant occurrence of medulloblastoma in more than one generation of a family do not appear to be available in the literature.

II.C.2.   OTHER GENERATIONS AND DISTANT RELATIVES WITH DISCORDANT TUMOUR

II.C.2.1. Biemond 1955 - The Netherlands
          (personal communication in Van der Wiel 1959) (90)

A father and daughter. Dutch.

In his monograph Van der Wiel (1959) reported a personal communication from
Biemond (1955) concerning a father with a not histologically verified cerebral
tumour and a daughter with a medulloblastoma. No further information concerning
these cases was available or could be obtained after inquiry by the author.

II.C.2.2. Van der Wiel 1980 - Gouda, The Netherlands
          (personal communication)

A grandfather and granddaughter. Dutch.

The granddaughter was an only child. She died at the age of 5 years as the
result of a medulloblastoma for which she was previously operated upon.
The grandfather was operated upon at the age of 47 years because of a brain
tumour. Histological diagnosis was glioblastoma multiforme. He died 6 months
postoperatively.

   Family: The grandfather had two sons, no daughters. One son (the father of
the granddaughter) had a large spina bifida occulta. His brother was healthy.
A daughter of this brother died shortly after birth of anencephaly. The
mother's family showed no abnormalities (see also VII.C.2.13).

1 = glioblastoma multiforme
2 = medulloblastoma
3 = spina bifida occulta
4 = died shortly after
    birth of anencephaly

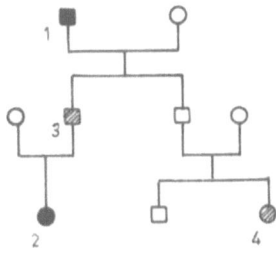

44

TABLE 1 - MONOZYGOTIC TWINS WITH CONCORDANT TUMOUR (II.A.1)

	case	gender	relationship	number of unaffected siblings	race or nationality	age at symptom occurrence	age at death	location of the tumour
II.A.1.1. Griepentrog 1957	1	f	s	1 s	Germ.	8 w	8 w	4th ventricle into R cerebellar hemisphere
	2	f	s	1 s	Germ.	birth	11 w	4th ventricle into cerebellum
II.A.1.2. Waldbaur 1976	1	f	s	2 br 1 s	Germ.	4 m	5 m	L cerebellum and 4th ventricle
	2	f	s	2 br 1 s	Germ.	16 m	16 m	epiphysis region and 3rd ventricle

TABLE 2 - MONOZYGOTIC TWINS WITH DISCORDANT TUMOUR (II.A.2)

	case	gender	relationship	number of unaffected siblings	race or nationality	age at symptom occurrence	age at death	location of the tumour
II.A.2.1. Leavitt 1928	1	m	br	?	Amer.	6 y	6 y	vermis of the cerebellum
	2	m	br	?	Amer.	8 y	8 y	cerebellar region
II.A.2.2. Sugita 1960	1	f	s	?	Japan.	10 y	?	cerebellum
	2	f	s	?	Japan.	?	8 y	posterior fossa

diagnosis	biopsy	autopsy	associated physical or mental conditions	family	comment
Medulloblastoma	-	+	Teratoid tumour of the breast with parts of medulloblastoma. Tumour in L adrenal and R kidney	Grand-aunt dwarf 1 m. Grand-aunt sudden death as a baby	Tumour in adrenal and kidney metastatic or primary tumour? Same twins as reported by Zülch 1956.
Medulloblastoma	-	+	-		
Medulloblastoma	-	+	Hip joint dysplasia on both sides	No nerve diseases. Mother had 4 abortions	
Pineoblastoma or undifferentiated pinealis tumour with medulloblastoma character	-	+	Hip joint dysplasia on both sides		

diagnosis	biopsy	autopsy	associated physical or mental conditions	family	comment
Medulloblastoma	-	+	-	?	Case 2: clinical diagnosis
Brain tumour	-	-	-		
Medulloblastoma	+	-	?	?	Case 2: clinical diagnosis. Personal communication in Metzel 1963
Brain tumour	-	-	?		

TABLE 3 - MONOZYGOTIC TWINS, ONE DEMONSTRATING MEDULLOBLASTOMA (II.A.3)

		case	gender	relationship	number of unaffected siblings	race or nationality	age at symptom occurrence	age at death	location of the tumour
II.A.3.1. Cushing 1930		1	f	s	?	Amer.	13 y	13 y	cerebellum
			f	s	?	Amer.		soon after birth	
II.A.3.2. Cushing 1930		1	f	s	?	Amer.	9 y	-	cerebellum midline
			f	s	?	Amer.			
II.A.3.3. Macklin 1934		1	m	br	?	Can.	14 y	-	cerebellum
			m	br	?	Can.			
II.A.3.4. Ende 1955		1	f	s	?	Amer.	still-born	intra-uterine	L hemisphere
			f	s	?	Amer.			
II.A.3.5. Norris 1970	A	1	m	br	?	?	?	3 y	
			m	br	?	?			
	B	1	m	br	?	?	?	11 y	
			m	br	?	?			
	C	1	f	s	?	?	?	13 y	
			f	s	?	?			
II.A.3.6. Bodor 1974		1	m	br	?	Swed.	5 y	-	vermis and R cerebellar hemisphere 4th ventricle
			m	br	?	Swed.			

diagnosis	biopsy	autopsy	associated physical or mental conditions	family	comment
Medulloblastoma	+	-	-	?	Mono- or dizygotic? Twin sister died soon after birth. No further information
			-		
Medulloblastoma	+	-	Slight internal squint of the left eye	?	
			Slight internal squint of the right eye		
Medulloblastoma	+	-	?	?	Twin brother had a sarcoma of the left scapula at the same age
			Sarcoma of the L scapula at 14 y		
Medulloblastoma or ependymoma	-	+	Hydrocephalus	?	Histological diagnosis uncertain. Medulloblastoma or ependymoma suggested
			Anaemia		
Medulloblastoma	?	?	?	?	Monozygotic twins? Mentioned in a study on childhood cancer deaths in a California twin-birth cohort
			?		
Medulloblastoma	?	?	?	?	
			?		
Medulloblastoma	?	?	?	?	
			?		
Medulloblastoma	+	-	?	?	
			?		

TABLE 4 - SIBLINGS WITH CONCORDANT TUMOUR (II.B.1)

	case	gender	relationship	number of unaffected siblings	race or nationality	age at symptom occurrence	age at death	location of the tumour
II.B.1.1. Bennett 1946	1	m	br	?	?	18 - 38 y	?	?
	2	m	br	?	?	?	?	?
II.B.1.2. Kjellin 1960	1	m	half br	?	Swed.	10 y	10 y	vermis of the cerebellum and 4th ventricle
	2	f	half s	2	Swed.	9 y	11 y	vermis of the cerebellum
II.B.1.3. Bickerstaff 1967	1	m	br	2 s 1 br	Engl.	2 y	2 y	vermis of the cerebellum and 4th ventricle
	2	m	br	2 s 1 br	Engl.	3 y	-	vermis of the cerebellum and 4th ventricle
II.B.1.4. Belamaric 1969	1	f	s	1 s 4 br	Chin.	15 d	68 d	vermis and cerebellar hemispheres
	2	f	s	1 s 4 br	Chin.	at birth	12 d	vermis and cerebellar hemispheres
II.B.1.5. Chen 1970	1	f	s	3 s 7 br	Guam.	?	13 y	-
	2	f	s	3 s 7 br	Guam.	?	7 y	-
	3	m	br	3 s 7 br	Guam.	?	5 y	L hemisphere
	4	m	br	3 s 7 br	Guam.	?	5 y	paraventricular and R hemisphere

diagnosis	biopsy	autopsy	associated physical or mental conditions	family	comment
Medulloblastoma	+	?	?	?	Case 1 was in the military age group (18-38 y)
Medulloblastoma	?	?	?		
Medulloblastoma	+	+	-	?	A half-brother and half-sister
Medulloblastoma	+	-	-		
Medulloblastoma	+	+	-	-	
Medulloblastoma	+	-	Traumatic skull fracture left parietal region		
Medulloblastoma	-	+	Obstructive hydro-cephalus, purulent meningitis, bronchopneumonia	The eldest sister died at 4 months with progressive hydrocephalus	Medulloblastoma occurrence in a third sister is suspected
Medulloblastoma	-	+	Cyanosis after de-livery, hepatomegaly, obstructive hydro-cephalus, purulent meningitis		
Medulloblastoma	?	+	Black naevi on the back, hypoplasia of corpus callosum	Two sibs with leukaemia, some sibs with black naevi and café-au-lait spots. Two grandfathers hepatoma; great-uncle laryngeal cancer; 2 rela-tives ALS	Relationship with phacomatoses complex and/or SBLA cancer syndrome
Medulloblastoma	?	+	Café-au-lait spots, haemangioma of leg and spleen		
Glioblastoma	?	+	Café-au-lait spots on the back		
Haemangioma	?	+	-		

TABLE 4 - continued

	case	gender	relationship	number of unaffected siblings	race or nationality	age at symptom occurrence	age at death	location of the tumour
II.B.1.6. Yamashita 1975	1	m	br	1 s	Japan.	2 y	3 y	vermis and cere-bellar hemispheres and 4th ventricle
	2	m	br	1 s	Japan.	1 y	1 y	vermis and cere-bellar hemispheres
II.B.1.7. Wakai 1980	1	m	br	?	Japan.	11 y	?	?
	2	m	br	?	Japan.	10 y	?	?

51

diagnosis	biopsy	autopsy	associated physical or mental conditions	family	comment
Medulloblastoma	+	-	-	-	
Medulloblastoma	+	-	-		
Medulloblastoma	?	?	?	?	
Medulloblastoma	?	?	?		

TABLE 5 - SIBLINGS WITH DISCORDANT TUMOUR (II.B.2)

	case	gender	relationship	number of unaffected siblings	race or nationality	age at symptom occurrence	age at death	location of the tumour
II.B.2.1. Turcot 1959	1	m	br	?	Can.	17 y	17 y	medulla spinalis
	2	f	s	?	Can.	21 y	21 y	L frontal lobe
II.B.2.2. Thomas 1977	1	f	s	?	Scot.	5 y	5 y	L cerebellar hemisphere
	2	f	s	?	Scot.	2 y	2 y	midline cerebellum and both cerebellar hemispheres
II.B.2.3. Blattner 1979	1	m	br	2 s	Amer.	33 y	-	R temporal
	2	m	br	2 s	Amer.	2 y	2 y	4th ventricle

diagnosis	biopsy	autopsy	associated physical or mental conditions	family	comment
Medulloblastoma	-	±	Polyposis colon with adeno-carcinoma	-	Glioma-polyposis or Turcot syndrome
Glioblastoma	-	+	Polyposis colon, chromophobe adenoma hypophysis		
Mixed ganglio-neuroma and neuroblastoma	+	-	-	?	Discordance open to discussion
Desmoplastic medulloblastoma	+	-	-		
Astrocytoma I-II	+	-	-	Sister: seizure; distant rel.: cerebellar tumour (metas-tatic?); many relatives with cancer: breast, sarcomas, leukaemia	Manifestation of SBLA cancer syndrome
Medulloblastoma	-	+	-		

GENERAL ASPECTS OF MEDULLOBLASTOMA

The term medulloblastoma was introduced into the neurological literature by
Bailey and Cushing in 1925 (2). In their opinion it was a highly malignant mid-
cerebellar tumour, generally demonstrating clinically during childhood, and
composed chiefly of undifferentiated cells of embryonic type (medulloblasts).
In their original description of 29 cases the great majority of the tumours was
located somewhere in the vermis overlying the posterior part of the fourth ventricle, but a few cases originated in the cerebral hemispheres. A later review
led to the reclassification of most of the cerebral cases in other categories
such as oligodendroglioma and other glioma (20).

The cell of origin of the medulloblastoma is still a matter of discussion in
modern pathology. Different sites of origin have been postulated. Some authors
maintain that it arises from the external granular layer of the cerebellar folia,
a fetal layer which gradually disappears in the infant cerebellum during the first

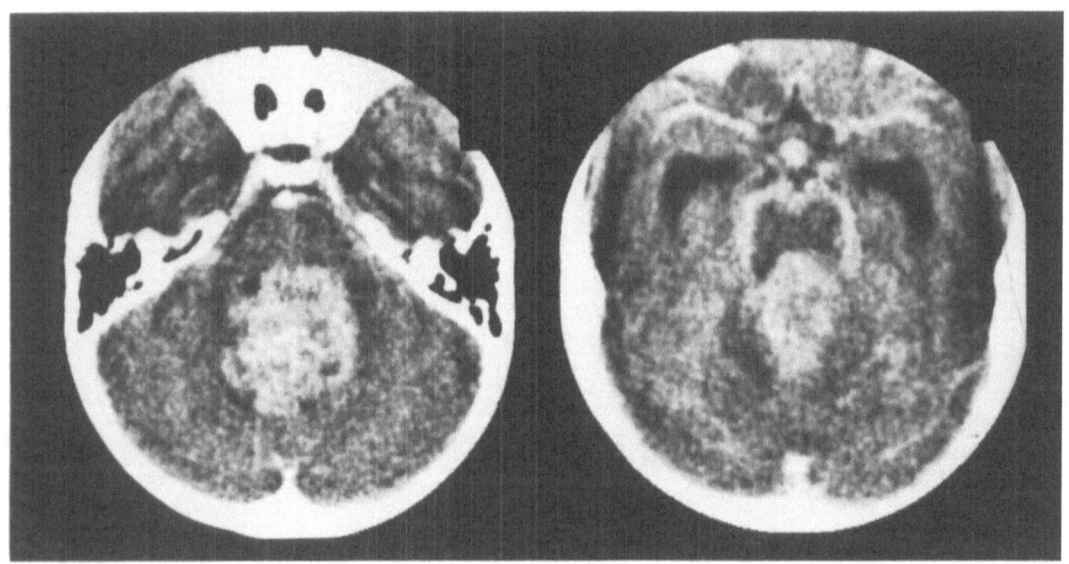

Fig. 1. CT-scan of a midline cerebellar medulloblastoma (enhanced)

year of life (39, 41, 51, 67, 72, 76, 77, 82, 86). A second possibility includes
a small foci of embryonal cell nests situated in the posterior medullary velum
(61, 64, 67, 95). Especially the numerous midline tumours are believed to arise
from these cells. On the basis of experimental induction and tissue culture
studies some authors propose the internal granular neurons as a possible source
of origin (47, 93, 94). Most authors, however, agree that the medulloblastoma is
an embryonic cell derived malignancy that develops by outgrowth of persisting
primitive cells.

Medulloblastomas are classified among the intracranial tumours of neuroepithelial origin and account for 4 to 10% of these tumours (75, 78, 86, 95).
In the new World Health Organization (WHO) classification they are subdivided
under the group of poorly differentiated and embryonal tumours (96). Other classifications have included medulloblastoma in the primary brain sarcoma group
(23, 32, 42) or the neuronal tumour group (63, 75).

Since the earliest reports a much higher frequency of medulloblastoma in
childhood has been noted, accounting for 20% of all intracranial tumours in
children (18, 80, 86). About 80% of these occur before the age of 15 years and
the frequency in males is higher than in females (19, 28a, 67, 72, 80, 95). These

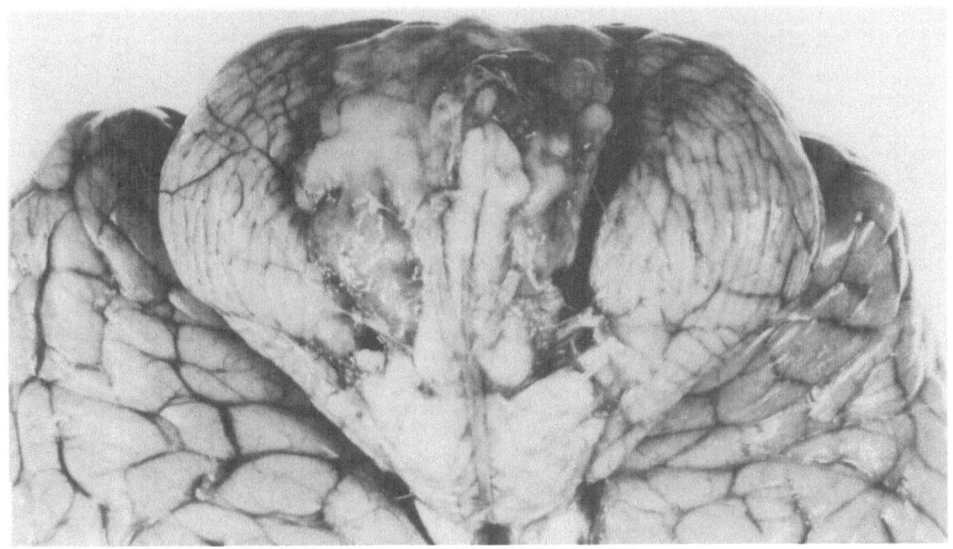

Fig. 2. Macroscopic appearance of a cerebellar medulloblastoma

childhood medulloblastomas are primarily located in the midline, while tumours
occurring in the adult group - approximately 15 to 20% of the medulloblastomas
occur in the 15 to 35 year age group - are primarily located in the lateral lobes
of the cerebellum (13, 20, 62, 67, 72, 74). In spite of the embryonal character
the occurrence of congenital medulloblastoma is surprisingly rare (1, 38, 39, 60).

Clinically the medulloblastoma often causes an increase in intracranial
pressure by obstructing the ventricular system, and the presenting symptoms are
mainly related to this obstruction: vomiting often without nausea, unsteadiness
of gait, headache, blurring of vision or diplopia, and dizziness (25, 53, 62, 72,
80). On neurological examination the dominating disorders are papilloedema,
nystagmus, abducens paresis and cerebellar disturbances. Seizures are rare although
they can occur as a late sign (25, 53, 62, 72, 80).

Macroscopically medulloblastomas are soft, friable and moderately well-
demarcated tumours with a grayish(-red) colour. Generally the tumours infiltrate
the floor of the fourth ventricle and extend into its cavity. The medulloblastoma
shows a marked tendency of seeding through the subarachnoid space of the brain
and the spinal cord. The leptomeningeal metastases can be diffuse or nodular (68,
71, 72, 75, 95).

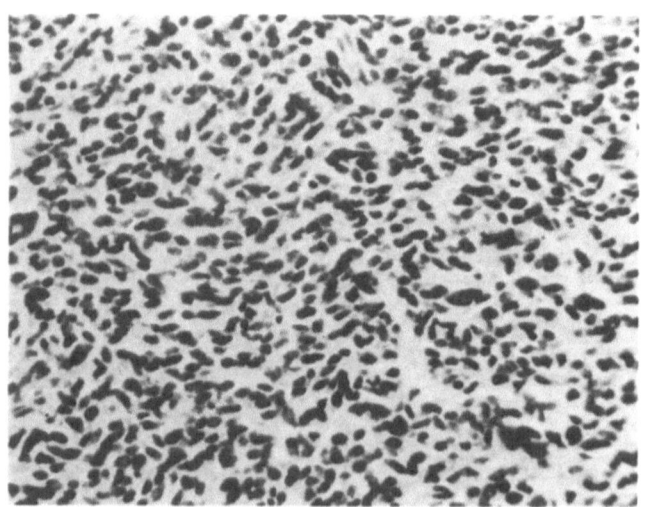

Fig. 3. Microscopic appearance of a cellular cerebellar medulloblastoma
HE, 200x

Extracranial metastases are rare but may occur, especially to the bone and lymph nodes, particularly after operation (partial removal or shunt operation), after intracranial spread and in the desmoplastic variety of medulloblastoma (12, 22, 62, 79).

Microscopically this cellular tumour generally consists of densely packed small, round to oval cells with hyperchromatic nuclei and scanty cytoplasm. Mitotic activity is variable. The formation of pseudo-rosettes - carrot-shaped cells around a blood vessel - that are found in approximately one-third of the cases, is highly characteristic for medulloblastoma (2, 68, 71, 72, 75, 95, 96). Differentiation of the medulloblastoma cells into mature ganglion cells (40, 72, 75) or spongioblastic, oligodendroglial and astrocytic cells can occur (2, 3, 72, 73, 74, 75, 91).

Some uncommon variants of medulloblastoma are: desmoplastic medulloblastoma (also called arachnoidal cerebellar sarcoma in the German literature) (33, 72, 74, 96), pigmented papillary medulloblastoma, and medullo-myoblastoma (72, 75, 96).

Surgical removal, complete irradiation of the central nervous system, and multiagent chemotherapy have been shown to improve the prognosis of medullo-blastoma (11, 25, 62, 80, 84).

FAMILIAL ASPECTS OF MEDULLOBLASTOMA

Case reports

The first report of possible familial occurrence of medulloblastoma dates from
Leavitt in 1927. At the Annual Meeting of the American Neurological Association
he presented the cases of two identical twin brothers who died of cerebellar
tumours (II.A.2.1). In the first twin who died at the age of 6 1/2 years, a
tumour was found at necropsy in the vermis of the cerebellum. Histologically a
diagnosis of medulloblastoma was made, a condition described two years earlier
by Bailey and Cushing. The second twin died at the age of 8 1/2 years having
shown symptoms consistent with the diagnosis of cerebellar tumour. Unfortunately
the consent of the parents for necropsy was not obtained and no histological
diagnosis of the tumour was available. This report has been registered among the
discordant occurrences.

Two (possibly three, if II.A.2.2. is included) reports of identical twins with
medulloblastoma followed in the literature, compared to five (possibly eight, if
II.A.3.4.a, b, c, are included) reports on identical twins of whom only one had
a medulloblastoma (tables 1, 2, and 3).

The report of Griepentrog and Pauly (II.A.1.1) is of special interest as one of
the twins also had a congenital teratoid tumour of the left clavicular region,
which after histological investigation showed to have parts of medulloblastoma
tissue. Furthermore, at necropsy tumours were found in the lymph nodules of the
neck, the right kidney and left adrenal, but unfortunately no microscopic study
of these tumours was performed. The unusually early age of manifestation, the
complete similarity of the tumours in these identical twins and finally the combination with a congenital teratoid malformation may point to the role of hereditary factors as a cause. The occurrence of a dwarf in the family may indicate
the presence of heredodegenerative traits. These twins reported by Griepentrog
and Pauly were also mentioned by Zülch in the 'Handbuch der Neurochirurgie' (67).
Waldbaur et al. (II.A.1.2) reported the occurrence of a cerebellar medulloblastoma
in a girl 5 months of age, and of a pineoblastoma in her identical twin sister at
the age of 16 months. It has been stressed that these tumours are cytologically
indistinguishable (50, 53), and this report on medulloblastoma and pineoblastoma
in identical twin sisters suggests an even more intimate relationship. The
authors stress in their article that the tumours in this case must be considered

as concordant tumours. As a choice they have been classified here among the
medulloblastomas.

Another possibly concordant occurrence of medulloblastoma in identical twins has
been reported by Metzel (54) as a personal communication from Sugita. One of
these Japanese twins underwent operation of a cerebellar medulloblastoma at the
age of 10 years, and her twin-sister died of a clinically diagnosed tumour of
the posterior fossa at the age of 8 years (II.A.2.2).

Familial aggregation of medulloblastoma in siblings has been reported in seven
families (table 4), all reported cases concerning occurrence in two siblings,
with the possible exception of the cases of Belamaric and Chau (II.B.1.4) where
a third sibling may have been involved. In the family described by these authors
two sisters died of medulloblastoma of the cerebellum. A third sister had died
at the age of 4 months of hydrocephalus, but details indicative of a possible
cerebellar tumour were not available. There were no other daughters in this
family and all the male children were in good health.

Investigating the clinical and genetic patterns of neurological diseases on Guam,
Chen et al. discovered a family demonstrating four siblings with brain tumours.
The brain tumours were diagnosed from material collected at autopsy and included
two sisters with medulloblastoma, one brother having a glioblastoma and another
brother a paraventricular haemangioma (II.B.1.5).

Another recent report of brain tumours in sisters merits special attention.
Thomas et al. (II.B.2.2) describe a case of two sisters; one died at the age of
5 years of a cerebellar tumour diagnosed as a mixed neuroblastoma and ganglioneuroma, while her younger sister died at the age of 2 years of desmoplastic
medulloblastoma of the cerebellum. This case has been registered here under discordant tumours, but this choice remains debatable. The authors stressed the
fact that in a medulloblastoma varying degrees of ganglionic differentiation may
be seen on occasion, *resulting in the appearance of atypical yet mature looking
ganglion cells, but that differentiation of this type would not lead to the type
of circumscribed nodule that was a conspicuous feature of this tumour*. It may be
argued that the appearance of these tumours in two sisters was purely fortuitous,
but taking into account the still dominant view that medulloblastoma may show
differentiation towards more mature ganglion cells, some authors even regarding
medulloblastoma as a form of neuroblastoma, the cases reported by Thomas et al.
might provide some proof of the debated possibility of divergent differentiation
in medulloblastoma.

Reports on familial occurrence of medulloblastoma in more than one generation
of a family do not appear to be available in the literature.

60

Examining the parameters of the reports on familial occurrence of medulloblastoma one finds:

Gender:

	female	male
twins	4	-
siblings	5	9

The number of reports on concordant familial medulloblastoma occurrence presently
available in the literature is too small to permit conclusions as to a male or
female predominance in these cases. In all but one report the tumours were found
in siblings of the same sex. In two reports there were no other healthy siblings
of that same sex. In the exceptional report of Kjellin et al. (II.B.1.2), who
describe a half-brother and half-sister with medulloblastoma, the occurrence
possibly represents a coincidental combination of similar brain tumours in two
close relatives.

Age:

In all but four cases of concordant tumour occurrence the age at which the
first symptoms of the tumour presented lay in the first decade of life. The
exceptions were the cases of a medulloblastoma occurring in a patient of military
service age in this case falling within the age group of 18 to 38 years reported
by Bennet (II.B.1.1), the 13-year-old girl reported by Chen et al. (II.B.1.5), and
the two brothers of 10 and 11 years mentioned by Wakai et al. (II.B.1.7). The
brother of the patient reported by Bennet has not been included in figure 1 as no
information as to his age was available. The majority of the cases occurred in the
first three years of life (58.8%) with a predominance in the first year (29.4%)
(fig. 1).

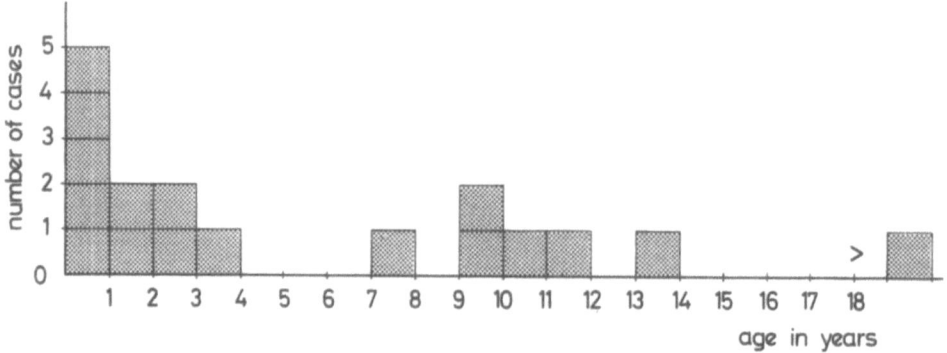

Fig. 1. Age at tumour manifestation in familial cases of medulloblastoma

In the cases of Griepentrog and Pauly (II.A.1.1) and Belamaric and Chau (II.B.1.4)
the inception of the neoplastic growth began either before birth or a short time
thereafter. In two of the patients the tumour must have originated during intra-
uterine life. External environmental factors could only have had a limited
influence in these cases.

Location of the tumour:

In most cases of familial medulloblastoma occurrence the tumour was located in
the vermis of the cerebellum with or without growth into the fourth ventricle
and the cerebellar hemispheres. The location was almost invariably in the midline
region, which is normal in childhood medulloblastomas.

Associated physical or mental conditions:

Associated physical or mental conditions in concordant tumour occurrence:

Twins:
- teratoid tumour of the breast and tumour
  in left adrenal and right kidney   1
- hip joint dysplasia   2

Siblings:
- traumatic skull facture   1
- purulent meningitis   2
- hepatomegaly   1
- black naevi   1
- hypoplasia corpus callosum   1
- café-au-lait spots   1
- haemangiomata   1

The report of Griepentrog and Pauly (II.A.1.1) who also found a teratoid tumour
of the left chest in one of their cases has been discussed earlier. Unfortunately
no microscopic study of the tumours in the lymph nodules of the neck, the right
kidney and left adrenal was performed. The question of the metastatic character
of the medulloblastoma remains open in this case. According to the authors it
seems more probable that these tumour elements were primary extracranial tumours
or primary components of the teratoid.

Of the sisters reported by Chen et al. (II.B.1.5) one had black naevi and hypoplasia of the corpus callosum, the other several café-au-lait spots and haemangiomata. These findings suggest a relationship with the phacomatoses.

Turcot et al. (II.B.2.1) described two siblings in both of which the brain tumour
was associated with polyposis of the colon, an association since then referred to
as the glioma-polyposis or Turcot syndrome (see associated diseases).

Family:

Thorough investigations of family histories have been either neglected or
scarcely mentioned in the reports on familial medulloblastoma. Although thorough
family studies are considered of great importance in the research on familial
brain tumours, information in this regard seems seldom to have been persued.

Members of the family investigated by Chen et al. (II.B.1.5) had clinical features
of phacomatosis such as café-au-lait spots and black naevi. Malignancies were also
found among relatives, such as leukaemia, hepatoma and laryngeal cancer. Similar
to the family reported by Blattner et al. (II.B.2.3), this family may be regarded
as a manifestation of the SBLA cancer syndrome (see associated hereditary diseases
and familial aspects of glioma).

Other parameters such as number of unaffected siblings, race or nationality,
pregnancy and birth, et cetera, are not discussed as the data on such parameters
are severely limited.

It is clearly difficult to draw conclusions regarding hereditary factors from
a small series of 18 (possibly 23) cases of medulloblastoma occurring in 9 (or 11)
families. As no reports are available in the literature of concordant occurrence
of medulloblastoma in more than one generation of a family, conclusions as to the
importance of hereditary factors remain speculative. Attention is drawn to the
fact that in two, possibly four, families the medulloblastomas were found in
identical twins, a fact which in itself might be interpreted as implying hereditary factors. In contradiction to this interpretation are the five, possibly
eight, reports on identical twins in which one member suffered from medulloblastoma and the other did not.

Serial studies

Norris and Jackson (59) studied childhood cancer deaths, other than from
leukaemia, in California-born twins. Seven twins - 4 dizygotic, 3 unspecified -
were found, demonstrating a medulloblastoma; their twin-partners had no cerebral
tumour (II.A.3.4).
Hauge and Harvald (34, 35) investigated the relatives of 27 patients with medulloblastoma. One of the probands was a dizygotic twin. In 282 relatives of these 27
probands no case of intracranial tumour was found. Only relatives over the age of
10 years, however, were included in the study.
In his extensive study on death from childhood cancer in siblings under 15 years
of age Miller (55) investigated the death certificates of 21,659 children and
reported two brothers, one having died at the age of 4 years of a medulloblastoma
and the other at the age of 5 years of a rhabdomyosarcoma in the maxillary area.
This same combination of tumours in two brothers has been found by Li and Fraumeni
(45) who studied 418 children who died from a rhabdomyosarcoma. These cases are of
special interest because of the identical chromosomal aberrations found in these
two tumours (16).
Choi et al. (15) performed a retrospective matched control study of 157 cases of

primary central nervous system tumours, based on interviews with family members.
For the verified tumour group including 126 subjects, 12 brain tumours were reported among 2104 relatives as compared to 3 brain tumours among 2404 relatives
of the 126 matched control subjects. For total tumours and all gliomas the dis-
parities in occurrence of central nervous system neoplasms among the families of
the study subjects and the control subjects were statistically significant. The
126 verified tumours included 6 medulloblastomas. Among their relatives two cases
of brain tumours and two 'other tumours' were found as compared to three 'other
tumours' in the control group. The number of patients within this category, however, was too small for statistical significance. Unfortunately in most of the
cases the specific histopathological type of the 'family tumour' was not available.

Associated hereditary diseases and congenital factors

Medulloblastomas have been described in association with autosomal dominant
disease entities. They can occur as a feature of multiple basal cell carcinoma
or Gorlin's syndrome (i.c. multiple basal cell carcinomas in early life, odonto-
genic cysts of the jaws, skeletal anomalies, intracranial calcifications of the
falx, medulloblastoma, ovarian fibroma, lymphomesenteric cysts and a characteristic facies with frontal and temporo-parietal bossing and well-developed supra-
orbital ridges). The occurrence was first noted by Herzberg and Wiskemann (37),
and subsequently by other authors (29, 30, 36, 65). Gorlin (29), who reviewed
more than 100 reports of this syndrome, noted that it is likely autosomal dominant
with high penetrance and variable expressivity. The medulloblastomas occurring
within this syndrome seem to appear early, 50% of the cases being under 2 years
of age when the diagnosis of medulloblastoma is made (58).
As stated earlier, medulloblastomas also occur within the SBLA cancer syndrome,
an autosomal dominantly inherited predisposition for sarcomas, breast cancer,
brain tumours, leukaemia, lung and laryngeal cancer, and adrenal cortical carcinoma (48, II.B.1.5. and II.B.2.3; see also familial aspects of glioma).
Medulloblastomas have also incidentally been reported in autosomal recessive
diseases. Shuster et al. (81) reported a child with medulloblastoma and Louis-Bar
syndrome or ataxia telangiectasia, a rare autosomal recessive disorder characterized by progressive cerebellar ataxia, oculocutaneous telangiectases and immuno-
deficiencies. Study of the chromosomal pattern of patients with this syndrome
showed that the chromosomes nrs 7 and 14 were preferentially involved (52).
As mentioned previously, medulloblastomas have been described within the glioma-
polyposis or Turcot syndrome, a rare disease with a probably autosomal recessive

mode of inheritance (26, 85) in which familial polyposis of the colon is associated with familial or isolated brain tumours (II.B.2.1, 17, 70; see also
familial aspects of glioma). Binder et al. (8) reported the occurrence of a
medulloblastoma in a large family with adenomatous colonic and gastric polyps
and sebaceous cysts, possibly suggesting a relationship with Gardner's syndrome
(21, 27). Rare cases of medulloblastoma have been described in xeroderma pigmen-
tosum (6) and the blue rubber-bleb nevus syndrome (66).

Rosano et al. (69) reported a child with an XYY karyotype, who showed a slight
psychomotor retardation and malformative signs and died at the age of 7 years
from a medulloblastoma.

The possible relationship between brain tumour occurrence (among the 110 patients
with brain tumours were 5 cases of medulloblastoma) and spina bifida, and also
the relation between mongoloid idiocy and the occurrence of brain tumours, were
studied by De Weerdt and Schut (89), but no correlation could be found between
these factors.

While there is general consensus as to the embryonal character of medulloblastoma,
congenital examples have been rarely reported. Nine cases were collected from the
literature by Ohta et al. (60). Females were more often affected than males, and
enlargement of the head (hydrocephalus) was the most prominent feature.

Cytogenetic aspects

Chromosomal patterns have been studied in sporadic cases of medulloblastoma
(16, 46). The karyotype of medulloblastoma cells is characterized by the presence
of several extra normal-appearing chromosomes in the 6-12, X or 4-5 group, and a
variable number of small duplicated fragments (double-minutes). In a patient with
a medulloblastoma Lubs et al. (46) found similar double fragments in cells of the
peripheral blood and bone marrow, and interpreted these to be metastatic cells.
The same disorders of chromosomes, however, have been seen in other tumours such
as glioma, neuroblastoma, rhabdomyosarcoma and bronchial carcinoma (16). The significance of these chromosomal abnormalities in malignant neoplasms is not completely understood. In their review Mulcahy and Harlan (57) summarize possible
interpretations of such chromosomal abnormalities, the possibilities being:
*1. the chromosomal changes are primary events resulting in malignancy; 2. the
chromosomal changes are secondary effects of the neoplastic process; 3. the
chromosomal changes and the malignancy are dual effects of a primary causative
factor; 4. the chromosomal changes, while not primary, lead to the establishment
of clones of malignant cells with a selective advantage for neoplastic progression.*
According to the authors ... *interpretation four has received considerable support*

in the literature.

The occurrence of a medulloblastoma in a patient with an XYY karyotype has been previously mentioned.

In view of the available data a definite conclusion in regard to the relationship between genetic factors and medulloblastoma occurrence is not possible. The available reports on familial aggregation of medulloblastoma may only suggest a genetic susceptibility in these families. The extent of genetic influence must be investigated. A detailed reporting of new cases of familial aggregation must be stressed, as well as the need for careful family studies of patients with medulloblastoma. Further search for possible chromosomal factors in the etiology of these neoplasms, especially in familial cases, appears essential.

REFERENCES

1. ARNSTEIN LH, BOLDREY E, NAFFZIGER HC 1951
    A case report and survey of brain tumours during the neonatal period.
    J Neurosurg 8:315-319
2. BAILEY P, CUSHING H 1925
    Medulloblastoma cerebelli. A common type of mid-cerebellar glioma of
    childhood.
    Arch Neurol Psychiatry (Chic) 14:192-224
3. BARNARD RO, PAMBAKIAN H 1980
    Astrocytic differentiation in medulloblastoma.
    J Neurol Neurosurg Psychiatry 43:1041-1044
4. BELAMARIC J, CHAU AS 1969
    Medulloblastoma in newborn sisters. Report of two cases.
    J Neurosurg 30:76-79
5. BENNETT WA 1946
    Primary intracranial neoplasma in military age group-world war II.
    Mil Surgeon 99:594-652
6. BIANCHI C, GIAMMUSSO V, BERTI N, VASSALLO A 1979
    Medulloblastoma in paziente con xeroderma pigmentoso.
    Pathologica 71:697-701
7. BICKERSTAFF ER, CONNOLLY RC, WOOLF AL 1967
    Cerebellar medulloblastoma occurring in brothers.
    Acta Neuropathol 8:104-107
8. BINDER MK, ZABLEN MA, FLEISCHER DE, SUE DY, DWYER RM, HANELIN L 1978
    Colon polyps, sebaceous cysts, gastric polyps, and malignant brain
    tumor in a family.
    Digest Diseases 23:460-466
9. BLATTNER WA, McGUIRE DB, MULVIHILL JJ, LAPKIN BC, HANANIAN J,
    FRAUMENI Jr JF 1979
    Genealogy of cancer in a family.
    JAMA 241:259-261
10. BODOR F, HAKANSSON CH, LINDGREN M 1974
    Irradiated cerebellar medulloblastoma in a monozygotic twin.
    Acta Radiol Ther Phys Biol 13:255-265
11. BONGARTZ EB, BAMBERG M, NAU HE, SCHMITT G, BAYINDIR C 1979
    Optimal therapy in medulloblastoma.
    Acta Neurochir 50:117-125
12. BOOHER Jr KR, SCHMIDTKNECHT TM 1977
    Cerebellar medulloblastoma with skeletal metastases. Case report and
    review of the literature.
    J Bone Joint Surg 59-A:684-686
13. CHATTY EM, EARLE KM 1971
    Medulloblastoma: a report of 201 cases with emphasis on the rela-
    tionship of histologic variants to survival.
    Cancer 28:977-983

14. CHEN K, BRODY JA, KURLAND LT, ELIZAN TS   1970
    Clinical and genetic patterns of neurological diseases other than
    amyotrophic lateral sclerosis on Guam.
    Neurology 20:954-964
15. CHOI NW, SCHUMAN LM, GULLEN WH   1970
    Epidemiology of primary central nervous system neoplasms. II: case-
    control study.
    Am J Epidemiol 91:467-485
16. COX D, YUNCKEN C, SPRIGGS AI   1965
    Minute chromatin bodies in malignant tumours of childhood.
    Lancet 2:55-58
17. CRAIL HW   1949
    Multiple primary malignancies arising in the rectum, brain and
    thyroid.
    Naval Med Bull 49:123-128
18. CRAIG W Mck, KEITH HM, KERNOHAN JW   1949
    Tumors of the brain occurring in childhood.
    Acta Psychiatr Neurol Scand 24:375-390
19. CRUE BL   1958
    Medulloblastoma.   .
    Charles C Thomas, Springfield, Ill
20. CUSHING H   1930
    Experiences with the cerebellar medulloblastomas. A critical review.
    Acta Pathol Microbiol Scand 7:1-86
21. DANES BS, KRUSH AJ, GARDNER EJ   1977
    Is Gardner syndrome a distinct genetic disorder?
    Lancet 2:925
22. DAS S, DALBY JE   1977
    Distant metastases from medulloblastoma.
    Acta Radiol Ther Phys Biol 16:117-123
23. DISTELMAIER P   1977
    Klinik, Differentialdiagnose und radiologisches Bild der primären
    Hirnsarkome.
    Nervenarzt 48:405-418
24. ENDE N   1955
    Congenital brain tumor in one of identical twins.
    Cancer 8:1057-1059
25. EYKENBOOM WMH   1976
    Medulloblastoma.
    Thesis, Rotterdam
26. FRAUMENI Jr JF   1981
    Glioma-polyposis syndrome (Turcot syndrome).
    In: Vinken PJ, Bruyn GW (eds) Handbook of Clinical Neurology.
    North-Holland Publ Co, Amsterdam vol 42:735-736
27. GARDNER EJ, RICHARDS RC   1953
    Multiple cutaneous and subcutaneous lesions occurring simulta-
    neously with hereditary polyposis and osteomatosis.
    Am J Human Genet 5:139-147
28. GEYER H, PEDERSEN O   1939
    Zur Erblichkeit der Neubildungen des Zentralnervensystems und
    seiner Hüllen.
    Z Ges Neurol Psychiatr 165:284-294

28a. GOLD EB, GORDIS L   1978
     Patterns of incidence of brain tumors in children.
     Ann Neurol 5:565-568
29. GORLIN RJ, SEDANO H   1971
     The multiple nevoid basal cell carcinoma syndrome revisited.
     Birth Defects 7(8):140-148
30. GORLIN RJ, VICKERS RA, KELLY E   1965
     The multiple basal-cell nevi syndrome: An analysis of a syndrome
     consisting of multiple nevoid basal-cell carcinoma, jaw cysts, skele-
     tal anomalies, medulloblastoma and hyporeponsiveness to
     parathormone.
     Cancer 18:89-104
31. GRIEPENTROG F, PAULY H   1957
     Intra- und extrakranielle, frühmanifeste Medulloblastome bei
     ergbleichen Zwillingen.
     Zentralbl Neurochir 17:129-140
32. GULLOTTA F   1967
     Vergleichende Untersuchungen zur Morphologie und Genese der soge-
     nannten Medulloblastome.
     Acta Neuropathol (Berl)8:76-83
33. GULLOTTA F, NEUMANN J   1980
     Medulloblastome und zerebelläre Sarkome. Eine histologische-
     katamnestische Untersuchung.
     Neurochirurgia 23:35-40
34. HAUGE M, HARVALD B   1957
     Genetics in intracranial tumours.
     Acta Genet 7:573-591
35. HAUGE M, HARVALD B   1960
     Studies in the etiology of intracranial tumours.
     Acta Psychiatr Neurol Scand 33:163-170
36. HAWKINS III JC, HOFFMAN HJ, BECKER LE   1979
     Multiple nevoid basal-cell carcinoma syndrome (Gorlin's syndrome):
     Possible confusion with metastatic medulloblastoma.
     J Neurosurg 50:100-102
37. HERZBERG JJ, WISKEMANN A   1963
     Die fünfte Phakomatose.
     Dermatologica 126:106-123
38. JELLINGER K, SUNDER-PLASSMANN M   1973
     Connatal intracranial tumours.
     Neuropaediatrie 4:46-63
39. KADIN ME, RUBINSTEIN LJ, NELSON GS   1970
     Neonatal cerebellar medulloblastoma originating from the fetal
     external granular layer.
     J Neuropathol Exp Neurol 29:583-600
40. KANE W, ARONSON SM   1967
     Gangliogliomatous maturation in cerebellar medulloblastoma.
     Acta Neuropathol (Berl) 9:273-279
41. KERSHMAN J   1938
     The medulloblasts and the medulloblastoma. A study of human embryos.
     Arch Neurol Psychiatr (Chic) 40:937-967
42. KERSTING G   1967
     Die Gewebszüchtung der Medulloblastome.
     Acta Neuropathol (Berl) 8:100-103

43. KJELLIN K, MÜLLER R, ASTRÖM KE   1960
    The occurrence of brain tumors in several members of a family.
    J Neuropathol Exp Neurol 19:528-537
44. LEAVITT FH   1928
    Cerebellar tumors occurring in identical twins.
    Arch Neurol Psychiatry (Chic) 19:617-622
45. LI FP, FRAUMENI Jr JF   1969
    Rhabdomyosarcoma in children: epidemiologic study and identification
    of a familial cancer syndrome.
    J Natl Cancer Inst 43:1365-1373
46. LUBS Jr HA, SALMON JH, FLANIGAN S   1966
    Studies of a glial tumor with multiple minute chromosomes.
    Cancer 19:591-599
47. LUMSDEN CE   1974
    Tissue culture of brain tumours.
    In: Vinken PJ, Bruyn GW (eds) Handbook of Clinical Neurology.
    North-Holland Publ Co, Amsterdam vol 17:42-104
48. LYNCH HT   1981
    SBLA Syndrome.
    In: Vinken PJ, Bruyn GW (eds) Handbook of Clinical Neurology.
    North-Holland Publ Co, Amsterdam vol 42:769-771
49. MACKLIN MT   1940
    An analysis of tumors in monozygous and dizygous twins.
    J Hered 31:277-290
50. MACKLIN MT   1941
    Tumours in monozygous and dizygous twins.
    Can Med Assoc J 44:604-606
51. MARBURG O   1931
    Zur Kenntnis der sog. Medulloblastome.
    Dtsch Z Nervenheilk 289:117-119
52. MARK J   1977
    Chromosomal abnormalities and their specificity in human neoplasms:
    an assessment of recent observations by banding techniques.
    Adv Cancer Res 24:165-222
53. MENKES GH   1974
    Textbook of child neurology.
    Lea and Febiger, Philadelphia
54. METZEL E   1963
    Über die familiär gehäuften Gliome.
    Arch Psychiatr Nervenkr 204:537-555
55. MILLER RW   1968
    Deaths from childhood cancer in sibs.
    N Eng J Med 279:122-126
56. MILLER RW   1971
    Deaths from childhood leukemia and solid tumors among twins and
    other sibs in the United States, 1960-1967
    J Natl Cancer Inst 46:203-209
57. MULCAHY GM, HARLAN WL   1976
    Occurrences of central nervous system tumors, with special reference
    to relative genetic factors.
    In: Lynch HT (ed) Cancer Genetics
    Charles C Thomas, Springfield, Ill, p 263-325

58. NEBLETT CR, WALTZ TA, ANDERSON DE 1971
Neurological involvement in the nevoid basal cell carcinoma
syndrome.
J Neurosurg 35:577-584
59. NORRIS FD, JACKSON EW 1970
Childhood cancer deaths in California-born twins. A further report
in types of cancer found.
Cancer 25:212-218
60. OHTA T, KAJIKAWA H, TAKEUCHI J 1977
Congenital tumours of the brain.
In: Vinken PJ, Bruyn GW (eds) Handbook of Clinical Neurology.
North-Holland Publ Co, Amsterdam vol 31:35-75
61. OSTERTAG B 1936
Einteilung und Charakteristik der Hirngewächse.
Gustav Fischer, Jena
62. PAILLAS JE, HASSOUN J, TORRES-GARCIA P, MICHOTEY P, VIALET G 1979
Les medulloblastomes de l'adulte.
Arch Anat Cytol Pathol 27:78-84
63. POLAK M 1967
On the true nature of the so-called medulloblastoma.
Acta neuropathol (Berl) 8:84-95
64. RAAF J, KERNOHAN J 1944
Relation of abnormal collections of cells in posterior medullary
velum of cerebellum to origin of medulloblastoma.
Arch Neurol Psychiatry (Chic) 52:163-169
65. RAYNER CRW, TOWERS JF, WILSON JSP 1977
What is Gorlin's syndrome? The diagnosis and management of the basal
cell naevus syndrome, based on a study of thirty-seven patients.
Br J Plast Surg 30:62-67
66. RICE JS, FISCHER DS 1962
Blue rubber-bleb nevus syndrome.
Arch Dermatol 86:503-511
67. RINGERTZ N, TOLA JH 1950
Medulloblastoma.
J Neuropathol Exp Neurol 9:354-372
68. ROBBINS SL 1974
Pathologic basis of disease.
WB Saunders Co, Phildapelphia p 1520-1521
69. ROSANO M, DELELLIS M, MASSARA B, DITONDO U, CASINI C 1970
Cariotipo xyy e medulloblastoma.
Acta Genet Med Gemellol 23:259-263
70. ROTHMAN D, KENDALL AB 1975
Dilemma in a case of Turcot's (Glioma-polyposis) syndrome: report of
a case.
Dis Colon Rectum 18:514-515
71. RUBINSTEIN LJ 1972
Tumors of the central nervous system. In: Atlas of Tumor Pathology.
2nd series, Fasc 6.
Armed Forces Inst of Pathol, Washington DC p 130-152
72. RUBINSTEIN LJ 1975
The cerebellar medulloblastoma: its origin, differentiation,
morphological variants, and biological behaviour.
In: Vinken PG, Bruyn GW (eds) Handbook of Clinical Neurology .
North-Holland Publ Co, Amsterdam vol 17:167-193

73. RUBINSTEIN LJ, HERMAN MM, HANBERY JW 1974
    The relationship between differentiating medulloblastoma and dedif-
    ferentiating diffuse cerebellar astrocytoma. Light electron
    microscopic, tissue and organ culture observations.
    Cancer 33:675-690
74. RUBINSTEIN LJ, NORTHFIELD DWC 1964
    The medulloblastoma and the so-called "arachnoidal cerebellar
    sarcoma". A critical re-examination of a nosological problem.
    Brain 87:379-412
75. RUSSELL DS, RUBINSTEIN LJ 1977
    Pathology of the tumours of the nervous system. 4th ed.
    Edward Arnold, London p 146-283
76. SACCONE A, EPSTEIN JA 1948
    Granuloblastoma, primary neuroectodermal tumor of the cerebellum.
    J Neuropathol 7:287-298
77. SCHEINKER JM 1939
    Zur Frage der Pathogenese und Pathologie der Medulloblastome.
    Monatschr Psychiatr Neurol 101:103-113
78. SCHOENBERG BS, CHRISTINE BW, WHISNANT JP 1976
    The descriptive epidemiology of primary intracranial neoplasms: the
    Connecticut experience,
    Am J Epidemiol 104:499-510
79. SCHNITZLER ER, RICHARDS MJS, CHUN RWM 1978
    Cerebellar medulloblastoma. An analysis of four cases of extraneural
    metastasis.
    Am J Dis Child 132:1004-1008
80. SCUCCIMARA A, CARTERI A, GIORDANO R, CROTTI FM, TOMEI G, ZAVANONE ML
    1979
    Medulloblastoma in children: review on 119 cases.
    J Neurosurg Sci 23:37-46
81. SHUSTER J, HART Z, STIMSON CW, BROUGH AJ, POULIK MD 1966
    Ataxia telangiectasia with cerebellar tumor.
    Pediatrics 37:776-786
82. STEVENSON L, ECHLIN F 1934
    Nature and origin of some tumours of the cerebellum.
    Medulloblastoma.
    Arch Neurol Psychiatry (Chic) 31:93-109
83. THOMAS M, ADAMS JH, DOYLE D 1977
    Neuroectodermal tumours in the cerebellum in two sisters.
    J Neurol Neurosurg Psychiatry 40:886-889
84. THOMAS PRM, DUFFNER PK, COHEN ME, SINKS LF, TEBBI C, FREEMAN AI 1980
    Multimodality therapy for medulloblastoma.
    Cancer 45:666-669
85. TODD DW, CHRISTOFERSON LA, LEECH RW, RUDOLF L 1981
    A family affected with intestinal polyposis and gliomas.
    Ann Neurol 10:390-392
86. TOLA JH 1951
    The histopathological and biological characteristics of primary
    neoplasms of the cerebellum and the fourth ventricle, with some
    aspects of their clinical picture, diagnosis, and treatment (on the
    basis of 71 verified cases).
    Acta Chir Scand (Suppl) 164:1-112

87. TURCOT J, DESPRÉS JP, StPIERRE F   1959
    Malignant tumors of the central nervous system associated with fami-
    lial polyposis of the colon. Report of two cases.
    Dis Colon Rectum 2:465-468
87a. WAKAI S, SEGAWA H, KITAHARA S, ASANO T, SANO K, OGIHARA R, TOMITA S
    1980
    Teratoma in the pineal region in two brothers. Case reports.
    J Neurosurg 53:239-243
88. WALDBAUR H, GOTTSCHALDT M, SCHMIDT H, NEUHÄUSER G   1976
    Medulloblastom des Kleinhirns und Pineoblastom bei eineiigen
    Zwillingen.
    Klin Pädiat 188:366-371
89. WEERDT CJ de, SCHUT T   1972
    Some aspects of heredity of brain tumours.
    Psychiatr Neurol Neurochir (Amst) 75:293-298
90. WIEL HJ van der   1959
    Inheritance of glioma.
    Thesis, Elsevier, Amsterdam
91. WILLIS RA   1967
    Pathology of tumours, 4th ed.
    Butterworth, London
92. YAMASHITA J, HANDA H, TOYAMA M   1975
    Medulloblastoma in two brothers.
    Surg Neurol 4:225-227
93. ZIMMERMAN HM   1967
    The histopathology of experimental "medulloblastoma".
    Acta Neuropath (Berl) 8:69-75
94. ZIMMERMAN HM   1969
    Brain tumors: their incidence and classification in man and their
    experimental production.
    Ann NY Acad Sci 159:337-359
95. ZÜLCH KJ   1956
    Biologie und Pathologie der Hirngeschwülste.
    In: Olivecrona H, Tönnis W (eds) Handbuch der Neurochirurgie, Bnd 3
    Springer, Berlin p 118-140
96. ZÜLCH KJ   1981
    Principles of the new World Health Organization (WHO) classifi-
    ciation of brain tumors.
    Neuroradiology 19:59-66

Chapter III

FAMILIAL MENINGIOMA

CASE REPORTS

CLASSIFICATION

A. *TWINS*

    1. Monozygotic twins with concordant tumour

    2. Monozygotic twins with discordant tumour

    3. Monozygotic twins, one demonstrating meningioma

    4. Dizygotic twins

B. *SIBLINGS*

    1. Siblings with concordant tumour

    2. Siblings with discordant tumour

C. *OTHER GENERATIONS AND DISTANT RELATIVES*

    1. Other generations and distant relatives with concordant tumour

    2. Other generations and distant relatives with discordant tumour

TABLES

III.A.   *TWINS*

III.A.1.   MONOZYGOTIC TWINS WITH CONCORDANT TUMOUR

III.A.1.1.   <u>Sedzimir et al. 1973 - Liverpool, England</u> (90)

Identical twins. Male. English.

<u>Case 1</u>

<u>History</u>: The patient was born after a normal pregnancy. *He developed normally, parallel to his twin brother* ... At the age of 16 months he developed a squint of the right eye and was found to have a congenital cataract. At the age of seven years it was stated that *the right eye was 'useless' because of a posterior polar congenital cataract and divergent squint. The left eye was proptosed and ophthalmoplegic.*

At the age of 8 years the patient developed *'abnormality of gait'. In the lower limbs, slight spasticity was found in both legs with bilaterally increased tendon reflexes and extensor plantar responses. He also had marked bilateral 'claw feet'.*

When the patient was nine years of age he was again admitted to hospital. At that time the following neurological signs were found: an almost complete spastic paraplegia, depression of sensation to pin prick from D7 to S2 dermatomes bilaterally, distention of the bladder, vibration sense depressed below the knees and joint position sense was lost in the toes, reflexes were clonic at both knees and ankles with bilateral extensor plantar responses. Marked clawing of both feet was noted.

Lumbar myelography demonstrated complete obstruction at the level of D11 vertebral body ... Laminectomy of dorsal 10, 11 and 12 vertebrae was performed ... A meningioma situated in front and to the left of the dorsal spinal cord was totally resected. The postoperative recovery was satisfactory.

At the age of 13 years the patient was reexamined in relation to illness of his twin brother. No new abnormalities were found at physical examination. *Skull radiographs ... showed evidence of right frontal enostosis. There was a Klippel-Feil anomaly with rather wide cervical canal. A brain scan showed evidence of a large right frontal falx meningioma.* No treatment of this neoplasm was undertaken.

<u>Microscopic study</u>: *The dorsal meningioma contained cellular syncytial and psammomatous areas. There were numerous calcispherites.*

Diagnosis: Spinal thoracic meningioma. Right frontal falx meningioma.
Congenital ophthalmological disorders of both eyes.

Case 2

History: Normal pregnancy, birth and early development. At the age of 12
years the patient had progressive pain in the neck, mainly left sided, and
developed a painful torticollis. *He woke up one morning with paresis of the
left arm and leg* and was admitted to hospital.
On examination *there was left-sided hemiparesis with increased tendon reflexes
and bilaterally extensor plantar responses. Vibration sense and joint position
sense were depressed in the left upper and lower limbs. Radiographs of the
skull showed changes in the region of the pituitary fossa consistent with
long-standing raised intracranial pressure and sclerosis in the region of the
tuberculum sellae and adjacent bony structures. Cervical spine radiography
showed considerable widening of the spinal canal throughout the upper cervical
segments consistent with an expanding process in this region.* Right carotid
angiography showed appearances *consistent with the presence of a meningioma of
the tuberculum sellae.*
At operation *an enormous meningioma was removed piece-meal. It appeared to
invade the posterior ethmoidal cells and surrounding bone on both sides and
extended as far as the right olfactory groove.*
Postoperatively the patient *developed weakness of the right upper limb and
gradually ... became entirely tetraplegic. There was in addition a loss to
pin-prick sensation bilaterally below C4 dermatome. Vibration and joint
position sense were lost in both lower limbs and depressed in the hands and
fingers. His breathing was entirely diaphragmatic. ... some bladder sensation
was preserved.*
Lumbar myelography disclosed another tumour in addition to the suspected
upper cervical meningioma. *The contrast medium was completely held up at
the level of the body of D11 vertebra ...*
Cervical laminectomy of C1 to C6 was performed and a large meningioma was
resected. *It was situated anterolaterally to the cord, which was displaced
posteriorly and to the right. The attachment of the meningioma to the dura
mater was over a very small area.*
Under the same anaesthetic a laminectomy of dorsal 9 to 12 vertebrae was
performed and another meningioma was found *also anterolaterally to the cord.*
Postoperatively the patient had a serious neurological deficit, especially on
the left side of his body, and was confined to a wheel-chair.
He died at the age of 14 years of unspecified cause.

Autopsy: Was not performed.

Microscopic study: *The frontal basal meningioma was very cellular with syncytial and psammomatous areas. ... very few mitoses were seen. The upper cervical ... and mid-dorsal meningioma showed outstandingly similar histological patterns in all fragments of syncytial and psammomatous type of meningioma with many calcispherites.*

On comparison the tumours of case 1 were somewhat more cellular and those of case 2 showed more calcification of psammomata and more calcispherites. *Otherwise all these tumours were remarkably similar.*

Diagnosis: Two spinal meningioma (cervical and thoracic). Tuberculum sellae meningioma.

Family: *The family history was unremarkable. The twins' paternal grandfather died at the age of 69 years of 'cardiac condition'. The grandmother is alive at the age of 68 years. The twins have one paternal aunt who emigrated many years ago to Canada where she had twin boys who died within days after birth. The boys' maternal grandfather is alive and well, aged 68 years; the grandmother parted from her husband and nothing is known about her. The mother and father of the twins and the third child, a boy aged 7 years, are well and have not suffered from any severe illness.*

COMMENT

No signs of neurofibromatosis were present in the two patients or in the family.

III.A.2.   MONOZYGOTIC TWINS WITH DISCORDANT TUMOUR

III.A.2.1. Hoppe 1952 - Berlin, Germany (41)

Identical twins. Male. German.

Case 1

History: The patient was the first born twin. There was a normal birth, growth and early development. The patient had never been seriously ill until the age of 35 years when he had a brain injury with concussion. A few weeks later he developed epileptic seizures which repeated at irregular intervals. The type of seizure was always the same: visual aura, turning of the head and eyes to the right, and shortly afterwards generalized convulsion with loss of consciousness.

At the age of 38 the patient was admitted to hospital, and by encephalographic study a left frontal tumour was diagnosed.

At operation no tumour was found and postoperatively the patient still had seizures, which became more frequent. The patient also complained of headaches and loss of memory. At the age of 40 years the patient was readmitted to hospital.

On examination a left-sided hyposmia, slight left-sided exophthalmus, slight papilloedema, more on the left than on the right, a slight loss of the right temporal visual field, a right central facial paresis, brisker reflexes on the right than on the left, and language disturbances were found. Radiographs of the skull showed a pointed head-form. Left carotid angiography showed a tumour mass as large as an apple with many small vessels presenting on the sphenoid bone.

At operation a tumour attached to the sphenoid was removed. The postoperative course was good and the patient was free of complaints.

A year afterward he had an attack with hemiparesis on the right side and complete aphasia from which he slowly recovered in the course of nine months.

Microscopic study: Meningioma.

Diagnosis: Left sphenoidal meningioma.

Case 2

History: The patient had a normal birth, growth and development. He had been healthy until the age of 53, when he began stumbling while walking. A few days afterwards he had a transient right-sided facial paresis and a speech disturbance. One month later he incurred a paresis of the right side of the body, again with speech disturbance, and was admitted to hospital.

On examination the following disorders were found: papilloedema on both sides, right central facial paresis, hypotonic paresis of the right arm and leg, lower tendon reflexes on the right than on the left, an expressive aphasia, and lowering of consciousness. Radiograph of the skull showed a pointed head-form with dura calcification at the dorsum sellae. Angiography showed a process in the left fronto-medial region without pathological vessels.

At operation a tumour the size of a mandarin was found with multiple cysts localized in the posterior fronto-median region.

The postoperative course was at first satisfactory and the patient was irra-diated. Fourteen days after operation the patient died suddenly.

    Autopsy: Was not permitted.

    Microscopic study: Glioblastoma fusiforme.

    Diagnosis: Glioblastoma, left fronto-central.

    Family: There were several twins in the family of the patients' mother. The mother herself was one of twins. She and her twin sister had asthma. The father of the patients had a brain injury with an impression fracture of the skull when he was 53 years of age. He died at the age of 60.

COMMENT

Case 1 was first reported in detail by Pedersen and Geyer in 1938. They also examined the patient of case 2 at that time but could not then find any abnormalities (III.A.3.2).

III.A.3.   MONOZYGOTIC TWINS, ONE DEMONSTRATING MENINGIOMA

III.A.3.1. Kuhnen 1953 - Münster, Germany (52)

Male monozygotic twin. German.

The author studied a series of seven twin-pairs, one twin of each pair having
a brain tumour.
He extensively described one of identical male twins who was operated upon
because of an endotheliomatous meningioma in the right temporo-parietal region
at the age of 15 years.

The patient's brother was healthy. No occurrence of nervous or mental disease
was found in 50 other relatives.

III.A.3.2. Pedersen and Geyer 1938 - Berlin, Germany (73)

Male monozygotic twin. German.

The authors report monozygotic male twins, one of whom had a left sphenoidal
meningioma at the age of 40 years.

His healthy twin brother underwent an extensive neurological examination at
that time but nothing could be found. At the age of 53 years a left fronto-
central glioblastoma fusiforme was discovered in this brother. This case is
reported in detail by Hoppe in 1952 (III.A.2.1).

III.A.4.   DIZYGOTIC TWINS

No reports on dizygotic twins with concordant meningioma are presently available.

Hauge and Harvald (35) describe a dizygotic female twin having a meningioma
and dying at the age of 61 years. Her twin sister was still alive and well
at the age of 74 years.

Kuhnen (52) reported dizygotic twins (male and female), the male having a
left fronto-parietal meningioma at the age of 41 years. His twin sister was
healthy.

III.B.   *SIBLINGS*

III.B.1.   SIBLINGS WITH CONCORDANT TUMOUR

III.B.1.1. Ectors and Van Bogaert 1953 - Brussels, Belgium (28)

A brother and sister. Belgian.

Case 1 (brother)

History: This engineer was admitted to hospital at the age of 40 years.
For several months he had complained of a painful torticollis, a numb feeling
in the fingers of both hands and feet, loss of position sense of the right
hand and fingers, and a loss of strength of the right hand and leg. He also
noticed an imperative miction and defaecation pattern.
On examination there was slight circumduction of the right leg while walking.
A slight paresis of the right arm and hypaesthesia of the right side of the
body with an upper level at C_3 were present. Deep tendon reflexes were brisker
on the left than on the right. At lumbar puncture a complete block was found.
The protein content of the CSF was 0.69 cg.
At operation an intra- and extradural tumour was found at the anterior side
of the bulbus attached to the dura and extending from the foramen magnum to C_2.
A fusion of the posterior arc of the atlas with the foramen magnum was discovered.
The postoperative course was good and neurological examination a few months
later revealed no abnormalities. A year after operation a small tumour was
discovered at the internal side of the right upper leg. Permission was not
obtained for removal of this tumour.
Microscopic study: showed a lobulated meningioma with numerous psammoma
bodies, many blood vessels, and some areas with xanthomatous transformation.
Diagnosis: Meningioma of the foramen magnum.

Case 2 (sister)

History: This female was admitted to hospital at the age of 40 years. Her
complaints began years before admission. At the age of 25 years she complained
of numb feelings in both hands, and difficulties with fine movements of the
left hand. Since 32 years of age she had intermittent dysuria. At the age of
35 years she deteriorated with vomiting, headaches, dizziness and pain in the
neck. In the year before admission her complaints progressed slowly. A month

before admission a small schwannoma was removed from her left fore-arm.

On examination she had disturbances of gait, a positive Romberg sign, limitation of the neck movements, hypaesthesia of the right side of the body with an upper level at C_2, hypaesthesia of the left C_2 and C_3 dermatome, a paresis of the left arm and leg, brisk tendon reflexes of the legs with a positive Babinski sign on the right, and a disturbance of coordination, more obvious on the left than on the right. At lumbar puncture a partial block was found. The protein content of the CSF was 1.0 cg.

At operation an intra- and extradural tumour was found attached to the dura and extending over the entire posterior surface and left lateral side of the foramen magnum. There was fusion of the posterior arc of the atlas with the foramen magnum.

The postoperative course was good and examination six months later showed only a slight neurological deficit.

  Microscopic study: showed a meningioma with numerous psammoma bodies.

  Diagnosis: Meningioma of the foramen magnum.

  Family: The father of these patients died at the age of 69 years of a heart attack. The mother was in good health. The patients had two sisters who were also in good health. Case 1 had five children. Case 2 had three children; she had also had two abortions. None of the family members showed congenital abnormalities or signs of neurofibromatosis.

COMMENT

The presence of a schwannoma in case 2 and an unverified small subcutaneous tumour in case 1 suggest a possible relationship with neurofibromatosis. According to the authors the evidence for such a relationship was insufficient.

85

III.B.1.2. Gaist et al. 1959 - Bologna, Italy (31)

A brother and sister. Italian.

Case 1 (sister)

History: At the age of 39 years this female was admitted to hospital. One
and a half years previously she had a first episode of sudden loss of consciousness. A similar episode occurred 6 months later. At that time she started complaining of frontal headaches and dizzy spells. One month before admission she
noticed that her vision was beginning to fail.
On examination the patient showed marked pyramidal signs on her right side ....
There was papilledema of the optic discs; visual acuity was 4/10 in the right
eye and 1/50 in the left. The electroencephalogram showed a slow-wave abnormality in the left hemisphere. Left carotid angiography showed two round areas of
abnormal vascularization in the frontopolar and ascending frontal regions. The
more anterior of these two areas ... seemed to be supplied mostly by a branch
of the middle meningeal artery.
A left frontal craniotomy revealed the presence of two large tumours embedded
in normal cerebral parenchyma and closely adherent to the dura mater. The
tumours were removed together with the dura mater.
The postoperative course was very good. Almost three years after operation the
patient showed some slight abnormalities in her behavior.
Microscopic study: The tumour consists of fibrocellular tissue, here and
there dissociated by hemorrhagic areas. The cells are arranged in sinusoid
streams running in different directions .... The nuclei are round or oval in
shape, rich in evenly distributed chromatin and without nucleolus. The vascular
component is well represented by capillary vessels or by larger blood spaces ....

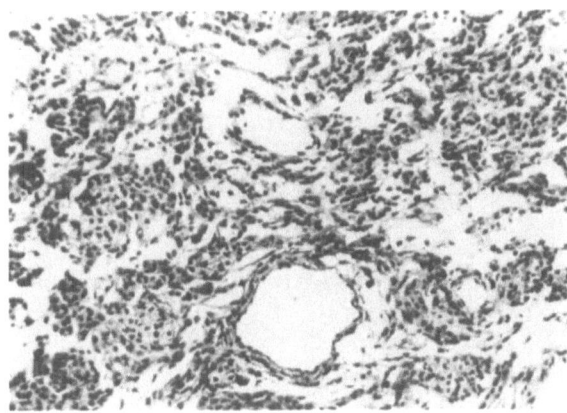

Fig. 1.
Microscopic appearance
of the tumour of case
1.
(Gaist G, Piazza G
1959 (31))

*In many areas the section consists of fibrocellular bundles arranged in whorls
around a small vessel. The stroma appears formed by connective-tissue strands
or by short fibrous tracts, partly showing hyaline degeneration.*

Diagnosis: Two meningiomas, left frontal.

Case 2 (brother)

History: At the age of 36 years this male was admitted to hospital. *Five
months previously he had a first generalized seizure with loss of consciousness
during sexual intercourse; a similar episode occurred 1 month later in the same
circumstances. Anticonvulsive therapy was prescribed, which he discontinued 1
month before admission, as seizures had not recurred.* Ten days before admission
he had a generalized seizure and another one 24 hours later.
On examination the patient showed a *slight left facial weakness and left hyper-
reflexia. Mild bilateral peripapillary edema was present; visual acuity was
10/10 bilaterally.* Cerebrospinal fluid pressure was normal, but protein content
elevated (80 mg). On electroencephalography a right frontal focus was present.
*... right carotid angiography showed a marked downward displacement of peri-
callosal and callosomarginal arteries.*
*Through a right frontal craniotomy, a large parasagittal tumor, closely
adherent to the dura mater, was exposed and removed.*
Postoperative course was good but the patient had *one seizure every 5 to 6
months.*

Microscopic study: The tumour *consists almost entirely of a layer of cells
closely packed into cords running in different directions, and showing active
proliferation. There is a loose connective stroma with a few blood vessels.
The cells are polygonal with clear cytoplasm; the nuclei are large, unequal
and vesicular, with chromatin in clumps. The loose connective stroma is partly
hyalinized.*

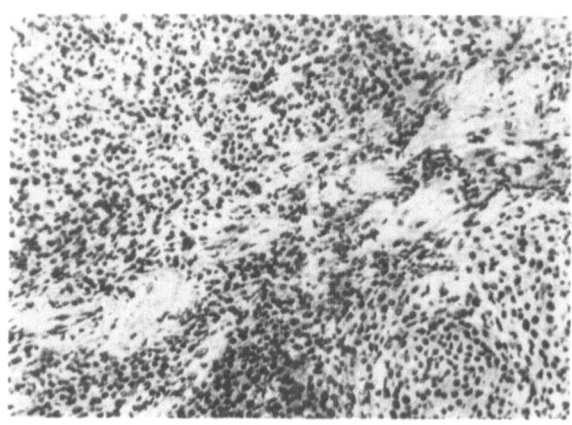

Fig. 2.
Microscopic appearance
of the tumour of case
2.
(Gaist G, Piazza G
1959 (31))

Diagnosis: Right parasagittal meningioma.

COMMENT

No data concerning the relatives of the two patients are given in this report. Probably the other members of the family have not been investigated as the authors state: *It is not entirely uncommon that members of the same family may be affected by similar intracranial expansive processes, particularly neurofibromas, as part of von Recklinghausen's disease.*

III.B.1.3. <u>Grunert et al. 1970 - Vienna, Austria</u> (34)

Two brothers. Greek.

<u>Case 1</u>

<u>History</u>: At the age of 53 years the patient was admitted to hospital because
of a since three months progressive bitemporal hemianopia.
Neurological examination revealed a bitemporal hemianopia but no other disorders. A left and right carotid angiogram and a pneumencephalogram were normal.
At operation a tumour which could be completely removed was found mainly
situated under and behind the chiasma opticum.
The postoperative course was good.

   <u>Microscopic study</u>: Endotheliomatous type of meningioma.

   <u>Diagnosis</u>: Meningioma in the chiasma region (suprasellar meningioma).

<u>Case 2</u>

<u>History</u>: At the age of 49 years the patient was admitted to hospital because
of a sudden hemiparesis on the right accompanied by headaches, dizziness and
diplopia. At the age of 38 the patient had been operated on because of an
aneurysm of the a. communicans anterior. Because of the broad base of this
aneurysm it could not be clipped. At the age of 46 years the patient had a
transient disturbance of speech which was treated conservatively.
Neurological examination revealed an organic psychosyndrome, expressive
aphasia, central facial paresis and hemiparesis on the right. A left and right
carotid angiogram showed the already diagnosed aneurysm of the a. communicans
anterior and signs of internal hydrocephalus. A pneumencephalogram revealed a
large tumour of the third ventricle extending into both lateral ventricles.
By a right frontal craniectomy the part of the tumour in the right lateral
ventricle and in the third ventricle was removed. The tumour portion in the
left lateral ventricle was not removed.
The postoperative course was satisfactory and the patient was discharged in
good condition.

   <u>Microscopic study</u>: Fibromatous-endotheliomatous type of meningioma.

   <u>Diagnosis</u>: Meningioma of the third ventricle.

   <u>Family</u>: According to the first brother (case 1), who was a medical doctor
by profession, a sister of theirs had died of a not identified brain tumour.
No further data are known about this case.

COMMENT

In this report the family members of the patients were not investigated. The blood type of the two brothers was different: O Rh + in case 1 and A_1 Rh + in case 2.

III.B.2.   SIBLINGS WITH DISCORDANT TUMOUR

III.B.2.1. <u>Koch 1954 - Münster, Germany</u> (50)

A brother and sister. German.

Koch investigated the families of a series of 350 female patients with a
brain tumour, mainly glioma and meningioma. Among these families a familial
aggregation of brain tumours was found six times, four cases of which could
be verified histologically. One of these cases was a 44-year-old female with
a parasagittal meningioma. Her brother had a tumour of the right temporal
lobe, and hemiparkinsonism, at the age of 47 years. This tumour was not
microscopically examined.

   <u>Family</u>:

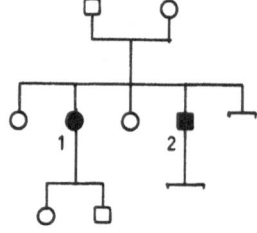

    1 = meningioma
    2 = brain tumour

III.B.2.2. <u>Chateau et al. 1971 - Lyon, France</u> (16)

A brother and sister. French.

<u>Case 1</u> (sister)

<u>History</u>: The patient was admitted to hospital at the age of 46 years. For a month she had complained of occipital headaches, paraesthesia in the right half of the body, clumsiness of the right hand, loss of function in the right leg, and osmatic hallucinations.

Neurological examination showed a right-sided hemiparesis, tendon reflexes on the right brisker than on the left, and a positive Romberg sign. The EEG showed a right parietal focus and a focus left temporo-occipital. The echo was displaced 6 mm to the right. A left carotid angiogram showed an expansive process parasagittal in the left parietal region.

At operation an extracerebral tumour was found with a diameter of 3 cm attached to the falx.

The postoperative course was good.

<u>Microscopic study</u>: Fibroblastic meningioma.

<u>Diagnosis</u>: Meningioma left parietal, parasagittal.

<u>Case 2</u> (brother)

<u>History</u>: At the age of 43 years the patient was admitted to hospital. Since three weeks he had complained about cervico-occipital headaches, vertigo and a drunkards gait.

On examination a cerebellar syndrome, a hypoacousis on the left and a horizontal bilateral nystagmus were found. Radiographs of the skull, and echo were normal. The EEG showed slow waves in the left temporal region spreading to the right. An angiogram was performed and raised suspicion of an *angio-reticulome kystique*. A ventriculogram showed an expansive process in the left posterior fossa.

At operation in the left cerebellar hemisphere a voluminous cyst was found containing xanthochromic fluid, and in the top of it a small tumour situated near the median line.

The postoperative course was good.

<u>Microscopic study</u>: Haemangioblastoma of the cerebellum.

<u>Diagnosis</u>: Haemangioblastoma of the left cerebellum.

<u>Family</u>: Examination of the entire family did not reveal any signs of neurofibromatosis or phacomatosis. No further data about the family are given in the article.

III.C.   *OTHER GENERATIONS AND DISTANT RELATIVES*

III.C.1.   OTHER GENERATIONS AND DISTANT RELATIVES WITH CONCORDANT TUMOUR

III.C.1.1. Wagman et al. 1960 - Philadelphia, U.S.A. (97)

A mother and daughter. American.

Case 1 (mother)

History: At the age of 69 years the patient was admitted to hospital
because of *terminal uremia .... There was a fifteen year history of diminishing
vision in the left eye, limitation of movement of the left eyeball and lid,
progressing to blindness and complete external ophthalmoplegia. This had been
accompanied by increasing prominence of bone in the left temporal region.*

Autopsy: *No evident cerebral neoplasm was found .... The dura at the base
in the left middle fossa was thickened, adherent to the tip of the left temporal
bone .... The floor of the left anterior fossa, extending into the sphenoid
bone, was densely thickened and eburnated. The cavity of the left orbit was
greatly reduced by bony overgrowth with a roof measuring 2 centimeters in
thickness. The contents of the orbit ... were compressed .... The sphenoid and
ethmoid sinuses on the left were obliterated by the bony process and were greatly
reduced in size on the right.*

Microscopic study: *revealed the abnormal bone to be infiltrated with typical
meningioma of arachnoidal type. Similar neoplastic cells infiltrated both
surfaces of the adjacent dura with a microscopic nodule invading the subarachnoid space at the tip of the left temporal lobe. Neoplastic infiltration
was also present in the contents of the orbit and within the anterior pituitary.*

Diagnosis: Intra-osseus meningioma in the left anterior and middle fossa.

Case 2 (daughter)

History: At the age of 43 years the patient was first admitted to hospital
because of *a firm tumor mass in the right fronto-parietal region of the skull.
... she had had a small nodule in that area for about 5 years after mild trauma
with rapid increase in its size for 2 months prior to this visit.
Neurological examination was negative. X-ray films demonstrated a 5½ centimeter
square area of increased density in the right fronto-parietal region ...
suggestive of a meningioma.
At operation, firm porous bone ... was removed. The underlying dura was gritty*

and thickened. Sections of the operative specimen disclosed typical meningioma of arachnoidal type involving both bone and dura.

Two years later X-ray revaluation showed on the opposite side a bony mass in the temporal region. *Review of the initial films suggested that this process might have been present at the time of the original operation.*

... 46 months after the first procedure, a left fronto-temporal craniectomy was performed because of proptosis and papilledema of the left eye with increasing size of the bony mass. ... bony thickening and gritty, indurated dura were encountered with no gross tumor. The extent of bony involvement precluded total removal.

Microscopic study: *Both bone and dura showed infiltration by arachnoid meningioma ....*

Diagnosis: Intra-osseus meningioma right fronto-parietal and left fronto-temporal.

COMMENT

The family members of the two patients have not been investigated.

III.C.1.2. <u>Joynt and Perret 1961 - Iowa, U.S.A.</u> (45)

A mother and daughter. American.

<u>Case 1</u> (mother)

   <u>History</u>: The patient was admitted to hospital at the age of 63 years. She had sustained an occipital skull fracture in an automobile accident at the age of 53 years. Following this injury she complained of mild but persistent head-aches. *The headaches had increased in severity ... in the six months prior to admission. Two days prior to admission, she had a convulsion which started in the right arm and spread to the right side of the face and ... lower extremity. Similar seizures occurred 4 times during the following two days, and the patient was incontinent of urine ....*
At physical examination there was a weakness of the right arm and leg. *Roentgenograms of the skull showed a downward displacement of the pineal body.* Left carotid angiography suggested the presence of a parasagittal tumour. *A left frontal craniotomy was performed. The tumor was located in the inter-hemispheral fissure and was attached to the falx predominantly on the left side. The tumor ... weighed 72 gm.*
Postoperatively the patient was doing very well. She had *spells of jerking of the right arm for which she was receiving anticonvulsants.*

   <u>Microscopic study</u>: The tumour consisted of *strands of elongated cells with plump and uniformly stained nuclei. The strands intertwined and occasionally ended in whorls. Some of the tissue strands presented more elongated cells and nuclei resembling fibrous tissue. Numerous psammoma bodies were present. The pathologic diagnosis was a mixed meningioma with syncytial, fibrous, and psammomatous elements present.*

   <u>Diagnosis</u>: Left parasagittal meningioma.

<u>Case 2</u> (daughter)

   <u>History</u>: The patient was admitted to hospital at the age of 36 years. She complained of *headaches accompanied by vomiting for two months.*
Physical examination revealed no abnormalities. *Roentgenograms of the skull were normal.* The headaches lessened while in the hospital and the patient was discharged. One week later *she experienced double vision. On her return to the hospital, mild bilateral sixth nerve paresis and early papilledema were evident. Ventriculography and right carotid angiography demonstrated a mass lesion in the right frontal region.*
Right frontal craniotomy disclosed a well-demarcated, partly cystic tumor

arising from the dura of the frontal pole and displacing the frontal lobe.
The tumor was totally removed ... and weighed 38 gm.
The postoperative period was uneventful.

Microscopic study: *The microscopic sections revealed approximately the*
same findings as that of case 1. However, there was more syncytial tissue,
and psammoma bodies ... were less numerous. The pathologic diagnosis was the
same as that of case 1.

Diagnosis: Meningioma right frontal.

Family: The mother had 3 brothers and 7 sisters. One brother died of heart
disease and one of cancer of the internal organs. A sister died in an accident.
There was no history of a brain tumour in the family.
The daughter had 3 brothers and 1 sister. The sister was suffering from
multiple sclerosis. The patient had had 3 normal pregnancies and 2 miscarriages.
The children were alive and well.

COMMENT
According to the authors, they have carefully attempted to eliminate the
possibility of neurofibromatosis. There were no known instances of consanguinity in the ancestors of the cases.

III.C.1.3. <u>Joynt and Perret 1965 - Iowa, U.S.A.</u> (46)

A mother and daughter. American.

<u>Case 1</u> (mother)

   <u>History</u>: The patient was admitted to hospital at the age of 59 years. She *suffered from headaches for several years* .... One day before her admission she complained of *extreme fatigue and vomiting.*
On examination, she was lethargic but answered questions when stimulated. She had bilateral ankle clonus but otherwise the extremities were flaccid. The spinal fluid was bloody ....
The patient died the day after admission. Clinical diagnosis was cerebral haemorrhage.

   <u>Autopsy</u>: At autopsy an encapsulated tumour, 6 cm in diameter was found *located under the left frontal lobe, firmly attached to the dura. It was 'pink-grey' in colour and 'rubbery' in consistency. The central portion of the tumour was soft and haemorrhagic. There was an extensive pontine haemorrhage.*

   <u>Microscopic study</u>: ... *the tumour consisted of spindle-shaped cells arranged in strands. There were frequent areas of whorl formation. The nuclei were round to elongated with vesicular nucleoplasm and small nucleoli. There were no psammoma bodies, and no calcification.* Histological diagnosis was meningothelial meningioma.

   <u>Diagnosis</u>: Meningioma left frontal. Pontine haemorrhage.

<u>Case 2</u> (daughter)

   <u>History</u>: The patient was admitted to hospital at the age of 36 years. She complained of *intermittent headaches for two years. They were most severe in the morning and were occasionally accompanied by nausea and vomiting. She also noted that a 'strange' taste accompanied the headaches. For one year before her admission she had increasing difficulty with her vision.*
On examination she had high grade papilloedema and hyperactive deep tendon reflexes. There was anosmia on the right side. Radiographs of the skull showed *enlargement of the sella turcica ... suggesting increased intracranial pressure. The right carotid angiogram was abnormal ... and showed a venous tumour stain deep in the right anterior fossa.*
At operation, a hard, nodular, encapsulated tumour was located under the right frontal lobe arising from the olfactory groove. The tumour was large, extending to the anterior tip of the anterior fossa, back to the sphenoid ridge, and medially beneath the falx.

*The patient made an excellent recovery and was asymptomatic six months after
the operation.*

Microscopic study: The tumour consisted of *polygonal and long spindle-
shaped cells in a reticular arrangement. The nuclei were quite uniformly round
with finely granular nucleoplasm. Numerous psammoma bodies in all stages of
development were seen. There were flecks of calcium throughout the tumour
which had large areas of degeneration.*

Diagnosis: Right frontal olfactory groove meningioma.

COMMENT

Relatives of the patients were not examined in this report.

III.C.1.4. <u>Sahar 1965 - Jerusalem, Israel</u> (85)

Two brothers and their second cousin. Israeli.

<u>Case 1</u> (second cousin)

<u>History</u>: At the age of 47 years this woman was admitted to hospital. *She complained of headaches localized in the right temporo-parietal region and a single episode of unconsciousness.* Neurological findings included *bilateral papilledema, left upper quadrant anopia and slight left hemiparesis. Skull roentgenograms showed displacement of the pineal body to the left and decalcification of the sella. Right carotid angiography demonstrated a right temporal lobe lesion.*

Through a right temporal craniotomy a meningotheliomatous meningioma of the convexity was removed. It was 5 cm. in diameter.

Sixteen months after this operation the patient was readmitted to hospital because of *frequent attacks of unconsciousness in spite of anti-convulsive treatment.*

Examination showed *recurrence of the same neurological signs as on the first admission. A repeat angiogram showed a vascular lesion in the right temporal region.*

At reoperation *a meningioma weighing 200 gm. originating in the upper surface of the tentorium was completely removed.*

The patient's recovery was uneventful, and she has had no further symptoms.

    <u>Microscopic study</u>: *showed a fibromatous type of meningioma.*

    <u>Diagnosis</u>: Right temporal convexity meningioma.

               Right temporal tentorium meningioma.

<u>Case 2</u> (brother)

<u>History</u>: At the age of 45 years the patient was admitted to hospital because of *blurred vision and pain in the neck on straining.*

On examination there was *bilateral papilledema, nystagmus on left lateral gaze, left peripheral facial paresis and weakness of the gag reflex on the left. There was also ataxia in the left arm and leg and mild left hemiparesis. Skull roentgenograms and EEG record were normal. Ventriculography showed symmetrical dilatation of the lateral and third ventricles with displacement of the aqueduct towards the right.*

Suboccipital craniectomy disclosed a meningioma anterior to the cerebellar hemisphere and the brain stem. Only a partial removal was possible.

The patient died 48 hours after the operation with signs of brain stem failure.

Autopsy: No reference to an autopsy is made in the article.

Microscopic study: *The tumor was identified as a meningotheliomatous meningioma.*

Diagnosis: Meningioma anterior to the cerebellar hemisphere and the brain stem.

Case 3 (brother)

History: At the age of 41 years the patient was admitted to hospital because of *headache and loss of vision in the left eye. The patient had been under psychiatric care for 15 years for headaches and depression.*
Neurological examination revealed *organic depression, with difficulty in certain mental functions. There was bilateral anosmia and temporal pallor of the left optic disc. Vision in the left eye was limited to counting fingers at a distance of 1 m. Skull roentgenograms showed decalcification of the dorsum sellae. The EEG showed slow wave activity in both frontal areas. A left carotid angiogram disclosed a subfrontal lesion crossing the midline.*
A bifrontal craniotomy revealed an olfactory groove meningioma which was completely removed.

Microscopic study: The meningioma was of the meningotheliomatous type.
Diagnosis: Olfactory groove meningioma.

Family:

1 = case 1
2 = case 2
3 = case 3

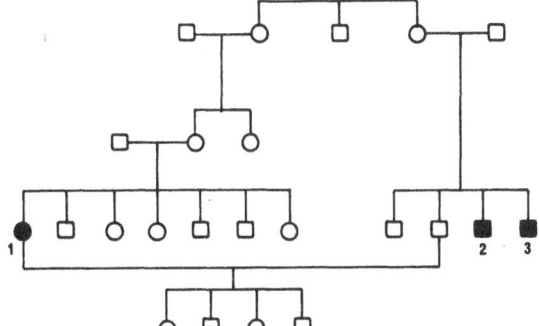

100

COMMENT

The blood types of the 3 cases were:

        Case 1: A_2 MM   Rh: cc dd ee

        Case 2: AB   Rh: cc dd ee

        Case 3: A_1 MM   Rh: cc dd ee

They did not differ in any meaningful manner from those in other members of the family. None of the patients reported showed any evidence of neurofibromatosis.

III.C.1.5. <u>Girard et al. 1977 - Lyon, France</u> (32)

A grandmother, mother and daughter. French.

Case 1 (grandmother)

<u>History</u>: This female was admitted to hospital at the age of 38 years with a 3-year-history of progressive exophthalmos of the right eye accompanied by a tumour of the left temporal bone. She was said to have had two recent left-sided hemiplegic attacks.

On examination severe papilloedema was found. The right eye was infected and painful, and had to be enucleated.

The patient died 48 hours after operation.

<u>Autopsy</u>: Multiple tumours (27 in number) were discovered, mainly located at the base of the brain.

<u>Microscopic study</u>: showed the tumours to be meningiomas.

<u>Diagnosis</u>: Multiple meningiomas.

Case 2 (mother)

<u>History</u>: This female was admitted to hospital because of an intracranial hypertension syndrome existing for six months, accompanied by severe papilloedema and a progressive blurring of vision. She was said to have demonstrated three periods of *hypersomnia*. A voluminous tumour of the right fronto-parietal bone, pre-existing for five years and progressive in size, was present. She was mentally retarded and bilaterally deaf.

On examination two tiny papilliform tumours of the left hand were found which were histologically identified as oedematous neurofibromas. In addition to the tumour of the right fronto-parietal bone radiographs of the skull revealed a tumour of the ala minor of the right sphenoid bone, and density abnormalities in the left occipital region and numerous other areas of the skull. Angiography showed numerous tumours on both the left and the right. Because of the multiplicity of the tumours and their extensive spread no operation was undertaken.

<u>Diagnosis</u>: The clinical diagnosis of multiple meningiomas was made.

Case 3 (daughter)

<u>History</u>: This female was admitted to hospital at the age of 24 years because of an intracranial hypertension syndrome with severe bilateral papilloedema, headaches and vomiting. In three months she had developed a tumour of the right frontal bone.

On examination the patient showed mental retardation. No neurological disorders

were found. In addition to the right frontal tumour radiographs of the skull
showed hyperostosis of the right os petrosum and the two anterior clinoid
processes, and several density abnormalities in the right and left frontal
areas. Angiography confirmed the existence of a large right frontal tumour
and several small vascular tumours.

At operation a parasagittal frontal meningioma was removed as well as one of
the small vascular tumours.

Postoperatively the patient was hemiplegic on the left, this condition disappearing almost entirely within a few months.

    Microscopic study: showed an epithelial type meningioma.

    Diagnosis: Multiple meningiomas.

    Family: No further information concerning the family is given in the
article.

COMMENT

Unfortunately no histological verification of the tumours in case 2 was
obtained. The presence of two tiny neurofibromas in this case and her bilateral deafness possibly suggest a relationship with neurofibromatosis. A
clinical form of expression of neurofibromatosis is suggested by the authors.

III.C.1.6. Delleman et al. 1978 - Amsterdam, The Netherlands (25)

A brother (proband), sister, father, uncle and aunt. Dutch.

Case 1 (brother, proband)
    History: This male had *gradually increasing left-sided exophthalmos and decreasing visual acuity that led to enucleation of the eye when he was 22. Over the next 5 years, he was twice operated on for recurrence of the tumor ....* Examination at the age of 32 years was *normal except for a loss of smell on the left. His left leg had been atrophic since he was 23, with negative reflexes and normal sensibility. Roentgenograms showed hyperostosis of the orbit.*
    Microscopic study: showed a psammomatous meningioma of the optic nerve sheath.
    Diagnosis: Meningioma of the left optic nerve sheath.

Case 2 (sister)
    History: *A spinal meningioma at T5-T6 was removed* at the age of 25 years. *Four years later trochlear paresis, torticollis, and elevation of the left eye were found; X-rays showed hyperostosis* and at the age of 31 years a *hyperostotic meningioma was found at craniotomy.*
    Microscopic study: Meningiomas.
    Diagnosis: Spinal and intracranial meningioma.

Case 3 (father)
    History: This male *underwent removal of a fist-sized left parasagittal meningioma* at the age of 63 years. *Subsequently, icterus and a right hemiparesis developed* and he died at the age of 64 years.
    Autopsy: *Multiple meningiomas were found. The two largest were at the base of the frontal pole and in the falx.*
    Microscopic study: Meningiomas.
    Diagnosis: Multiple meningiomas.

Case 4 (uncle, brother of case 3)
    History: At the age of 70 years this male *was operated on ... for intracranial tumor and multiple meningiomas were found, three on the dura in the frontoparietotemporal region and a very large one on the sphenoidal ridge. He died 1 month postoperatively.*
    Autopsy: Not mentioned.
    Microscopic study: Meningiomas.
    Diagnosis: Multiple meningiomas.

Case 5 (aunt, sister of case 3)

   History: At the age of 42 years this female *showed bilateral papilledema,*
left sensory and motor trigeminal abnormalities, total deafness on the left,
diminished hearing on the right, left glossopharyngeal paresis, right-sided
atrophy of the tongue, and a slight difference in myotatic reflexes. Skull
films showed destruction of the tip of the left temporal bone.
Operation was not deemed advisable and she died one year later.

   Autopsy: *Bilateral acoustic neurinomas and multiple meningiomas were found.*

   Microscopic study: As by autopsy.

   Diagnosis: Bilateral acoustic neurinomas and multiple meningiomas.

   Family: A sister of the proband (6) *had undergone a clinical examination*
by a neurologist .... She was diagnosed as having bilateral paresis of the
cricoarytenoid muscles and right-sided motor radiculopathy at L4-L5, myelo-
graphy was negative. She had multiple café-au-lait spots on the back and
legs ... and also reported *that her daughter and an aunt and uncle on the*
paternal side had brown pigmented spots. No evidence of meningioma or neurofibromatosis was found among the other family members.

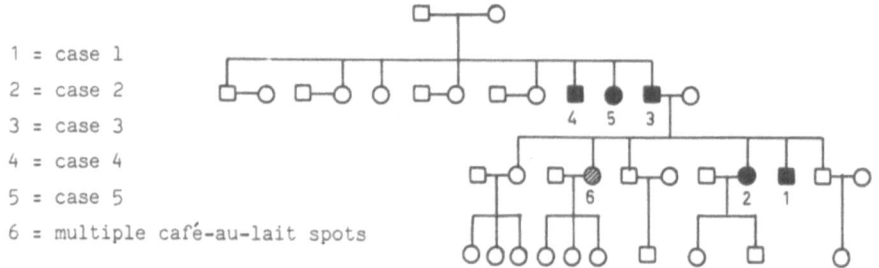

1 = case 1
2 = case 2
3 = case 3
4 = case 4
5 = case 5
6 = multiple café-au-lait spots

COMMENT

The bilateral acoustic neurinomas in case 5 and the presence of multiple
café-au-lait spots and brown pigmented spots in other family members makes
a relationship with neurofibromatosis very likely. The authors also state
we are impelled to regard all of our cases as manifestations of von Reckling-
hausen disease, a syndrome well known for its extreme variability.

III.C.1.7. Memon 1980 - New York, U.S.A. (61)

A mother and son. American.

Case 1 (mother)

History: This female was admitted to hospital at the age of 63 years *with the complaints of increased frequency of seizures, headache, and confusion. She had undergone a craniotomy for the removal of a meningioma of the para-sagittal region on the right side* 20 years earlier. *She had been left with a weakness of her left foot and a seizure disorder for which she was taking Dilantin.*

Examination showed *that the patient was confused and disoriented.* There was *a minimal left hemiparesis with foot drop, increased deep tendon reflexes on the left side, and an extensor plantor response. A skull x-ray film showed the site of the previous craniectomy in the right parasagittal region* ... *An isotope* ... *brain scan revealed a large uptake in the right sphenoid ridge area. A right brachial angiogram revealed a shift of the right middle cerebral artery superiorly and medially.*

At craniotomy a *large lateral sphenoid ridge meningioma, which was buried in the sylvian fissure close to the bone, was removed.*

During the postoperative course there was increased weakness of the left upper extremity, which improved gradually over a period of 3 weeks.

Microscopic study: *showed ovoid to elliptical nuclei and fibrous cytoplasm. There were no psammoma bodies and no calcification. Mitotic figures or bizarre giant cells were not observed in the tumor.*

Diagnosis: Right sphenoid ridge meningioma. Postoperative state resulting from previous right parasagittal meningioma removal.

Case 2 (son)

History: This 35-year-old male was admitted to hospital *with a history of seizures that had begun 6 months before admission. The seizures were of the tonic-clonic type.*

Examination *was essentially negative except for decreased pain sensation in both lower extremities. X-ray films of the skull were negative. A brain scan and an angiogram showed a mass lesion in the midfrontal region involving the sagittal sinus.*

At craniotomy *the excision of a bifrontal parasagittal meningioma was carried out.*

The postoperative course was uneventful ....

Microscopic study: *showed moderate to marked cellularity and relatively large, round to elliptical nuclei with a delicate chromatin pattern. The cytoplasm was ill-defined and fibrous in appearance with occasional whorl formation and xanthomatous changes. In some areas the nuclei were small and hyperchromatic, although mitotic figures were not present.*

Diagnosis: Bifrontal parasagittal meningioma.

Family: The living family consisted of the mother, a daughter and a son, and the children of the son and daughter. ... *upon examination none of the above-mentioned family members showed any stigma of neurofibromatosis, nor did they recall any evidence of this disease in previous generations.*

COMMENT

The patient in case 1 suffered a second meningioma in a different location than that of the first meningioma after an unusual delay of 20 years.

III.C.2. OTHER GENERATIONS AND DISTANT RELATIVES WITH DISCORDANT TUMOUR

III.C.2.1. Patterson and Anderson 1940 - Los Angeles, U.S.A. (71)

A father and two sons. American.

Case 1 (father)

History: The patient was admitted to hospital at the age of 49 years. Ten years earlier he was operated upon because of *a large cyst in the left cerebellar hemisphere. The cyst was drained but no tumor tissue was found.* A haemangioblastoma had been suspected. The years following surgery, *his symptoms of headache, ataxia, and instability of gait improved greatly.* Four years before admission all symptoms gradually recurred. *His blindness, which was present at the time he was operated upon, persisted.*
Neurological examination on admission revealed that *the patient was completely blind, with high-grade papilledema bilaterally and large fixed pupils. Nystagmus was present in all directions, and there was considerable ataxia and dysmetria in the left arm and leg; the Babinski and Gordon signs were noted bilaterally.* At operation *a dark colored highly vascular tumor was disclosed occupying the site of the left cerebellar hemisphere and extending across the midline.* During operation *there was a rather free bleeding; the patient's condition became poor and he died abruptly.*

Autopsy: Not mentioned in the article.

Microscopic study: ... *numerous vascular spaces were observed, which in certain areas were classical of hemangioblastoma showing many closely and regularly placed thin walled vessels. Many foam cells were identified under high power examination.*

Diagnosis: Haemangioblastoma of the left cerebellum.

Case 2 (son)

History: At the age of 23 years the patient was admitted to hospital. Symptoms had been experienced by the patient three years previously, presenting as *an abrupt onset of numbness in the left foot. ... the next morning the leg was weak, the foot beginning to drop.* In the next years gradually, *jacksonian convulsions made their appearance, beginning with numbness in the foot and leg, rapidly including the trunk, the left arm and the face. These attacks gradually increased in number up to six or eight each day and weakness in the left leg became prominent. The headaches grew very severe and periods of drowsiness accompanied by bradycardia were frequent.*
On examination there was a *tremendous vascularity of the scalp ....*

Papilledema was present bilaterally, more on the right, and a left hemiparesis was noted ... with considerable loss of touch discrimination in the left hand. The deep reflexes were all increased, and greater on the left with bilateral Babinski signs ....

Four operative stages and numerous blood transfusions were necessary before a mass the size of a small orange could finally be enucleated.

Postoperatively the patient was well except *for minor convulsions at about six week intervals.*

Microscopic study: *The tumour was shown ... to be an angioblastic meningioma. Many large vascular spaces in areas resembling meningiotheliomatous tissue were in evidence, and suggested the group of combined meningiotheliomatous-angioblastic meningiomas.*

Diagnosis: Angioblastic meningioma right parietal, parasagittal.

Case 3 (son)

History: The patient was admitted to hospital at the age of 29. For two months he complained of *progressive blurring of vision ... and occipito-frontal headaches which grew increasingly more intense. Vomiting ..., became very frequent .... He became dizzy to the point that even sitting up in bed was greatly disturbing. The patient was ... prone to sleep as much as fifteen hours in a day. On admission, the patient was in a profound stupor, from which he could be aroused only by means of strongly painful stimulation.*

Further neurological examination revealed *bilateral tenderness in the sub-occiput; there was marked choking of the optic discs ....* The vestibular portion of the eighth cranial nerve was practically inert on the right. *Hypotonia and ataxia were marked in the lower extremities, both more pronounced on the right; the upper extremities were ... mildly ataxic, with dysdiadokokinesia in the hand. The deep reflexes were equally hyperactive ....* At ventriculography a *marked internal hydrocephalus was disclosed, with complete filling of the third ventricle.*

A suboccipital craniotomy was ... performed. At a depth of 2 cm. a cyst was punctured in the right lobe of the cerebellum, *and clear yellow coagulable fluid obtained. The cyst was opened ..., but no tumor nodule could be seen grossly. The patient's convalescence was uneventful, and for twelve months he has remained symtom free.*

Diagnosis: Cyst in the right cerebellum (haemangioblastoma?).

Family: There were three children in the family, the third being a girl of 22 years who was completely normal. The mother died in her thirties of pulmonary tuberculosis. Little is known about her parents. The paternal grandfather and grandmother presented no symptoms which might lead one to believe that they had intracranial tumours, both died at the age of 70 years or older, of unrelated causes.

COMMENT

Histologically there is a striking resemblance between angioblastic meningioma and cerebellar haemangioblastomas as seen in Von Hippel-Lindau's disease. The authors note that *meticulous re-examination of the optic fundi in both sons demonstrated no retinal abnormalities of any kind*. According to the authors, this report cannot be considered as other than a form of Von Hippel-Lindau's disease.

110

III.C.2.2. __Blickenstorfer 1951 - Zürich, Switzerland__ (10)

A brother and sister, grandmother and aunt. Swiss.

The author reports a brother (proband) who died of a histologically verified
right occipital glioblastoma multiforme at the age of 69 years, and his eldest
sister who had a frontal meningioma. Their maternal grandmother and aunt also
died of brain tumours at respectively 71 and 65 years of age.
Fifty-nine members of the family were investigated but aside from mental disorders no other important diseases were found (VII.C.2.3).

III.C.2.3. __Kemper 1964 - Münster, Germany__ (48)

An aunt and nephew. German.

This author studied 371 male and 296 female patients having brain tumours.
Among these patients six occurrences of familial brain tumours were noted,
including a 47-year-old female who died of a histologically verified right
temporal glioblastoma multiforme and her 19-year-old nephew who was operated
upon because of a left temporo-parieto-occipital fibromatous meningioma
(VII.C.2.10).

TABLES

TABLE 1 - MONOZYGOTIC TWINS WITH CONCORDANT TUMOUR (III.A.1)

	case	gender	relationship	number of unaffected siblings	race or nationality	age at symptom occurrence	age at death	location of the tumour
III.A.1.1. Sedzimir 1973	1	m	br	1 br	Engl.	8 y	-	1. spinal T10-T12 2. R frontal falx
	2	m	br	1 br	Engl.	12 y	14 y	1. spinal C1-C6 2. spinal T9-T12 3. tuberculum sella

TABLE 2 - MONOZYGOTIC TWINS WITH DISCORDANT TUMOUR (III.A.2)

	case	gender	relationship	number of unaffected siblings	race or nationality	age at symptom occurrence	age at death	location of the tumour
III.A.2.1. Hoppe 1952	1	m	br	?	Germ.	35 y	-	L sphenoidal
	2	m	br	?	Germ.	53 y	53 y	L fronto-central

TABLE 3 - MONOZYGOTIC TWINS, ONE DEMONSTRATING MENINGIOMA (III.A.3)

	case	gender	relationship	number of unaffected siblings	race or nationality	age at symptom occurrence	age at death	location of the tumour
III.A.3.1. Kuhnen 1953	1	m	br	5	Germ.	13 y	-	R temporo-parietal
		m	br	5	Germ.			

diagnosis	biopsy	autopsy	associated physical or mental conditions	family	comment
Transitional meningioma	+	-	Congenital cataract + divergent squint OD proptosis + ophthal-moplegia OS; claw feet; Klippel-Feil anomaly	-	Case 1: clinical diagnosis of intra-cranial meningioma. Case 2: cause of death unknown
Transitional meningioma	+	-	-		

diagnosis	biopsy	autopsy	associated physical or mental conditons	family	comment
Meningioma	+	-	Pointed head form. Head injury at age of 35 y	Several twins in the family of the mother	Case 1 first reported by Pedersen & Geyer in 1938. Case 2 healthy at that time
Glioblastoma	+	-	Pointed head form		

diagnosis	biopsy	autopsy	associated physical or mental conditions	family	comment
Endotheliomatous meningioma	+	-	-	-	

114

TABLE 4 - SIBLINGS WITH CONCORDANT TUMOUR (III.B.1)

	case	gender	relationship	number of unaffected siblings	race or nationality	age at symptom occurrence	age at death	location of the tumour
III.B.1.1. Ectors 1953	1	m	br	2 s	Belg.	39 y	-	foramen magnum
	2	f	s	2 s	Belg.	25 y	-	foramen magnum
III.B.1.2. Gaist 1959	1	f	s	?	Ital.	38 y	-	L frontal (2)
	2	m	br	?	Ital.	36 y	-	R parasagittal
III.B.1.3. Grunert 1970	1	m	br	?	Greek	53 y	-	suprasellar
	2	m	br	?	Greek	47 y	-	3rd and lateral ventricles

TABLE 5 - SIBLINGS WITH DISCORDANT TUMOUR (III.B.2)

	case	gender	relationship	number of unaffected siblings	race or nationality	age at symptom occurrence	age at death	location of the tumour
III.B.2.1. Koch 1954	1	f	s	5	Germ.	44 y	?	parasagittal
	2	m	br	5	Germ.	47 y	?	R temporal
III.B.2.2. Chateau 1971	1	f	s	?	French	46 y	-	L parietal, parasagittal
	2	m	br	?	French	43 y	-	L cerebellum

diagnosis	biopsy	autopsy	associated physical or mental conditions	family	comment
Psammomatous meningioma	+	-	Fusion atlas-foramen magnum; small tumour R upper leg	-	Relationship with neurofibromatosis
Psammomatous meningioma	+	-	Fusion atlas-foramen magnum; schwannoma L fore-arm		
Transitional meningioma	+	-	-	?	
Meningothelioma-tous meningioma	+	-	-		
Endotheliomatous meningioma	+	-	Blood-group O, Rh +	A sister died of a brain tumour	
Transitional meningioma	+	-	Blood-group A_1, Rh + Aneurysm of the a. communicans anterior		

diagnosis	biopsy	autopsy	associated physical or mental conditions	family	comment
Meningioma	?	?	?	-	Study on 350 female patients having a brain tumour
Brain tumour	?	?	?		
Fibroblastic meningioma	+	-	-	-	
Haemangio-blastoma	+	-	-		

TABLE 6 - OTHER GENERATIONS AND DISTANT RELATIVES WITH CONCORDANT TUMOUR (III.C.1)

	case	gender	relationship	number of unaffected siblings	race or nationality	age at symptom occurrence	age at death	location of the tumour
III.C.1.1. Wagman 1960	1	f	m	?	white Amer.	54 y	69 y	L anterior and middle fossa
	2	f	d	?	white Amer.	43 y	-	1. R. fronto-parietal 2. L fronto-temporal
III.C.1.2. Joynt 1961	1	f	m	3 br 7 s	white Amer.	63 y	-	L parasagittal
	2	f	d	3 br 1 s	white Amer.	36 y	-	R frontal
III.C.1.3. Joynt 1965	1	f	m	?	Amer.	59 y	59 y	L frontal
	2	f	d	?	Amer.	34 y		R frontal
III.C.1.4. Sahar 1965	1	f	cous	6	Isr.	47 y	-	1. R temporal convexity 2. R temporal tentorium
	2	m	br	2	Isr.	45 y	45 y	anterior to cerebellar hemisphere and brain stem
	3	m	br	2	Isr.	41 y (26 y ?)	-	Olfactory groove
III.C.1.5. Girard 1977	1	f	grand-m	?	French	35 y	38 y	multiple tumours (27) mainly at the brain base
	2	f	m	?	French	?	-	multiple
	3	f	d	?	French	24 y	-	multiple

diagnosis	biopsy	autopsy	associated physical or mental conditions	family	comment
Arachnoidal meningioma	-	+	-	?	Intra-osseus meningiomas without gross tumour
Arachnoidal meningioma	+	-	Mild head injury at 38 y		
Mixed meningioma	+	-	Head injury with occipital skull fracture at 53 y	Brother case 1 cancer of the internal organs; sister case 2 multiple sclerosis	
Mixed meningioma	+	-	-		
Meningothelial meningioma	-	+	Pontine haemorrhage	?	Case 1: tumour diagnosed at autopsy
Psammomatous meningioma	+	-	-		
Fibromatous meningioma	+	-	Blood-group A_2, Rh -	-	Case 1 second cousin of the two brothers (cases 2 and 3)
Meningotheliomatous meningioma	+	-	Blood-group AB, Rh -		
Meningotheliomatous meningioma	+	-	Blood-group A_1, Rh -		
Meningioma	-	+		?	Relationship with neurofibromatosis
Brain tumours	-	-	Mental retardation, 2 tiny neurofibromas, bilateral deafness		
Epithelial meningioma	+	-	Mental retardation		

118

TABLE 6 - continued

	case	gender	relationship	number of unaffected siblings	race or nationality	age at symptom occurrence	age at death	location of the tumour
III.C.1.6. Delleman 1978	1	m	br	2 br 2 s	Dutch	22 y	–	L optic nerve
	2	f	s	2 br 2 s	Dutch	25 y	–	spinal T_5-T_6 cerebral
	3	m	f	1 br 4 s	Dutch	63 y	64 y	multiple
	4	m	uncle	1 br 4 s	Dutch	70 y	70 y	multiple
	5	f	aunt	1 br 4 s	Dutch	42 y	43 y	multiple
III.C.1.7. Memon 1980	1	f	m	?	Amer.	43 y 63 y	–	R parasagittal R sphenoid ridge
	2	m	s	1 s	Amer.	35 y	–	bifrontal parasagittal

diagnosis	biopsy	autopsy	associated physical or mental conditions	family	comment
Psammomatous meningioma	+	-	-	Sister of case 1 multiple café-au-lait spots. Her daughter and an aunt and uncle brown pigmented spots	Relationship with neurofibromatosis
Meningioma	+	-	-		
Meningioma	+	+	-		
Meningioma	+	-	-		
Meningioma	-	+	Bilateral acoustic neurinomas		
Fibromatous meningioma	+	-	-	-	Case 1: 20-year interval between two meningiomas
Transitional meningioma	+	-	-		

TABLE 7 - OTHER GENERATIONS AND DISTANT RELATIVES WITH DISCORDANT TUMOUR (III.C.2)

	case	gender	relationship	number of unaffected siblings	race or nationality	age at symptom occurrence	age at death	location of the tumour
III.C.2.1. Patterson 1940	1	m	f	?	white Amer.	39 y	49 y	L cerebellar hemisphere
	2	m	s	1 s	white Amer.	20 y	-	R parietal, parasagittal
	3	m	s	1 s	white Amer.	29 y	-	R cerebellar hemisphere
III.C.2.2. Blickenstorfer 1951	1	m	br	1 s	Germ.	68 y	69 y	R occipital
	2	f	s	1 s	Germ.	?	?	frontal
	3	f	grand-m	?	Germ.	60 y	71 y	?
	4	f	aunt	?	Germ.	64 y	65 y	?
III.C.2.3. Kemper 1964	1	f	aunt	?	Germ.	47 y	47 y	R temporal
	2	m	neph	2 s	Germ.	19 y	-	L temporo-parieto-occipital

diagnosis	biopsy	autopsy	associated physical or mental conditions	family	comment
Haemangio-blastoma	+	-	Cyst in L cerebellum 10 y earlier	Mother of cases 2 and 3 died of tuberculosis	Manifestation of Von Hippel-Lindau's disease
Angioblastic meningioma	+	-	-		
Cyst (haemangio-blastoma?)	+	-	-		
Glioblastoma	+	-	-	59 relatives investigated. Apart from mental disorders no other relevant diseases	No histological diagnoses of cases 3 and 4
Meningioma	+	-	-		
Brain tumour	?	?	-		
Brain tumour	?	?	-		
Glioblastoma multiforme	-	+	-	Mother of case 1 died at 80 y of apoplexy	Study of 453 patients with brain tumour; 6 cases of familial brain tumour occurrence were found
Fibromatous meningioma	+	-	Head injury at 5 y		

GENERAL ASPECTS OF MENINGIOMA

In series reports in the literature meningiomas have accounted for 9 to 27% of all primary tumours occurring intracranially (7, 21, 88, 99, 109) and for 20 to 30% of the intraspinal tumours (4, 66, 93, 109). Percentages of intracranial meningioma occurrence of up to 38% have been recorded in series having high autopsy rates, meningiomas often being found incidentally at autopsy (75, 99, 102). A higher incidence of meningioma occurrence in negroes as compared to caucasians, and Africans as compared to Europeans has been noted (1, 37). While incidence rates increase with increasing age (37, 75, 88), many clinical series report a peak occurrence between the ages of 30 and 60 years (7, 22, 53, 109). Intracranial meningiomas occurring in infants under one year of age (possibly congenital) are extremely rare and only 16 cases have been reported in the literature (5, 68). There is a clear predeliction for meningioma occurrence in females as compared to males, a ratio of approximately 2 : 1 being found (7, 37, 75, 88, 109). The

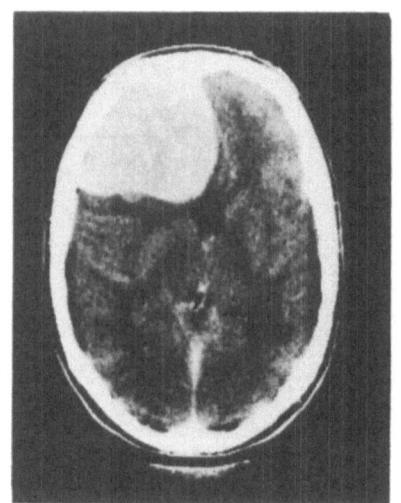
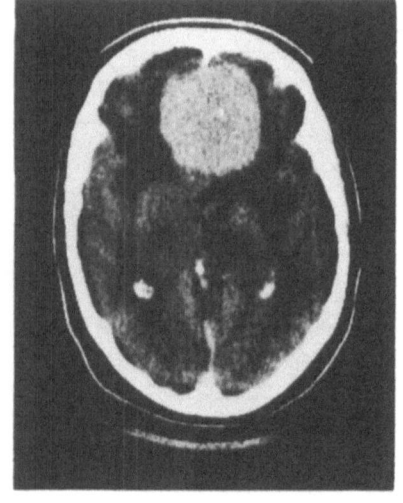

A   B

Fig. 1. CT-scans of large right frontal (A) and olfactory (B) meningiomas (enhanced)

increased frequency of meningiomas in women and the sometimes rapidly progressive course of these tumours during pregnancy may suggest a hormonal influence.
Estrogen and progesterone receptors have been found in meningioma tumour tissue
(27, 76). Other possible etiological factors in the occurrence of meningioma are
head injuries (22, 78, 98), exposure to therapeutic or diagnostic irradiation (2,
8, 11, 64, 78, 96), and consumption of foods containing high levels of nitrite (78).

Meningiomas were at one time thought to arise from the dura mater and hence were
known as dural endotheliomas (21). The cell of origin of the meningioma is, however,
the arachnoid cell of the arachnoid villi, which penetrate the dura and project
into the dural venous sinuses (83, 84, 109). For this reason the meningiomas are
commonly found along the course of the intracranial venous sinuses. The sites of
greatest predeliction are the parasagittal regions, the lateral cerebral convexi-
ties, the sphenoid ridge, the olfactory groove area, and the sella turcica region
(tuberculum sellae) (15, 22, 69, 84, 109). Meningiomas are less frequent below the
tentorium and may arise from the tentorium, especially around the Torcular Herophili
(confluens sinuum) and along the transverse sinus, or in the region of the foramen
magnum. Intraventricular meningiomas, when occurring, are mainly found in the lateral ventricles. Spinal meningioma are most frequently found in the thoracic region
(4, 66, 93) and are usually closely related to a nerve root as it emerges from the
subarachnoid space.
Occasionally meningiomas are multiple. Multiple meningiomas (cranial or spinal)

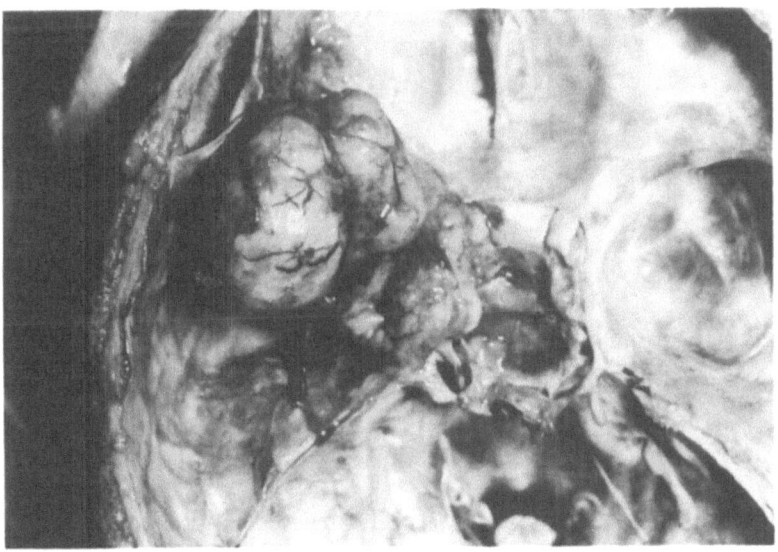

Fig. 2. Macroscopic appearance of a left sphenoidal ridge meningioma.

combined with neurinomas can occur in the central form of neurofibromatosis (23, 81). Meningioma can also be associated with glioma (51, 95) and pituitary adenoma (14, 24).

Clinically many different symptoms may occur in relation to the location and growth of the tumour. The most common complaints are headaches, visual impairment and focal seizures. There is often a striking discongruency between the size of the tumour and the extent of clinical symptoms, large convexity meningioma some-times causing few complaints while small meningiomas, especially at the base of the brain, may be associated with extensive symptomatology.

While there is considerable variance in appearance, meningioma are grossly grayish and nodular, well circumscribed and demarcated from the brain tissue. They are generally firmly attached to the inner surface of the dura (83, 84, 109), or less frequently form a flat plaque spreading over the dura inner surface ('meningioma en plaque') (15, 83, 84, 109). Calcification is sometimes found due to the presence of psammoma bodies and may be demonstrated by roentgenography of the skull. Hyperostosis may occur in the bone overlying the meningioma due to reactive new bone formation or osteoblastic differentiation of the tumour cells, eventually associated with invasion of the bone by meningioma cells (6, 19, 22, 30).

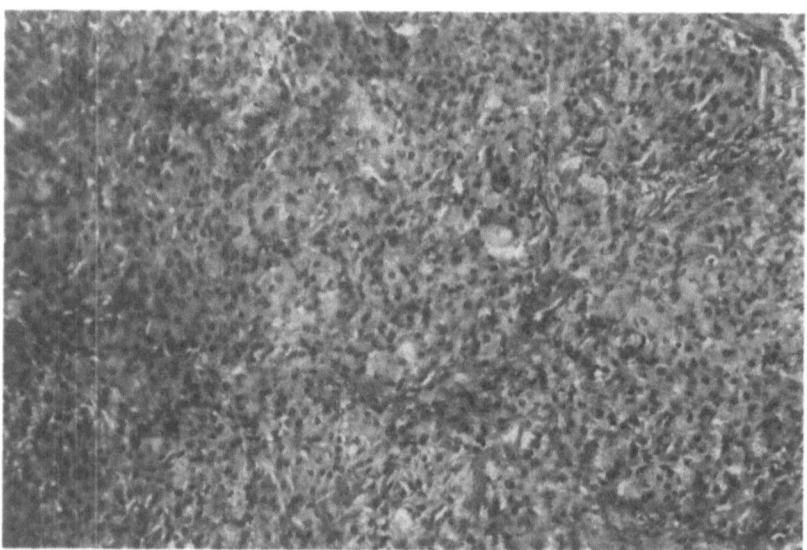

Fig. 3. Microscopic appearance of a meningotheliomatous meningioma
HE, 100x

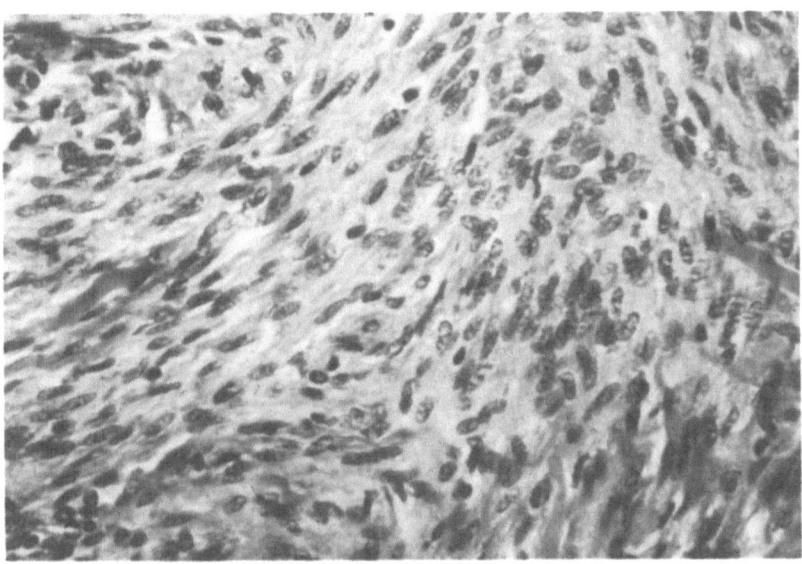

Fig. 4. Microscopic appearance of a fibroblastic meningioma
HE, 250x

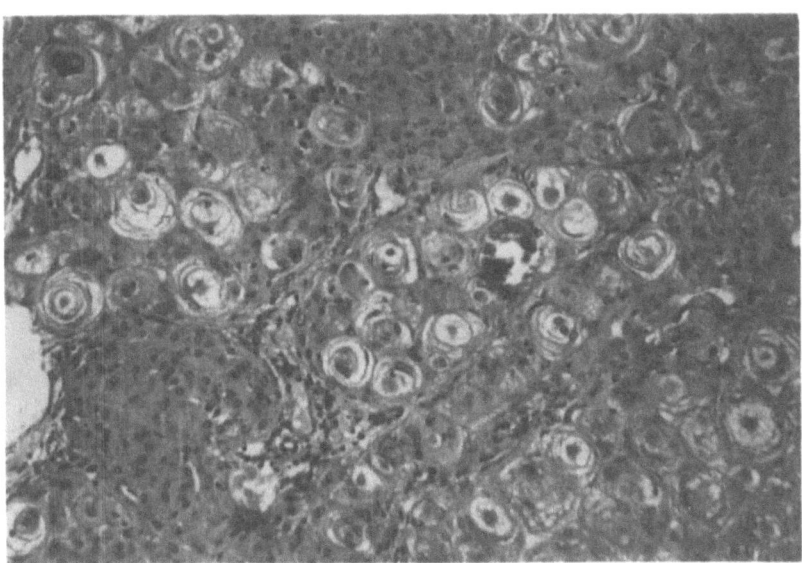

Fig. 5. Microscopic appearance of a psammomatous meningioma
HE, 100x

On microscopic examination a number of histological subtypes can be distinguished based on variation in the shape and size of the cells, their organization,
their vascularity and the presence of secondary structures including pigment,
calcium salts and lipid. As a result of this diversity a large number of classifications have been proposed in the literature including: meningotheliomatous,
angioblastic, psammomatous, fibroblastic, osteoblastic, xanthomatous, transitional,
mixed, melanoblastic and sarcomatous types. At present, aided by the use of the
electronmicroscope, meningioma have been classified into meningotheliomatous
(synonyms: syncytial, endotheliomatous, epithelial), fibroblastic (fibrous, fibromatous), transitional (mixed), psammomatous, angioblastic (angiomatous), papillary
and anaplastic (malignant) types (44, 84, 110). These types are all derived from
a single cell type, the mesenchymal arachnoid cell, which must have a potentiality
for differentiation.

The meningotheliomatous meningioma consists of clusters of cells in a whorling
pattern divided into distinct lobules by variable amounts of fibrous stroma. The
cells are polygonal with an epithelial-like arrangement ill-defined cell borders,
a pale cytoplasm and the frequent presence of a conspicuous nucleolus in the
nucleus (83, 84, 109). The stroma contains many blood vessels.

In fibroblastic meningioma the cells resemble fibroblast cells (elongated fusiform
cells). The most distinctive feature is the presence of numerous collagen and
reticulin fibres in the interstitial tissue (44, 83, 109).

Transitional forms can be seen between the meningotheliomatous and fibroblastic
meningioma, but variance in histological arrangement may also be seen within the
same meningioma (mixed) (44). Psammoma bodies, consisting of 'concentric laminae
of calcium salts that have been laid down in degenerating tumour cells' (83, 84)
are mainly encountered in transitional forms. When found occurring frequently some
authors use the term psammomatous meningioma (110).

The designation of the angioblastic type as a distinct subtype of meningioma is
controversial. Some authors (18, 74, 77) have regarded this neoplasm as being of
vascular origin, and labelled it a haemangiopericytoma. According to Horten et al.
(42) and others (83, 84), however, the angioblastic meningioma 'deserves to be
retained as a generic term to include craniospinal haemangiopericytomas and
transitional forms between haemangiopericytoma, haemangioblastoma and classic
meningioma'. These tumours are highly cellular and vascular. The structure is
highly similar to capillary haemangioblastomas, differing mainly in localization
and gross features (42, 84). Supratentorial cerebral capillary haemangioblastomas
have also been reported (60), which indicates that topographical location may not
be a truly differentiating factor between these two tumours.

Rarely, malignant (sarcomatous) change occurs in meningiomas, particularly in the angioblastic type (83). In general distant metastases from meningiomas are rare. Angioblastic meningioma, although infrequent, account for 15% of all metastasizing meningiomas (70, 91). Recurrence of meningioma after total extirpation is seen in approximately 10% of the cases. There is no obvious relationship between recurrence and the histological character of the meningioma (92). Metastasis of extraneural carcinoma, especially breast carcinoma, to intracranial meningioma have recently been described in the literature (12, 38, 39, 67, 86).

FAMILIAL ASPECTS OF MENINGIOMA

Case reports

The first report on the familial aggregation of meningiomas was made by
Ectors and Van Bogaert in 1953 (III.B.1.1), who described a brother and sister
with meningioma of the foramen magnum. In both patients a small subcutaneous
tumour was discovered, which in one case was histologically investigated and
identified as a schwannoma. Both patients also demonstrated fusion of the posterior arc of the atlas to the foramen magnum. The authors concluded that evidence
was insufficient to classify these cases among Von Recklinghausen's disease but
*elle indique cependant dans quel sens il faut envisager le groupement de ces
tumeurs familiales avec une signature malformative des gaînes mesenchymateuses
de l'axe spinal* (it indicates, however, in which sense one should regard this
group of familial tumours with a malformative character of the mesenchymatous
sheath of the spinal axis).

Girard et al. (III.C.1.5) reported three cases of multiple intracranial meningiomas affecting a grandmother, her daughter and granddaughter. The daughter had two
small papillomas on two fingers of the left hand, histologically identified as
neurofibromas. She was also bilaterally deaf but the presence of acoustic neurinomas could not be proven.

Delleman et al. (III.C.1.6) reported a family in which four members of two generations, a father, his brother, a son and daughter, had meningiomas without evidence
of neurofibromatosis. A sister of the father, however, died at the age of 43 years
with signs of a brain tumour, and at autopsy bilateral acoustic neurinomas and
multiple meningiomas were found. Another daughter had multiple café-au-lait spots
on the back and legs, and other blood-relatives were said to have brown pigmented
spots. The association of meningioma with, generally bilateral, acoustic neurinoma
and other signs of Von Recklinghausen's disease was noted by Cushing and Eisenhardt
(22) and confirmed by subsequent observations (3, 23, 54, 80, 81, 103, 104). The
neurofibromatosis syndrome consists of at least two forms: a peripheral form, as
described by Von Recklinghausen in 1882 being the most common type, and a central
form marked by bilateral acoustic neurinoma and rare peripheral signs such as
café-au-lait spots and neurofibromas. Overlap between the two forms of neurofibromatosis (mixed form) can occur. Meningioma, commonly multiple, are particularly
related to the central form of neurofibromatosis, which has an autosomal dominant

inheritance pattern with high penetrance (40, 43, 47, 55, 79, 82, 104).
The three reports mentioned (III.B.1.1, III.C.1.5, III.C.1.6) probably must be
regarded as manifestations of the central form of neurofibromatosis.

Familial occurrence of meningioma without the implication of neurofibromatosis
also has been reported.
One report of identical twins with multiple intracranial and spinal meningiomas
has been made (III.A.1.1). One of these twins also had congenital ophthalmological
disorders of both eyes and a Klippel-Feil anomaly on skull radiographs. One twin
died at the age of 14 years of unknown cause but autopsy was not performed. The
authors note the lack of indications in this family supportive of the view of
genetically transmitted meningiomatosis as a variant of Von Recklinghausen's
disease.
Another report on twins is that by Hoppe (III.A.2.1) who described identical male
twins, one twin having a meningioma and the other a glioblastoma. The twin with
the meningioma had been reported earlier by Pedersen and Geyer in 1938. At that
time the twin brother was also examined, but no abnormalities were then found.

Familial meningioma occurrence in siblings has been reported in three families;
in two families concerning a brother and a sister, and in one family two affected
brothers (table 4). In the report by Grunert et al. (III.B.1.3) a third sibling
may have been involved as one of the affected siblings, a medical doctor by profession, stated that his sister had died of an unidentified brain tumour. Signs
of neurofibromatosis were not reported in these cases, but extensive examination
of the families was not performed.
Two reports have been made of discordant familial tumour occurrence in siblings,
one sibling demonstrating a meningioma (table 5), the report by Chateau et al.
(III.B.2.2) of a sister with a fibroblastic meningioma and a brother with a
haemangioblastoma of the cerebellum being of special interest in regards to the
possibility of a relationship with Von Hippel-Lindau's disease.

The familial aggregation of meningioma in more than one generation or in distant relatives has been reported in seven families. Two of these families showed
stigmata of neurofibromatosis and have been discussed earlier (III.C.1.5,
III.C.1.6). The other five families comprised three cases involving a mother
and daughter, one case of a mother and son, and one case involving two brothers
and their cousin (table 6). No signs of neurofibromatosis were found in these
cases but careful examination of their relatives was not performed. In the report
by Joynt and Perret (46) the authors suggest that *there may be evidence of multiple neurofibromatosis which will become manifest at some future time, or may
have been overlooked in the original examinations.*

The occurrence of discordant intracranial tumours in three members of a family, one member having a meningioma, has been reported by Patterson and Anderson (III.C.2.1): the father in this family had a haemangioblastoma of the cerebellum; the eldest son was operated upon, demonstrating a parasagittal angioblastic meningioma *corresponding closely in structure with the hemangioblastoma of the father*; and a younger son had a cyst of the cerebellum of which the precise nature could not be determined but which resembled the type of cyst found in multiple hereditary haemangioblastomas or Von Hippel-Lindau's disease. The distinction between angioblastic meningioma and haemangioblastoma can be difficult and transitional forms between haemangioblastoma and angioblastic meningioma exist (see general aspects). These cases should be considered a manifestation of Von Hippel-Lindau's disease, which has a dominant hereditary pattern.
A report of brain tumour occurrence in three generations of a family has been made by Blickenstorfer (III.C.2.2); in two generations, however, the brain tumour type could not be established.

A number of parameters in familial meningioma occurrence can be examined:
Gender:
Fifteen women and twelve men have been reported in cases demonstrating a familial aggregation of meningioma occurrence. In comparison, in non-familial cases a higher frequency of meningioma occurrence in females as compared to males has been found with a female : male ratio of 1 1/2 or 2 : 1 for cranial meningiomas and a somewhat higher ratio for spinal meningiomas.
Age:
The average age in the encountered cases of familial meningioma was 40 years. In general, meningioma occur between the ages of 30 and 60 years (see general aspects), the findings in the familial cases registered being similar to that of non-familial occurrences.

Location of the tumour:

single meningioma	14 cases
multiple meningioma	13
cranial meningioma	22 cases
craniospinal meningioma	2
cranial and spinal meningiomas	3
cranial meningioma:	
- cerebral convexity	6 tumours
- parasagittal	4
- falx	3
- sphenoid ridge	2
- chiasma region	2
- olfactory groove	2
- intraosseus	2

- cerebellopontine angle	1 tumour
- tentorium	1
- optic nerve	1
- intraventricular	1

spinal meningioma:

- thoracic	3 tumours
- cervical	1

Relatively more multiple occurrences of meningioma were found in familial cases
as compared to non-familial. The site of tumour occurrence in familial and non-
familial cases did not essentially differ. The site of tumour occurrence in
affected persons within one family was identical in six of the twelve reports.
The ratio of intracranial as compared to spinal meningiomas was approximately the
same in both familial and non-familial cases.

Histological diagnosis:

meningotheliomatous meningioma	7
fibroblastic meningioma	2
psammomatous meningioma	4
transitional (mixed) meningioma	8

Histological features in familial cases did not differ from that of non-familial
cases, and there was no obvious predeliction for one subtype of meningioma.
Meningioma subtypes encountered in affected persons within one family were identical in five reports, different in four, and of uncertain similarity in two
reports.

Associated physical or mental conditions:

congenital ophthalmological disorders	1 case
Klippel-Feil anomaly	1
claw feet	1
fusion atlas-foramen magnum	2
small subcutaneous tumour	1
schwannoma	1
two neurofibromas	1
bilateral acoustic neurinomas	1
bilateral deafness	1
mental retardation	2
aneurysm of the a. communicans anterior	1
pontine haemorrhage	1
head injury	2
depression	1

The occurrence of some of these symptoms as stigmata of neurofibromatosis has
been mentioned. The presence of multiple congenital abnormalities in one of twins
with meningioma (ophthalmological disorders of both eyes, Klippel-Feil anomaly
and claw feet, III.A.1.1) is of interest. In two cases a previous head injury was
noted, in one case accompanied by skull fracture.

Blood-types, when reported, revealed no relevant data.

132

Family:

The families with associated neurofibromatosis, (III.B.1.1, III.C.1.5,
III.C.1.6) or Von Hippel-Lindau's disease (III.C.2.1, perhaps also III.B.2.2)
have been discussed.

Blickenstorfer (III.C.2.2) reporting a brother with a glioblastoma multiforme and
a sister with a meningioma, investigated 59 members of this family and found a
grandmother and a maternal aunt who died of unspecified brain tumours. Apart from
mental disorders no other important diseases were found in this family.

In the report by Joynt and Perret (III.C.1.2) a brother of the mother (case 1)
had cancer of the internal organs, and a sister of the daughter (case 2) had
multiple sclerosis.

Other reports did not mention disorders among the relatives of the patients,
associated conditions not being found or the families not extensively investigated.

Serial studies

Koch (50) investigated a series of 350 female patients having a brain tumour,
mainly gliomas and meningiomas, and found six occurrences of familial aggregation,
four of which were histologically verified. In one of these families the proband
had a meningioma and her brother an unspecified brain tumour (III.B.2.1). From
the same clinic in Münster Meyer (62) studied a series of 459 male patients having
a brain tumour, including 28 patients with a histologically verified meningioma.
The father of a patient with a parasagittal meningioma was found to have a neurinoma of the spinal cord and several cutaneous fibromas, a cyst and a fibroma of
the right kidney, and carcinoma of the stomach. This occurrence should be regarded
as a form of neurofibromatosis. In a follow-up study on 371 male and 296 female
patients having a brain tumour Kemper (48) found one case of familial brain tumour
occurrence among 18 male and 35 female patients having meningiomas: an aunt of a
male patient was found having a glioblastoma (III.C.2.3).

Hauge and Harvald (35, 36) investigated 1552 relatives of 155 patients with meningioma and found two cases of cerebral tumour, whereas five would have been expected
on the basis of prevalence rates. Of the two one was a histologically verified
glioblastoma multiforme and the other a cerebral tumour found at autopsy, no
microscopic examination of which was performed.

In a study based on interviews with family members of 24 meningioma patients
Choi et al. (17) found two brain tumours and 11 'other tumours' as compared to
three brain tumours and eight 'other tumours' among relatives of 24 members of a
matched control group.

Associated hereditary diseases and congenital factors

The importance of the association of meningioma occurrence with neurofibromatosis, especially the central form, has been stressed. Rarely, meningioma also
occur in other phacomatoses such as Von Hippel-Lindau's disease (III.C.2.1),
tuberous sclerosis (26), and Sturge-Weber disease (33).
Meningiomas have been described in Werner's syndrome, an autosomal recessive disorder marked by a characteristically small stature, premature senility,
scleroderma-like changes and other manifestations (29, 49). They may also be
found in patients with the multiple hamartoma syndrome or Cowden's disease, a
condition with an autosomal dominant inheritance pattern and such distinctive
features as multiple papillomas of the lip and mouth, breast cancer, thyroid
adenoma and carcinoma, bone and liver cysts, lipoma and polyps (65, 89, 100).
Of special interest is the association of meningioma with breast cancer (87, 94).
Schoenberg et al. (87) investigated 135 patients with multiple primary tumours in
whom at least one of the primary tumours was situated within the nervous system,
and found eight patients having a meningioma in association with breast cancer,
this number significantly exceeding the number of expected cases. The association
of breast cancer and meningiomas is most likely due to hormonal influences but
the possibility of genetic factors cannot be excluded.
A statistically significant association between meningiomas and extraneural
primary malignancies in general also has been demonstrated (9).
The simultaneous occurrence of meningioma and other primary brain tumours such as
glioma, craniopharyngioma and pituitary adenoma has been reported (14, 24). The
coexistence of meningioma and acromegaly may suggest the facilitation or stimulation of meningioma development by growth hormone (14).
De Weerdt and Schut (101) studied the families of 18 meningioma patients in order
to establish whether a correlation existed between the occurrence of these brain
tumours, spina bifida and mongoloid idiocy, but no correlation between these
factors could be demonstrated.
Intracranial (possibly congenital) meningiomas in infants younger than one year
of age are extremely rare, and only 16 cases have been reported in the literature
(5, 13, 68). They occur predominantly in males, and demonstrate a high incidence
of cyst formation and predominance of a fibroblastic type on histological examination.

Cytogenetic aspects

Chromosomal patterns of meningioma cells have been studied. The basic aber-
ration is monosomy of chromosome nr 22 in group G or a deletion of a terminal

part of varying size from one chromosome nr 22 (56, 57, 59, 63, 72, 105, 108).
The deleted chromosomal material is not translocated to another chromosome but
loss occurs of a definite part of the genome of these meningioma cells (58, 107).
In addition to the typical loss of a chromosome nr 22, involvement of other
chromosome types has been observed by some authors. Mark (58, 59) found a non-
random involvement of chromosome types in group A (nr 1), group C (nrs 8 and 9)
and group D (nrs 14 and 15). Cytological and cytogenetic studies of meningioma
cells by Zankl et al. (106) indicated the relatively frequent loss of sex
chromosomes in human meningiomas. In tumours of females one X-chromosome was lost,
whereas in tumours of males the Y-chromosome was frequently missing. The importance
of such chromosomal aberrations in meningioma cells is not as yet understood.

Proof of the heritability of meningiomas seems lacking. Efforts to demonstrate
significant familial brain tumour occurrence in family members of meningioma
patients have been unsuccessful and evidence of primary genetic causation in
meningioma development cannot be concluded from the cytogenetic studies. The
reports on familial occurrence of meningioma could suggest an influence of hereditary factors. More extensive examination of the reported cases and their relatives, however, might have revealed signs of neurofibromatosis, or such signs
might have manifested at a later date. The meningiomas occurring in these families
might also be a manifestation of a monosymptomatic form of neurofibromatosis, a
syndrome known for its extreme variability, or the familial aggregation might be
the result of chance alone.

REFERENCES

1. ADELOYE A 1979
   Neoplasms of the brain in the African.
   Surg Neurol 11:247-255
2. ALBERT RE, OMRAN AR 1968
   Follow-up study of patients treated by X-ray epilation for tinea
   capitis. I Population characteristics, posttreatment illnesses and
   mortality experience.
   Arch Environ Health 17:899-918
3. ALLIEZ J, MASSE JL, ALLIEZ B 1975
   Tumeurs bilatérales de l'acoustique et maladie de Recklinghausen
   observées dans plusieurs générations. Considérations sur les tumeurs
   de l'acoustique héréditaires (1).
   Rev Neurol (Paris) 131:545-558
4. ALTER M 1975
   Statistical aspects of spinal cord tumors.
   In: Vinken PJ, Bruyn GW (eds) Handbook of Clinical Neurology
   North-Holland Publ Co, Amsterdam vol 19:1-22
5. AMANO K, MIURA N, TAJIKA Y, MATSUMORI K, KUBO O, KOBAYASHI N,
   KITAMURA K 1980
   Cystic meningioma in a 10-month-old infant. Case report.
   J Neurosurg 52:829-833
6. BAILEY OT 1940
   Histologic sequences in meningioma with consideration of the nature
   of hyperostosis cranii.
   Arch Pathol 30:42-69
7. BEHREND RC 1974
   Epidemiology of brain tumours.
   In: Vinken PJ, Bruyn GW (eds) Handbook of Clinical Neurology.
   North-Holland Publ Co, Amsterdam vol 16:56-88
8. BELLER AJ, FEINSOD M, SAHAR A 1972
   The possible relationship between small dose irradiation to the
   scalp and intracranial meningiomas.
   Neurochirurgia 15:135-143
9. BELLUR SN, CHANDRA V, McDONALD LW 1979
   Association of meningiomas with extracranial primary malignancy.
   Neurology 29:1165-1168
10. BLICKENSTORFER E 1951
    Sieben Fälle operierter Okzipitalhirntumoren unter besonderer
    Berücksichtigung der psychischen Symptomatologie und deren Zusam-
    menhänge mit der Familienkonstitution.
    Wien Z Nervenheilk 4:94-119
11. BOGDANOWICZ W, SACHS Jr E 1974
    The possible role of radiation in oncogenesis of meningioma.
    Surg Neurol 2:379-383

12. BONITO L Di, BIANCHI C 1979
    Métastase d'un cancer mammaire dans un méningiome.
    Sem Hop Paris, 55:171-172
13. BUENO JG, ESTEBAN HM, LÓPEZ CB, PUENTES MLF 1977
    Congenital meningioma.
    Childs Brain 3:304-308
14. BUNICK EM, MILLS LC, ROSE LI 1978
    Association of acromegaly and meningiomas.
    JAMA 240:1267-1668
15. CASTELLANO F, GUIDETTI B, OLIVECRONA H 1952
    Pterional meningiomas "en plaque".
    J Neurosurg 9:188-196
16. CHATEAU R, ROUGEMONT J de, GROSLAMBERT R, BARGE M, PASQUIER H, FAURE H
    1971
    A propos des tumeurs cérébrales familiales (méningiome fibroblasti-
    que et hémangioblastome solitaire du cervelet).
    J Med Lyon 52:657-678
17. CHOI NW, SCHUMAN LM, GULLEN WH 1970
    Epidemiology of primary central nervous system neoplasms. II: case
    control study.
    Am J Epidemiol 91:467-485
18. CHOUX R, CHRESTIAN MA, TRIPIER MF, GAMBARELLI D, HASSOUN J, TOGA M
    1976
    Hémangiopéricytome cérébral. Étude ultrastructurale d'un cas.
    J Neurol Sci 28:361-371
19. COURVILLE CB, MARSH C, DEEB P 1952
    Massive deforming meningiomatous hyperostosis.
    Bull Los Angeles Neurol Soc 17:179-191
20. CUSHING H 1922
    The meningiomas (Cavendish lecture).
    Brain 45:282-316
21. CUSHING H 1932
    Intracranial tumors.
    Charles C Thomas, Springfield, Ill
22. CUSHING H, EISENHARDT L 1938
    The meningiomas.
    Charles C Thomas, Springfield, Ill
23. DAVIDOFF LM, MARTIN J 1955
    Hereditary combined neurinomas and meningiomas.
    J Neurosurg 12:375-384
24. DEEN Jr HG, LAWS Jr ER 1981
    Multiple primary brain tumors of different cell types.
    Neurosurgery 8:20-25
25. DELLEMAN JW, JONG JGY de, BLEEKER GM 1978
    Meningiomas in five members of a family over two generations, in one
    member simultaneously with acoustic neurinomas.
    Neurology 28:567-570
26. DONEGANI G, GRATTAROLA FR, WILDI E 1972
    Tuberous sclerosis (Bourneville disease).
    In: Vinken PJ, Bruyn GW (eds) Handbook of Clinical Neurology.
    North-Holland Publ Co, Amsterdam vol 14:340-389
27. DONNELL MS, MEYER GA, DONEGAN WL 1979
    Estrogenreceptor protein in intracranial meningiomas.
    J Neurosurg 50:499-502

28. ECTORS L, BOGAERT L van 1953
    Ablation d'un méningiome du trou occipital chez un frère et une soeur.
    Acta Neurol Psychiatr (Belg) 53:193-204
29. EPSTEIN CJ, MARTIN GM, SCHULTZ AL, MOTULSKY AG 1966
    Werner's syndrome.
    Medicine (Baltimore) 45:177-221
30. FREEDMAN H, FORSTER FM 1948
    Bone formation and destruction in hyperostosis associated with meningiomas.
    J Neuropathol Exp Neurol 7:69-80
31. GAIST G, PIAZZA G 1959
    Meningiomas in two members of the same family (with no evidence of neurofibromatosis).
    J Neurosurg 16:110-113
32. GIRARD PF, TRILLET M, CONFAVREUX C, CHAZOT G 1977
    Méningiomatose multiple et familiale. Un syndrome voisin de la neurofibromatose de Recklinghausen.
    Rev Neurol (Paris) 133:359-362
33. GÖKALP HZ, OZKAL E, ERDOGAN A, SELCUKI M 1981
    A giant meningioma of the fourth ventricle associated with Sturge-Weber disease.
    Acta Neurochirurgica 57:115-120
34. GRUNERT V, HORCAJADA J, SUNDER-PLASSMANN M 1970
    Familiäres Auftreten intrakranieller Meningeome.
    Wien Med Wochenschr 120:807-808
35. HAUGE M, HARVALD B 1957
    Genetics in intracranial tumours.
    Acta Genet 7:573-591
36. HAUGE M, HARVALD B 1960
    Studies in the etiology of intracranial tumours.
    Acta Psychiatr Neurol Scand 35:163-170
37. HESHMAT MY, KOVI J, SIMPSON C, KENNEDY J, FAN KJ 1976
    Neoplasms of the central nervous system. Incidence and population selectivity in the Washington DC, Metropolitan area.
    Cancer 38:2135-2142
38. HO KL 1980
    Metastasis of carcinoma to meningioma.
    Arch Pathol Lab Med 104:394-395
39. HOPE DT 1978
    Metastasis of carcinoma to meningioma.
    Acta Neurochir (Wien) 40:307-313
40. HOPE DG, MULVIHILL JJ 1981
    Malignancy in neurofibromatosis.
    Adv Neurol 29:33-56
41. HOPPE HJ 1952
    Diskordantes Auftreten von Hirntumoren bei erbgleichen Zwillingen.
    Zentralbl Neurochir 12:34-36
42. HORTEN BC, URICH H, RUBINSTEIN LJ, MONTAGUE SR 1977
    The angioblastic meningioma: a reappraisal of a nosological problem. Light-, electron-microscopic, tissue and organ culture observations.
    J Neurol Sci 31:387-410

138

43. HORTON WA 1976
    Genetics of central nervous system tumors.
    Birth defects: original article series XII:91-97
44. HUMEAU C, VIC P, SENTEIN P, VLAHOVITCH B 1979
    The fine structure of meningiomas: an attempted classification.
    Virchows Arch (Pathol Anat) 382:201-216
45. JOYNT RJ, PERRET GE 1961
    Meningiomas in a mother and daughter. Cases without evidence of
    neurofibromatosis.
    Neurology 11:164-165
46. JOYNT RJ, PERRET GE 1965
    Familial meningiomas.
    J Neurol Neurosurg Psychiatry 28:163-164
47. KANTER WR, ELDRIDGE R, FABRICANT R, ALLEN JC, KOERBER T 1980
    Central neurofibromatosis with bilateral acoustic neuroma: genetic,
    clinical and biochemical distinctions from peripheral neurofibroma-
    tosis.
    Neurology 30:851-859
48. KEMPER K 1964
    Vorkommen von Hirntumoren bei Zwillingen und in Familien.
    Thesis, Münster, Germany.
49. KOBAYASHI S, GIBO H, SUGITA K, KOMIYA I, YAMADA T 1980
    Werner's syndrome associated with meningioma.
    Neurosurgery 7:517-520
50. KOCH G 1954
    Beitrag zur Erblichkeit der Hirngeschwülste (vorläufige Mitteilung).
    Acta Genet Med Gemellol 3:170-191
51. KRAJEWSKI R 1979
    Simultaneous occurrence of meningioma and astrocytoma.
    Neurol Neurochir Pol 13:455-458
52. KUHNEN B 1953
    Beobachtungen an sieben Zwillingspaaren mit Hirntumoren.
    Acta Genet Med Gemellol 2:407-430
53. LAPRESLE J, NETZKY MG, JÜNEMANN HM 1952
    The pathology of meningiomas.
    Am J Pathol 28:757-791
54. LEE DK, ABBOTT ML 1969
    Familial central nervous system neoplasia. Case report of a family
    with von Recklinghausen's neurofibromatosis.
    Arch Neurol 20:154-160
55. LOTT IT, RICHARDSON Jr EP 1981
    Neuropathological findings and the biology of neurofibromatosis.
    Adv Neurol 29:23-32
56. MARK J 1970
    Chromosomal patterns in human meningiomas.
    Eur J Cancer 6:489-498
57. MARK J 1971
    Chromosomal aberrations and their relation to malignancy in
    meningomas: a meningoma with ring chromosomes.
    Acta Pathol Microbiol Scand (A) 79:193-200
58. MARK J 1973
    Karyotype patterns in human meningiomas.
    Comparison between studies with G- and Q-banding techniques.
    Hereditas 75:213-220

59. MARK J   1977
    Chromosomal abnormalities and their specifity in human neoplasms: an
    assessment of recent observations by banding techniques.
    Adv Cancer Res 24:165-222
60. McDONNELL DE, POLLOCK P   1978
    Cerebral cystic hemangioblastoma.
    Surg Neurol 10:195-199
61. MEMON MY   1980
    Multiple and familial meningiomas without evidence of neurofibroma-
    tosis.
    Neurosurgery 7:262-264
62. MEYER R   1956
    Vorkommen von Hirntumoren bei Zwillingen und in Familien.
    Thesis, Münster, Germany
63. MITELMAN F, LEVAN G   1976
    Clustering of aberrations to specific chromosomes in human
    neoplasms. II: A survey of 287 neoplasms.
    Hereditas 82:167-174
64. MODAN B, BAIDATZ D, MART H, STEINITZ R, LEVIN SG   1974
    Radiation-induced head and neck tumours.
    Lancet 1:277-279
65. MULVIHILL JJ, McKEEN EA   1977
    Discussion: genetics of multiple primary tumors.
    Cancer 40:1867-1871
66. NITTNER K   1976
    Spinal meningiomas, neurinomas and neurofibromas and hourglass
    tumours.
    In: Vinken PJ, Bruyn GW (eds) Handbook of Clinical Neurology.
    North-Holland Publ Co, Amsterdam vol 20:177-322
67. NUNNERY Jr E   1980
    Breast carcinoma metastatic to meningioma.
    Arch Pathol Lab Med 104:392-393
68. OHTA T, KAJIKAWA H, TAKEUCHI J   1977
    Congenital tumours of the brain.
    In: Vinken PJ, Bruyn GW (eds) Handbook of Clinical Neurology.
    North-Holland Publ Co, Amsterdam vol 31:35-74
69. OLIVECRONA H   1947
    The parasagittal meningiomas.
    J Neurosurg 4:327-341
70. PALACIOS E, AZAR-KIA B   1975
    Malignant metastasizing angioblastic meningiomas.
    J Neurosurg 42:185-188
71. PATTERSON GH, ANDERSON FM   1940
    Intracranial tumors occurring in three members of a family.
    Bull Los Angeles Neurol Soc 5:218-223
72. PAUL B, PORTER IH, BENEDICT WF   1973
    Giemsa banding in an established line of a human malignant
    meningioma.
    Humangenetik 18:185-187
73. PEDERSEN O, GEYER H   1938
    Diskordantes Auftreten von Hirntumoren bei erbgleichen Zwillingen.
    Zentralbl Neurochir 2:53-63

74. PEÑA CE 1975
    Intracranial hemangiopericytoma.
    Acta Neuropathol (Berl) 33:279-284
75. PERCY AK, ELVEBACK LR, OKAZAKI H, KURLAND LT 1972
    Neoplasms of the central nervous system. Epidemiologic con-
    siderations.
    Neurology 22:40-48
76. POISSON M, MAGDELENAT H, FONCIN JF, BLEIBEL JM, PHILIPPON J,
    PERTUISET B, BUGE A 1980
    Récepteurs d'oestrogènes et de progestérone dans les méningiomes.
    Étude de 22 cas.
    Rev Neurol (Paris) 136:193-203
77. POPOFF NA, MALININ TI, ROSOMOFF HL 1974
    Fine structure of intracranial hemangiopericytoma and angiomatous
    meningioma.
    Cancer 34:1187-1197
78. PRESTON-MARTIN S, PAGANINI-HILL A, HENDERSON BE, PIKE MC, WOOD C
    1980
    Case-control study of intracranial meningiomas in women in Los
    Angeles County, California.
    J Natl Cancer Inst 65:67-73
79. RICCARDI VM 1981
    Von Recklinghausen neurofibromatosis.
    N Engl J Med 305:1617-1627
80. RODRIGUEZ HA, BERTHRONG M 1966
    Multiple primary intracranial tumors in von Recklinghausens's
    neurofibromatosis.
    Arch Neurol 14:467-475
81. ROVINE BW, MULFORD EH 1960
    Bilateral acoustic neurinomas with multiple meningiomas.
    Neurology 10:323-324
82. RUBENSTEIN AE, MYTILINEOAU C, YAHR MD, REVOLTELLA RP 1981
    Neurological aspects of neurofibromatosis.
    Adv Neurol 29:11-21
83. RUBINSTEIN LJ 1972
    Tumors of the central nervous system. In: Atlas of Tumor Pathology,
    2nd series, Fasc 6.
    Armed Forces Inst of Pathol, Washingston DC p 169-190
84. RUSSELL DS, RUBINSTEIN LJ 1977
    Pathology of the tumours of the nervous system, 4th ed.
    Edward Arnold, London p 65-100
85. SAHAR A 1965
    Familial occurrence of meningiomas. Case report.
    J Neurosurg 23:444-445
86. SAVOIARDO M, LODRINI S 1980
    Hypodense area within a meningioma: metastasis from breast cancer.
    Neuroradiology 20:107-110
87. SCHOENBERG BS, CHRISTINE BW, WHISNANT JP 1975
    Nervous system neoplasms and primary malignancies of other sites.
    The unique association between meningiomas and breast cancer.
    Neurology 25:705-712
88. SCHOENBERG BS, CHRISTINE BW, WHISNANT JP 1976
    The descriptive epidemiology of primary intracranial neoplasms: the
    Connecticut experience.
    Am J Epidemiol 104:499-510

8y. ُLEDANO HO   1981
    Multiple hamartoma and neoplasia syndrome (Cowden syndrome)
    In: Vinken PJ, Bruyn GW (eds) Handbook of Clinical Neurology.
    North-Holland Publ Co, Amsterdam vol 42:754-755
90. SEDZIMIR CB, FRAZER AK, ROBERTS JR   1973
    Cranial and spinal meningiomas in a pair of identical twin boys.
    J Neurol Neurosurg Psychiatry 36:368-376
91. SHUANGSOTI S, HONGSAPRABHAS C, NETSKY MG   1970
    Metastasizing meningioma.
    Cancer 26:833-841
92. SIMPSON D   1957
    The recurrence of intracranial meningiomas after surgical treatment.
    J Neurol Neurosurg Psychiatry 20:22-39
93. SLOOFF JL, KERNOHAN JW, MacCARTY CS   1964
    Primary intramedullary tumors of the spinal cord and filum ter-
    minale.
    WB Saunders, Philadelphia
94. SMITH FP, SLAVIK M, MacDONALD JS   1978
    Association of breast cancer with meningioma. Report of two cases
    and review of the literature.
    Cancer 42:1992-1994
95. STRONG AJ, SYMON L, MacGREGOR BJL, O'NEILL BP   1976
    Coincidental meningioma and glioma. Report of two cases.
    J Neurosurg 45:455-458
96. WAGA S, HANDA H   1976
    Radiation-induced meningioma with review of literature.
    Surg Neurol 5:215-219
97. WAGMAN AD, WEISS EK, RIGGS HE   1960
    Hyperplasia of the skull associated with intra-osseus meningioma in
    the absence of gross tumor.
    J Neuropathol Exp Neurol 19:111-115
98. WALSH J, GYE R, CONNELLEY TJ   1969
    Meningioma: a late complication of head injury.
    Med J Aust 1:906-908
99. WARZOK R, GÜTHERT H   1978
    Die Tumoren des Zentralnervensystems im Biopsie- und Autopsiegut.
    I Mitteilung: Häufigkeit, Alters- und Geschlechtsverteilung.
    Zentralbl Allg Pathol 122:462-474
100. WEARY PE, GORLIN RJ, GENTRY Jr WC, COMER JE, GREER KE   1972
     Multiple hamartoma syndrome (Cowden's disease).
     Arch Dermatol 106:682-690
101. WEERDT CJ de, SCHUT T   1972
     Some aspects of heredity of brain tumours.
     Psychiatr Neurol Neurochir (Amst) 75:293-298
102. WOOD MW, WHITE RJ, KERNOHAN JW   1957
     One hundred intracranial meningiomas found incidentally at necropsy.
     J Neuropathol Exp Neurol 16:337-340
103. YOUNG DF, ELDRIDGE R, GARDNER WJ   1970
     Bilateral acoustic neuroma in a large kindred.
     JAMA 214:347-353
104. YOUNG DF, ELDRIDGE R, NAGER GT, DELAND FH, McNEW J   1971
     Hereditary bilateral acoustic neuroma (central neurofibromatosis).
     Birth Defects VII:73-86

105. ZANG KD, SINGER H   1967
     Chromosomal constitution of meningiomas.
     Nature 216:84-85
106. ZANKL H, SEIDEL H, ZANG KD   1975
     Cytological and cytogenetical studies on brain tumors. V: Preferen-
     tial loss of sex chromosomes in human meningiomas.
     Humangenetik 27:119-128
107. ZANKL H, WEISS AF, ZANG KD   1975
     Cytological and cytogenetical studies on brain tumors. VI: No evi-
     dence for a translocation in 22-monosomic meningiomas.
     Humangenetik 30:343-348
108. ZANKL H, ZANG KD   1971
     Cytological and cytogenetical studies on brain tumors. III: Ph'-like
     chromosomes in human meningiomas.
     Humangenetik 12:42-49
109. ZÜLCH KJ   1956
     Biologie und Pathologie der Hirngeschwülste.
     In: Olivecrona H, Tönnis W (eds) Handbuch der Neurochirurgie.
     Springer, Berlin Bd III:399-455
110. ZÜLCH KJ   1980
     Principles of the new World Health Organization (WHO) classification
     of brain tumors.
     Neuroradiology 19:59-66

Chapter IV

FAMILIAL CHOROID PLEXUS PAPILLOMA

CASE REPORTS

CLASSIFICATION

A. *TWINS*

1. Monozygotic twins with concordant tumour
2. Monozygotic twins with discordant tumour
3. Monozygotic twins, one demonstrating choroid plexus papilloma
4. Dizygotic twins

B. *SIBLINGS*

1. Siblings with concordant tumour
2. Siblings with discordant tumour

C. *OTHER GENERATIONS AND DISTANT RELATIVES*

1. Other generations and distant relatives with concordant tumour
2. Other generations and distant relatives with discordant tumour

TABLES

IV.A.   *TWINS*

IV.A.1.   MONOZYGOTIC TWINS WITH CONCORDANT TUMOUR

No reports on this occurrence are available in literature.

IV.A.2.   MONOZYGOTIC TWINS WITH DISCORDANT TUMOUR

No reports on this occurrence are available in literature.

IV.A.3. MONOZYGOTIC TWINS, ONE DEMONSTRATING CHOROID PLEXUS PAPILLOMA

IV.A.3.1. Koch 1953 - Münster, Germany (17)

In this report Koch describes thirteen pairs of twins, one twin in each pair
having a brain tumour. Three of the thirteen twin pairs were dizygotic; it
was uncertain at that time whether the other ten pairs were mono- or dizygotic.
Within these thirteen twin pairs no concordant occurrence of brain tumours was
established. One of the twins (male) had a plexus papilloma of the fourth
ventricle at the age of 32 years, histologically verified. His twin brother
was alive and well at the age of 35 years.
It must be stressed that it is uncertain whether this twin was monozygotic or
dizygotic. No further data are given in the article.

IV.A.4. DIZYGOTIC TWINS

Perhaps the case of Koch (1953) could be classified here, but as a choice it
is registered among monozygotic twins (IV.A.3.1). No other reports are available in literature.

IV.B.   *SIBLINGS*

IV.B.1.   SIBLINGS WITH CONCORDANT TUMOUR

IV.B.1.1. <u>De la Torre et al. 1963 - Winston-Salem, U.S.A.</u> (34)

A brother and sister. American.

<u>Case 1</u> (sister)

<u>History</u>: The patient was admitted to hospital at the age of nine months.
Her symptoms were: generalized weakness and irritability, failure to gain
weight and enlargement of the head.
On examination the suture lines were open. She had ataxia, papilloedema,
areflexia and generalized weakness. Cerebrospinal fluid pressure was 150 mm
H_2O and the protein content was 108 mg %. Roentgenograms of the skull showed
separation of cranial sutures. Radiographs of the spinal column revealed an
area of increased density in the left thoracic paravertebral region. Ventriculography (air) showed dilatation of both lateral ventricles, more on the
right, and a filling defect of the right lateral ventricle in the region of
the trigonum.
A right parieto-temporal craniotomy was performed and the tumour totally
removed. The patient died on the operating table of cardiac arrest.

<u>Autopsy</u>: *disclosed a neuroblastoma in the left paravertebral region and
another in the left adrenal gland; a pheochromocytoma was found in the right
adrenal gland.*

<u>Microscopic study</u>: Choroid plexus papilloma.

<u>Diagnosis</u>: Choroid plexus papilloma of the right lateral ventricle.
Neuroblastoma left adrenal and left paravertebral region. Pheochromocytoma
right adrenal.

<u>Case 2</u> (brother)

<u>History</u>: The patient was admitted to hospital at the age of 5 1/2 months
because of irritability, decrease in appetite and progressive enlargement of
the head.
On examination an enlarged head with bulging fontanels was found. He had
papilloedema, divergent strabismus and 'sluggish' pupils. CSF pressure was
420 mm H_2O and the protein content 157 mg %. Roentgenograms of the skull
showed separation of cranial sutures. Ventriculography (air) demonstrated

dilatation of both lateral ventricles with a filling defect of the left lateral ventricle and a shift to the right.

By a left parieto-temporal craniotomy a partial excision of the tumour was performed. The patient died on the operating table of cardiac arrest.

Autopsy: Not performed.

Microscopic study: Ependymoma.

Diagnosis: Ependymoma of the left lateral ventricle.

Family: A third sibling of these children had died a few years earlier at another hospital of *an undifferentiated tumour, compatible with the histologic diagnosis of neuroblastoma*, in the deep portion of the pterygomaxillary fossa. Permission for autopsy was not granted. No further data about the family are given in the article. The gender of the third sibling is not mentioned in the report.

COMMENT

The microscopic diagnosis of case 1 was choroid plexus papilloma and of case 2 ependymoma. The differential diagnosis between these tumours, however, can sometimes be very difficult. They are obviously closely related, originating from ependyma and its homologues, and therefore classified among the subgroup of ependymal brain tumours according to the present classification of brain tumours of the World Health Organization. These cases have been regarded here as manifestations of concordant tumours, and as a choice registered among the choroid plexus papilloma.

In case 1 the choroid plexus papilloma was associated with multiple neuro-blastomas and a pheochromocytoma, both tumours derived from elements of the neural crest (neurocristopathies), which have a heritable component. Unfortunately no autopsy of case 2 was performed.

IV.B.1.2. <u>Komminoth et al. 1965 - Paris, France</u> (19)

A brother and sister. French.

<u>Case 1</u> (brother)

<u>History</u>: The patient demonstrated a normal birth and development up to the age of two years. He was then admitted to hospital because - according to the parents - he would no longer walk, refused his food and had suffered from headaches during a three month period. A few months earlier he had experienced a mild head trauma.

On neurological examination the patient showed obvious meningeal symptoms and a decrease of the movements of his legs, especially on the left side, where he also had high tendon reflexes. The circumference of his head was increased, measuring 50 centimetres. Ophthalmological examination revealed papilloedema on the right side. A lumbar puncture showed xanthochromic cerebrospinal fluid with an elevated protein content of 1.32 mg %. Radiographs of the skull showed diastasis of the sutures. The EEG demonstrated focal disturbances in the right temporo-parieto-occipital region. On pneumencephalography a dilatation of the third and lateral ventricles was seen with a process occupying the occipital and posterior temporal horn at the right side.

At operation a tumour the size of a lemon was discovered in the right lateral ventricle extending into the frontal and temporal horn and inserted at the level of the glomus. It was totally removed.

The postoperative course was good and the patient received radiotherapy.

Seven months postoperatively the child was in good health. He had no neuro-logical or psychological symptoms.

<u>Microscopic study</u>: showed a typical papilloma of the choroid plexus with conservation of the epithelial structure of the choroid plexus. Numerous areas with angiomatosis were present. There were no signs of malignancy.

<u>Diagnosis</u>: Choroid plexus papilloma of the right lateral ventricle.

<u>Case 2</u> (sister)

<u>History</u>: The patient had a normal birth and development during the first years of life. At the age of three years she had experienced a mild head trauma. A few months later she developed disturbances in walking, followed by a hemiparesis on the left side. At the age of four years she was admitted to hospital.

On neurological examination the patient was somnolent. She had a hemiparesis of the face and body, brisk tendon reflexes and a positive Babinski sign on the left side. The circumference of the head measured 51.5 centimetres and there was an asymmetrical head shape. Ophthalmological examination revealed bilateral papilloedema. The EEG showed disturbances in the posterior part of both hemispheres with delta waves especially on the right side. A right carotid angiogram demonstrated an expansive process in the ventricles occupying the temporal region.

At operation a haemorrhagic tumour was removed from the right temporal horn of the lateral ventricle.

The postoperative course was complicated by meningeal symptoms and fever, but the patient gradually improved and after two weeks had only a regressive hemiparesis of the left arm and leg.

At discharge the child had a remnant left hemiparesis. The EEG showed a focal disturbance of the right posterior hemisphere.

A few months later the patient died at home of an infectious process of which no precise diagnosis could be made.

Autopsy: Not performed.

Microscopic study: showed fibrovascular papillary formations in a choroid epithelium with some angiomatosis in the stroma. No signs of malignancy were present.

Diagnosis: Choroid plexus papilloma of the right lateral ventricle.

Family: No data concerning the relatives of the two siblings are mentioned in the article.

152

IV.B.2.   SIBLINGS WITH DISCORDANT TUMOUR

IV.B.2.1. Faber 1934 - Pécs, Hungary (11)

Two brothers and one sister. Hungarian.

Case 1 (brother; proband)
    History: The patient was admitted to hospital at the age of 29 years. He
had complained of progressive headaches, dizziness and disturbances of gait
for three weeks prior to admission. A few days before admission he began
vomiting.
On physical examination no abnormalities could be found. Cerebrospinal fluid
pressure was 200 mm H$_2$O, and Pandy reaction ++. During his stay in hospital
the headaches, dizziness and vomiting progressed and he also complained of
diplopia. Once he had an epileptic seizure. Ophthalmological examination
showed no disorder. On repeated neurological examination the patient was seen
to be in a soporific, apathetic state and there was a facial nerve paresis,
anisocoria and paresis of the right internal rectus muscle.
Ten days after admission the patient developed respiratory disturbances with
general cyanosis and died within a few minutes.
    Autopsy: In the posterior part of the dilatated right lateral ventricle an
irregular papillomatous tumour mass was found with a red-grey colour. The
tumour was attached to the base of the lateral ventricle.
    Microscopic study: A carcinomatous degenerated choroid plexus papilloma
was seen.
    Diagnosis: Carcinomatous degenerated choroid plexus papilloma of the right
lateral ventricle.

Case 2 (brother)
    History: A brother of the proband died at the age of 5 years of a brain
tumour. No further data are known.

Case 3 (sister)
    History: A sister of the proband died at the age of 15 years after operation
of a brain tumour. No further data are mentioned in the article.

    Family: The mother of the proband died at the age of 32 years of a lung
carcinoma with metastases in the lymph nodes and the brain. There were also
two other sisters. One of them had two children, one of whom had hypertension.
The other sister was under treatment because of vertigo. She had one child

(a daughter) that was operated upon because of a glioma of the eye.

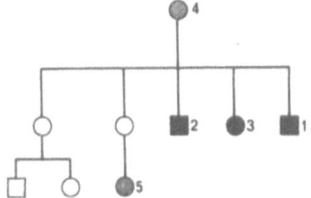

1 = case 1
2 = case 2
3 = case 3
4 = lung carcinoma
5 = glioma of the eye

COMMENT

Unfortunately no histological diagnosis of the brain tumours in cases 2 and 3 was made.

154

IV.B.2.2. <u>Peyser and Beller 1951 - Jerusalem, Israël</u> (29)

Two brothers. Israëli.

<u>Case 1</u>

   <u>History</u>: *Pregnancy and delivery of this child had been normal, and his weight was 3,200 g at birth. He developed normally in the first year of life. ... at the age of four months he had pertussis and at eight months bilateral otitis ....* The boy was admitted to hospital at the age of 20 months. *During the six months prior to admission the child lost weight and became thin and pale. ... his head grew abnormally big, ... he frequently vomited and slept much more than usual. He could not longer walk and was finally unable to sit up ....* He also developed convulsions.

At examination on admission a *very apathetic undernourished child* was seen *who apparently could not see. The head was abnormally large, the circumference being 50 cm and the anterior fontanelle open .... The cranial sutures were separated. All extremities were very spastic, more so on the left side, and reflexes were hyperactive. There were nystagmoid movements of both eyeballs. Ophthalmoscopic examination revealed blurred disks with signs of secondary atrophy ....* Ventriculography showed *a clear shift of the whole ventricular system to the left, probably due to a huge tumor in the right cerebral hemisphere. A catheter was inserted into the left lateral ventricle for ventricular drainage. After this procedure the child ran a very high temperature ... and was in a very bad state, so that craniotomy could not be risked. He died two days later with signs of respiratory failure.*

   <u>Autopsy</u> *revealed a huge soft tumor in the right cerebral hemisphere originating from the choroid plexus.*

   <u>Microscopic study</u>: The tumour was defined as a papilloma of the choroid plexus.

   <u>Diagnosis</u>: Choroid plexus papilloma of the right cerebral hemisphere.

<u>Case 2</u>

   <u>History</u>: The patient was admitted to hospital at the age of 14 years. *He had been healthy until three months prior to admission, when he began complaining of frontal headache which eventually grew worse and was accompanied by projectile vomiting. During the last few days before entering the hospital he complained of a feeling of numbness in the right half of his face.*
On examination the boy was *undernourished and groaned frequently. His neck was very stiff with marked opisthotonus .... There was slight paresis of both sixth*

cranial nerves. Hypaesthesia ... of the right half of the face was found.
There was papilledema of both optic nerves .... Both legs showed marked motor
weakness with loss of patellar reflexes. The Babinski toe sign was positive
on both sides. ... X-ray of the skull revealed no abnormality. Ventriculography showed *filling of the right ventricle only, which was pushed to the*
right and downwards. The right frontal horn did not fill. The left ventricle
was apparently obliterated.

A left fronto-temporo-parietal craniotomy was performed and a *cystic gliomatous*
tumor, 4 cm deep, was found and partially removed.

After operation there was no improvement and because of a gradually increasing
intracranial pressure five weeks later a secondary craniotomy was carried out.
After resection of the left frontal pole the soft, greyish-red tumor, the size
of an orange, was found in the frontal horn of the left lateral ventricle,
attached to its roof.

Postoperatively the patient was given X-ray treatment and he left the hospital
three months after admission.

Eight months later he died at home.

    Autopsy: Not performed.

    Microscopic study: Glioblastoma multiforme.

    Diagnosis: Glioblastoma multiforme of the left frontal horn.

    Family: The parents of the two brothers were healthy. They had four older
healthy children. No further data about the family are mentioned in the
article.

IV.C.   *OTHER GENERATIONS AND DISTANT RELATIVES*

Familial aggregation of choroid plexus papilloma in other generations and distant relatives have not been reported in the literature.

TABLES

TABLE 1 - SIBLINGS WITH CONCORDANT TUMOUR (IV.B.1)

	case	gender	relationship	number of unaffected siblings	race or nationality	age at symptom occurrence	age at death	location of the tumour
IV.B.1.1. De la Torre 1963	1	f	s	?	Amer.	?	9 m	R lateral ventricl
	2	m	br	?	Amer.	?	5 m	L lateral ventricl
VI.B.1.2. Komminoth 1965	1	m	br	?	French	2 y	-	R lateral ventricl
	2	f	s	?	French	3 y	4 y	R lateral ventricl

TABLE 2 - SIBLINGS WITH DISCORDANT TUMOUR (IV.B.2)

	case	gender	relationship	number of unaffected siblings	race or nationality	age at symptom occurrence	age at death	location of the tumour
IV.B.2.1. Faber 1934	1	m	br	2 s	Hung.	29 y	29 y	R lateral ventricl
	2	m	br	2 s	Hung.	?	5 y	?
	3	f	s	2 s	Hung.	?	15 y	?
IV.B.2.2. Peyser 1951	1	m	br	4	Isr.	14 m	20 m	R cerebral hemi-sphere
	2	m	br	4	Isr.	14 y	15 y	L frontal horn

diagnosis	biopsy	autopsy	associated physical or mental conditons	family	comment
Choroid plexus papilloma	+	+	Neuroblastoma L adrenal and L para-vertebral region. Pheochromocytoma R adrenal	A 3rd sibling died of a neuroblastoma of the ptery-gomaxillary fossa. No autopsy.	Concordant ependymal tumours. Association with tumours derived from neural crest.
Ependymoma	+	-	-		
Choroid plexus papilloma	+	-	Hydrocephalus. Mild head trauma	?	
Choroid plexus papilloma	+	-	Hydrocephalus. Mild head trauma		

diagnosis	biopsy	autopsy	associated physical or mental conditions	family	comment
Choroid plexus papilloma	-	+	-	One sister: vertigo. Mother: lung carcinoma with brain metastases. Niece: glioma of the eye.	No histological diagnosis of brain tumours in cases 2 and 3
Brain tumour	-	?	?		
Brain tumour	?	?	?		
Choroid plexus papilloma	-	+	Pertussis at 4 m and bilateral otitis at 8 m	-	
Glioblastoma multiforme	+	-	-		

GENERAL ASPECTS OF CHOROID PLEXUS PAPILLOMA

Papilloma of the choroid plexus are relatively rare and account for 0.4 to 0.6% of all primary intracranial tumours (3, 7, 33, 39).

The first case was reported by Guérard in 1832 and by 1970 more than 450 cases had been reported in the literature (20). These neoplasms can occur at any age but are most frequently encountered in the first decade of life, 74% of the occurrences according to Laurence (20), and account for 3.9% of intracranial tumours in children under 12 years of age (25).

Choroid plexus papilloma *are composed of adult epithelial cells that cover the ventricular choroid plexuses* (31), so these tumours occupy the sites of the ventricular system in which choroid plexus is normally found. They occur mainly in each of the lateral ventricles, in the fourth ventricle and in the cerebello-pontine angle. Less frequently they have been found in the third ventricle and rarely in various other sites (3, 20, 25, 31, 38, 39). In children the choroid

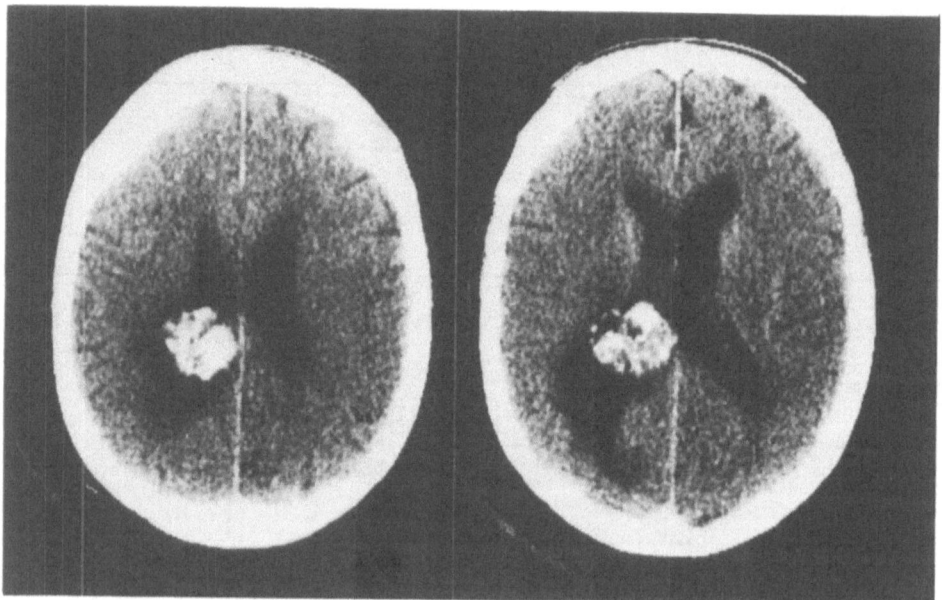

Fig. 1. CT-scan of a choroid plexus papilloma of the right lateral ventricle (not enhanced)

plexus papillomas are most frequently localized in the lateral ventricle where they are most commonly situated in the region of the trigone (3). In adults the fourth ventricle becomes the predominant site (3, 31, 38).

Progressive hydrocephalus is the most prominent as well as commonest clinical feature, especially in younger patients. The association of choroid plexus papillomas and communicating hydrocephalus has been variously ascribed to an overproduction of cerebrospinal fluid by the tumour (1, 26, 35), obstruction of the subarachnoid pathways secondary to intraventricular bleeding from the tumour (21), or both (20, 26, 31). Choroid plexus papillomas may also cause hydrocephalus of the destructive type as a result of blocking a portion of a lateral ventricle, the third, or the fourth ventricle by the tumour (38). The presenting symptoms in these cases are headaches, vomiting, an enlarging head and decreasing activity (3, 20, 25, 38). Other symptoms and signs arise as a result of involvement of adjacent structures by the tumour and include: dizziness, cerebellar signs, ataxic gait, nystagmus, tinnitus, diplopia and decreased vision (3, 20, 38). These symptoms mainly occur in the third and fourth ventricle examples of choroid plexus papillomas. On ophthalmological examination papilloedema is often present. The cerebrospinal fluid is usually under pressure and frequently is xanthochromic

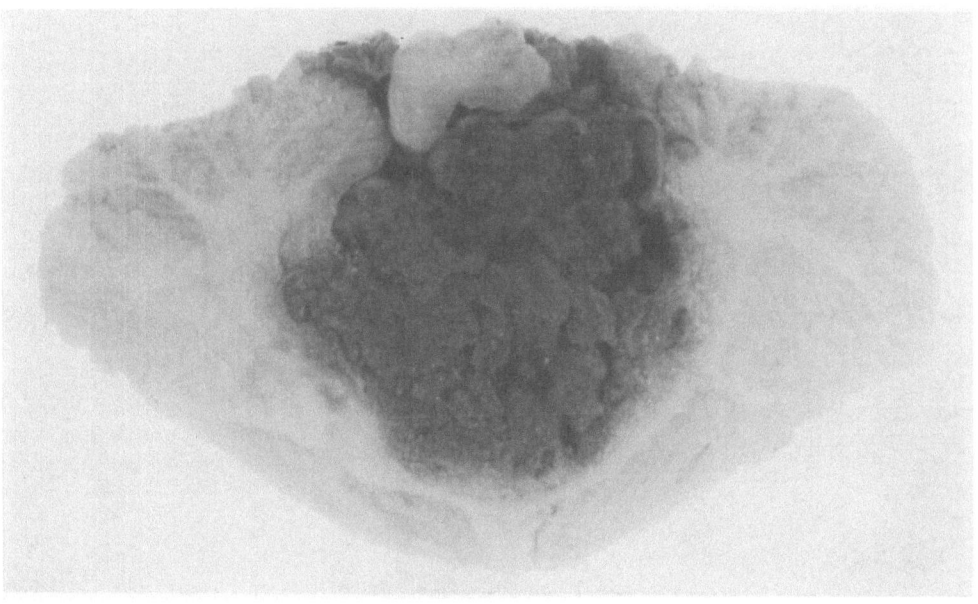

Fig. 2. Macroscopic appearance of a choroid plexus papilloma of the fourth ventricle

with a markedly elevated protein content. Attention must be paid to the fact that a disastrous reaction to lumbar puncture can occur with a rapidly progressive hydrocephalus and often progressive coma, a condition which may be irreversible (20).

Choroid plexus papillomas may vary in size from 1 cm to very large tumours of 7 cm or larger, completely filling an undilated or dilated lateral ventricle. Grossly they have a typical appearance. They usually arise from the glomus of the choroid plexus. The surface may be roughly globular, coarsely nodular, finely granular or even smooth. The colour is usually pinkish-purple, gray or red. The tumour is friable, very vascular and may contain a thin capsule. Calcifications are sometimes present (3, 20, 25, 31, 38).

Microscopically the histological picture closely resembles that of the normal choroid plexus with papillary formations composed of vascular stroma covered by a single layer of columnar or cuboidal epithelium. Electronmicroscopically cilia can be seen on the epithelial cells of papilloma (5, 28), but these are not seen by light microscopy. This and the absence of blepharoplasts distinguish them from papillary ependymoma (20, 28, 31). The differential diagnosis between these two tumours can sometimes be difficult, both originating from ependymal cells and

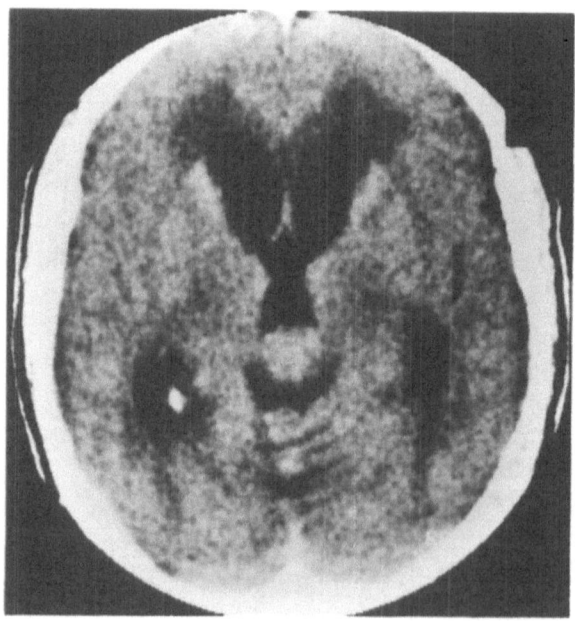

Fig. 3. Microscopic appearance of a choroid plexus papilloma
HE, 75x

therefore classified among the ependymal tumours in the classification of the
World Health Organization (40). The ultrastructural picture of choroid plexus
papillomas shows typical cytoplasmic inclusions similar to Biondi's bodies in
the normal choroid plexus (28).

Leptomeningeal dissemination of the choroid plexus papilloma along the cerebrospinal fluid pathways can occur (10, 39).

Malignant choroid plexus papilloma or choroid plexus carcinoma is an extremely
rare neoplasm. Only 22 well documented examples could be found in the literature
up to 1975 (8). This neoplasm most frequently arises in the lateral ventricles
and predominantly affects young children (13, 23, 36). In adults most of these
tumours are located in the fourth ventricle (8). It is not certain whether the
choroid plexus carcinoma originate primarily as a carcinoma or that there is
secondary malignant change of choroid plexus papillomas (13). The microscopic
structure shows evidence of infiltration and destruction of brain tissue with
necrosis. The tumour cells are pleomorphic and mitoses are common (6, 13, 20, 31).
Very few examples of extracranial metastasis of malignant choroid plexus
papilloma have been reported (36, 37).

FAMILIAL ASPECTS OF CHOROID PLEXUS PAPILLOMA

Reports on familial aggregation of choroid plexus papilloma have been infrequent. Literature on familial occurrence in twins, mono- or dizygotic, is
not available. The occurrence of a plexus papilloma in one member of a pair of
twins has been reported by Koch (IV.A.3.1). He describes a male twin having a
plexus papilloma of the fourth ventricle, histologically verified, at the age
of 32 years, while his twin brother was alive and well at the age of 35 years.
It is uncertain whether these twins were mono- or dizygotic.

In siblings two familial occurrences of choroid plexus papilloma have been
reported (IV.B.1.1. and IV.B.1.2). De la Torre et al. (IV.B.1.1) described three
siblings, one (a 9 month old female) having a choroid plexus papilloma of the
right lateral ventricle. She died at operation of cardiac arrest. Autopsy in
this case also *disclosed a neuroblastoma in the left paravertebral region and
another in the left adrenal gland; a pheochromocytoma was found in the right
adrenal gland*. Her brother underwent operation of a histologically diagnosed
ependymoma of the left lateral ventricle at approximately the same age (5 months
old); he also died of cardiac arrest during operation. As noted in the section
on general aspects, the differential diagnosis between choroid plexus papillomas
and ependymomas can be difficult. They are closely related, and classified under
the same subdivision of brain tumours by most authors and also according to the
classification of the World Health Organization (40). These cases may be considered
an example of concordant occurrence of ependymal tumours and have as a choice been
registered here among the choroid plexus papillomas. The choroid plexus papilloma
in the first sibling was associated with multiple neuroblastomas and a pheochromocytoma, both tumours being derived from the neural crest (neurocristopathies),
and having a heritable component (27, 32). A third sibling died of *an undifferentiated tumour, compatible with the histologic diagnosis of neuroblastoma* in the
pterygomaxillary fossa region. Unfortunately autopsy was not permitted for either
of the male siblings.

The second familial occurrence in siblings was reported by Komminoth et al. who
describe a two-year-old boy and his four-year-old sister, both operated upon
because of a choroid plexus papilloma (IV.B.1.2). The boy was in good health
seven months after operation, but his sister died a few months postoperatively.
of an obscure infectious process of which no precise diagnosis could be made.

Discordant neoplasm occurrence with papilloma involvement in siblings has been reported in two families. Faber reported a carcinomatous choroid plexus papilloma in a 29-year-old male, whose brother and sister also died of brain tumours at the ages of 5 and 15 years. Unfortunately no histological diagnosis of these tumours was made. A cousin of these siblings was operated upon because of a glioma of the eye and the mother died of a lung carcinoma with brain metastases at the age of 32 years (IV.B.2.1).

Peyser and Beller reported two brothers (20 months and 14 years of age) demonstrating respectively a choroid plexus papilloma and a glioblastoma multiforme (IV.B.2.2).

Familial aggregation of choroid plexus papilloma in other generations has not been reported.

Association of choroid plexus papilloma with other hereditary disease entities has been described in very rare cases. Lauritsen (22) investigated 68 relatives of a patient with Lindau's disease and found one member of the family with a papilloma of the choroid plexus of the fourth cerebral ventricle, *a finding not previously described in association with Lindau's disease*. Hamanaka et al. (14) reported a ten-month-old boy with a histologically verified papilloma of the choroid plexus who also suffered from Sturge-Weber disease, a syndrome with a heterogeneous inheritance (16, 18).

Congenital examples of choroid plexus papilloma have been reported, located especially in the lateral ventricles (4, 9, 24, 28a, 30).

As observations have been minimal it is clearly difficult to conclude familial or hereditary factor involvement in the etiology of these neoplasms. Only two concrete reports have been made of concordant tumour occurrence in siblings, and reports of the tumour occurrence in twins or more generations of a family have been lacking. Congenital occurrence and the association with other hereditary disease entities on the other hand, may imply involvement of chromosomal factors. These cases, however, are not numerous and chromosomal patterns of papillomas have not as yet been studied.

A possible etiological factor involved in the occurrence of this neoplasm has been suggested by Bastian (2). On electronmicroscopic examination of choroid plexus papilloma cells he discovered the presence of electron-dense particles within the tumour cells having the morphological characteristics of the papova group of viruses. These were not found in five normal choroid plexuses. A causal relationship between the viral group and this neoplasm may therefore exist, but has not as yet been confirmed by other authors.

166

REFERENCES

1. BARGE M, BENABID AL, ROUGEMONT J de, CHIROSSEL JP 1976
   L'hyper-production de LCR dans les papillomes du plexus choroide de
   l'enfant.
   Neurochirurgie 639-644
2. BASTIAN FO 1971
   Papova-like virus particles in a human brain tumor.
   Lab Invest 25:169-175
3. BOHM E, STRANG R 1961
   Choroid plexus papillomas.
   J Neurosurg 18:493-500
4. BRAUNSTEIN H, MARIN Jr F 1952
   Congenital papilloma of choroid plexus. Report of a case, with
   observations on pathogenesis of associated hydrocephalus.
   Arch Neurol Psychiatr (Chic) 68:475-480
5. CARTER LP, REGGS J, WAGGENER JD 1972
   Ultrastructure of three choroid plexus papillomas.
   Cancer 30:1130-1136
6. CASENTINI L, RIGOBELLO L, GEROSA M, PARDATSCHER K, ANDRIOLI GC 1979
   Choroid plexus carcinoma. Case report.
   Zentralbl Neurochir 40:239-244
7. CUSHING H 1932
   Intracranial tumours.
   Charles C Thomas, Springfield, Ill
8. DOHRMANN GJ, COLLIAS JC 1975
   Choroid plexus carcinoma. Case report.
   J Neurosurg 43:225-232
9. DRUCKER GA 1939
   Papillary tumor of the choroid plexus in a newborn infant.
   Arch Pathol 28:390-395
10. ERDOHAZI M 1969
    A clinical and pathological study of 43 cases of hydrocephalus not
    associated with spina bifida.
    Dev Med Child Neurol (Suppl) 20:31-37
11. FABER V 1934
    Fall von carcinomatös entartem Papillom des Seitenventrikels.
    Frankfurt Z Pathol 47:168-172
12. GUÉRARD G 1932
    Tumeur fungeuse dans le ventricule droit du cerveau chez une petite
    fille de trois ans.
    Bull Soc Anat (Paris) 8:211-214
13. GULLOTTA F, MELO AS de 1979
    Das Karzinom des Plexus choriodeus. Klinische, lichtmikroskopische
    und elektronenoptische Untersuchungen.
    Neurochirurgia 22:1-9

14. HAMANAKA Y, MORI S, KANOH M, UOZUMI T, MATSUOKA K, INOUE E, YOKOI H,
    YOSHITATSU S 1970
    A case of bilateral Sturge-Weber's disease with a plexuspapilloma at
    the left lateral ventricle.
    Brain Nerve (Tokyo) 22:99-103
15. HAWKINS III JC 1980
    Treatment of choroid plexus papillomas in children: a brief analysis
    of twenty years' experience.
    Neurosurgery 6:380-384
16. KOCH G 1940
    Beitrag zur Erblichleit der Sturge-Weberschen Krankheit.
    Z Ges Neurol Psychiatr 168:614-631
17. KOCH G 1954
    Beitrag zur Erblichkeit der Hirngeschwülste (Vorläufige Mitteilung).
    Acta Genet Med Gemellol 3:170-191
18. KOCH G 1972
    Genetic aspects of the phakomatoses.
    In: Vinken PJ, Bruyn GW (eds) Handbook of Clinical Neurology.
    North-Holland Publ Co, Amsterdam vol 14:488-562
19. KOMMINOTH R, WORINGER E, BAUMGARTER J, BRAUN JP, LE MAISTRE D 1965
    Papillome intraventriculaire familial. Caractéristiques
    angiographiques.
    Neurochirurgie 11:267-272
20. LAURENCE KM 1974
    The biology of choroid plexus papilloma and carcinoma of the lateral
    ventricle.
    In: Vinken PJ, Bruyn GW (eds) Handbook of Clinical Neurology.
    North-Holland Publ Co, Amsterdam vol 17:555-595
21. LAURENCE KM, HOARE RD, TILL K 1961
    The diagnosis of the choroid plexus papilloma of the lateral
    ventricle.
    Brain 84:628-641
22. LAURITSEN JG 1973
    Lindau's disease. A study of one family through six generations.
    Acta Chir Scand 139:482-486
23. LEWIS P 1967
    Carcinoma of the choroid plexus.
    Brain 90:177-186
24. MATSON DD 1953
    Hydrocephalus in a premature infant caused by papilloma of the
    choroid plexus. With report of surgical treatment.
    J Neurosurg 10:416-420
25. MATSON DD, CROFTON FDL 1960
    Papilloma of the choroid plexus in childhood.
    J Neurosurg 17:1002-1027
26. MILHORAT TH, HAMMOCK MK, DAVIS DA, FENSTERMACHER JD 1976
    Choroid plexus papilloma. I. Proof of cerebrospinal fluid overpro-
    duction.
    Childs Brain 2:273-289
27. MYRIANTHOPOULOS NC 1981
    Neuroblastoma.
    In: Vinken PJ, Bruyn GW (eds) Handbook of Clinical Neurology.
    North-Holland Publ Co, Amsterdam vol 42:758-759

28. NAVAS JJ, BATTIFORA H 1978
    Choroid plexus papilloma: light and electron microscopic study of
    three cases.
    Acta Neuropathol (Berl) 44:235-239
28a. OHTA T, KAJIKAWA H, TAKEUCHI J 1977
    Congenital tumours of the brain.
    In: Vinken PJ, Bruyn GW (eds) Handbook of Clinical Neurology.
    North-Holland Publ Co, Amsterdam vol 31:35-74
29. PEYSER E, BELLER AJ 1951
    Brain tumors in two brothers.
    Acta Med Orient (Tel-Aviv) 10:229-232
30. RASKIND R, BEIGEL F 1964
    Brain tumors in early infancy - probably congenital in origin.
    J Pediatr 65:727-732
31. RUBINSTEIN LJ 1972
    Tumors of the choroid plexus and related structures.
    In: Atlas of Tumor Pathology, 2nd series, Fasc 6.
    Armed Forces Inst of Pathol, Washington DC p 257-267
32. SCHIMKE RN 1981
    Pheochromocytoma.
    In: Vinken PJ, Bruyn GW (eds) Handbook of Clinical Neurology.
    North-Holland Publ Co, Amsterdam vol 42:764-766
33. STANLEY P 1968
    Papillomas of the choroid plexus.
    Br J Radiol 4:848-857
34. TORRE E de la, ALEXANDER Jr E, DAVIS II Jr C, CRANDELL DL 1963
    Tumors of the lateral ventricles of the brain. Report of eight
    cases, with suggestions for clinical management.
    J Neurosurg 20:461-470
35. TURCOTTE JF, COPTY M, BÉDARD F, MICHAUD J, VERRET S 1980
    Lateral ventricle choroid plexus papilloma and communicating hydro-
    cephalus.
    Surg Neurol 13:143-146
36. VALLADARES JB, PERRY RH, KALBAG RM 1980
    Malignant choroid plexus papilloma with extraneural metastasis. Case
    report.
    J Neurosurg 52:251-255
37. VRAA-JENSEN G 1950
    Papilloma of the choroid plexus with pulmonary metastases.
    Acta Psychiatr Scand 25:299-306
38. WILKINS H, RUTLEDGE BJ 1961
    Papillomas of the choroid plexus.
    J Neurosurg 18:14-18
39. ZÜLCH KJ 1956
    Biologie und Pathologie der Hirngeschwülste.
    In: Olivecrona H, Tönnis W (eds) Handbuch der Neurochirurgie.
    Springer, Berlin Bd III:335-346
40. ZÜLCH KJ 1981
    Principles of the new World Health Organization (WHO) classification
    of brain tumors.
    Neuroradiology 19:59-66

Chapter V

FAMILIAL CEREBRAL FIBROSARCOMA

CASE REPORTS

CLASSIFICATION

A. *TWINS*

    1. Monozygotic twins with concordant tumour

    2. Monozygotic twins with discordant tumour

    3. Monozygotic twins, one demonstrating cerebral fibrosarcoma

    4. Dizygotic twins

B. *SIBLINGS*

    1. Siblings with concordant tumour

    2. Siblings with discordant tumour

C. *OTHER GENERATIONS AND DISTANT RELATIVES*

    1. Other generations and distant relatives with concordant tumour

    2. Other generations and distant relatives with discordant tumour

TABLES

172

V.A.   *TWINS*

Case reports of cerebral fibrosarcoma occurrence in twins are not available
in the literature.

V.B.   *SIBLINGS*

V.B.1.   SIBLINGS WITH CONCORDANT TUMOUR

V.B.1.1. <u>Gainer et al. 1975 - Morgantown, U.S.A.</u> (8)

Two sisters. American.

Case 1

<u>History</u>: At the age of 64 years this woman was admitted to hospital. She complained of progressive deterioration of vision and diplopia since twelve months.
On examination *she was mildly confused and disoriented. Bilateral optic atrophy and a left third nerve palsy were present. She had no useful vision in the right eye. The EEG showed evidence of a left frontotemporal destructive lesion. Brain scan and arteriography showed a left frontotemporal mass extending to the midline.*
At operation *a firm rubbery tumor* was found *involving the inferior frontal and medial temporal lobes, about 5 cm in diameter. A subtotal resection was carried out.*
Postoperatively *the patient developed uncontrollable ... edema and died on the fourth postoperative day.*

<u>Autopsy</u>: *no neoplastic process was found in the body organs. Severe cerebral edema ... was found. The residual tumor did not infiltrate the brain.*

<u>Microscopic study</u>: The tumour consisted of *spindle-shaped cells with uniform oval dark-staining nuclei and frequent mitoses. Rich networks of reticulin and collagen fibers were present. The tumor had spread throughout the subarachnoid space, and did not infiltrate the brain.*

<u>Diagnosis</u>: Left frontotemporal fibrosarcoma.

Case 2

<u>History</u>: This woman was seen in the hospital at the age of 69 years with a *history of mild confusion and progressive left hemiparesis for eight weeks. She complained of moderate headache.*
On examination *she had a left hemiparesis, left homonymous hemianopsia, and was moderately confused. The EEG showed right hemispheric slow waves. Brain scan and arteriography showed a right frontotemporal tumor.*
At operation *a firm granular tumor in the right temporal area was found. The tumor was well demarcated except for the inferomedial aspect, where it was*

attached to the leptomeninges. It was approximately 7 cm in diameter. A wide resection was carried out.

Postoperatively the patient did well and she was discharged for home care. She died at home several months later.

Microscopic study: *the tumour showed large spindle-shaped cells with elongated oval nuclei. Abnormal mitoses, multinucleated giant cells, and areas of focal necrosis were present. There was a dense proliferation of collagen fibers that formed thick bundles streaming along tumor cells. The molecular layer of adjacent brain showed marginal gliosis, but no tumor invasion. The tumor was confined to the subarachnoid space.*

Autopsy: Was not obtained.

Diagnosis: Right temporal fibrosarcoma (or meningeal sarcoma or malignant meningioma).

Family: Data concerning other members of the family are not given in the article.

V.B.1.   SIBLINGS WITH DISCORDANT TUMOUR

Siblings with discordant tumour have not as yet been reported in the literature.

V.C.   *OTHER GENERATIONS AND DISTANT RELATIVES*

V.C.1.   OTHER GENERATIONS AND DISTANT RELATIVES WITH CONCORDANT TUMOUR

V.C.1.1. Gainer et al. 1975 - Morgantown, U.S.A. (8)

A father and a daughter. American.

Case 1 (father)
   History: This man was admitted to hospital at the age of 73 years. He complained of progressive frontal and occipital headaches since eight months. *He had experienced three episodes of loss of consciousness, and had recently become lethargic and confused.*
On examination, he was lethargic and mildly confused; no other deficits were found. The electroencephalogram showed right hemispheric abnormalities consistent with a destructive lesion. Arteriography and ventriculography showed a right occipitoparietal mass.
At operation a firm rubbery tumor was present in the right occipital lobe with reactive edema around it. A subtotal resection was done.
Postoperatively he remained comatose and died four days later.
   Autopsy: Was not obtained.
   Microscopic study: *the tumor showed spindle-shaped, elongated tumor cells with dark-staining nuclei. Moderate pleomorphism and frequent mitoses were present, as were rare giant cells. Scattered areas of necrosis within the tumor and a margin of reactive astrocytosis around the tumor were seen. The tumor had infiltrated into the pia-arachnoid.*
   Diagnosis: Right occipital fibrosarcoma.

Case 2 (daughter)
   History: This woman was admitted to hospital at the age of 59 years. She complained of progressive weakness of the right arm and leg since four months. On examination *a mild right spastic hemiparesis* was found without other abnormalities. *An EEG showed focal left fronto-temporal slow waves. A brain scan and arteriography showed evidence of two left frontotemporal masses. She was treated with radiation therapy and improved for four months. She then showed signs of progressive left hemisphere involvement and died in a nursing home four months later.*
   Autopsy: showed one area of tumour in the left inferior frontal gyrus and another area of tumour in the left precentral and postcentral gyri. There was

no connection between those two areas. *The general autopsy disclosed no malignant processes in other body organs.*

Microscopic study: Both tumour foci were identical and showed *spindle-shaped cells with elongated dark-staining nuclei exhibiting marked pleomorphism. Many giant cells were present. The tumor had infiltrated through the subarachnoid space and in one area had grown through the pia-arachnoid. Appropriate stains demonstrated dense proliferation of reticulin and collagen fibrils. The white matter between the tumors showed interstitial edema and reactive astrocytosis.*

Diagnosis: Two fibrosarcomas, one left frontal and another left fronto-parietal. The possibility of gliosarcomas was not excluded.

Family: Data concerning other members of the family are not given in the article.

COMMENT

The authors state correctly that no cases of familial occurrence of primary sarcomas of the central nervous system have previously been reported. On the other hand familial occurrence of sarcoma elsewhere in the body has been reported in literature.

V.C.2.   OTHER GENERATIONS AND DISTANT RELATIVES WITH DISCORDANT TUMOUR

V.C.2.1. Distelmaier 1977 - Bonn, Germany (6)

Grandfather, child, grandchild. German.

Reference is made to the occurrence of a cerebral fibrosarcoma in a patient
whose father and whose child had previously died as a result of brain tumours.

COMMENT

No other information is given in this report regarding the cases mentioned.
The reference has been included here as representing an occurrence of brain
tumour in 3 generations. As only one tumour was identified (as a fibrosarcoma),
the case has been placed in the category of discordant tumours.

TABLES

TABLE 1 - SIBLINGS WITH CONCORDANT TUMOUR (V.B.1)

	case	gender	relationship	number of unaffected siblings	race or nationality	age at symptom occurrence	age at death	location of the tumour
V.B.1.1. Gainer 1975	1	f	s	?	Amer.	63 y	64 y	L frontotemporal
	2	f	s	?	Amer.	69 y	69 y	R temporal

TABLE 2 - OTHER GENERATIONS AND DISTANT RELATIVES WITH CONCORDANT TUMOUR (V.C.1)

	case	gender	relationship	number of unaffected siblings	race or nationality	age at symptom occurrence	age at death	location of the tumour
V.C.1.1. Gainer 1975	1	m	f	?	Amer.	72 y	73 y	R occipital
	2	f	d	?	Amer.	59 y	60 y	One L frontal and another L fronto-parietal

TABLE 3 - OTHER GENERATIONS AND DISTANT RELATIVES WITH DISCORDANT TUMOUR (V.C.2)

	case	gender	relationship	number of unaffected siblings	race or nationality	age at symptom occurrence	age at death	location of the tumour
V.C.2.1. Distelmaier 1977	1	m	gf	?	Germ.	?	?	?
	2	?	ch	?	Germ.	?	?	?
	3	?	gch	?	Germ.	?	?	?

diagnosis	biopsy	autopsy	associated physical or mental conditions	family	comment
Fibrosarcoma	+	+	-	?	-
Fibrosarcoma	+	-	-		

diagnosis	biopsy	autopsy	associated physical or mental conditions	family	comment
Fibrosarcoma	+	-	-	?	Case 2: possibility of gliosarcomas not excluded
Fibrosarcomas	-	+	-		

diagnosis	biopsy	autopsy	associated physical or mental conditions	family	comment
?	?	?	?	?	?
Fibrosarcoma	?	?	?		
?	?	?	?		

GENERAL ASPECTS OF CEREBRAL FIBROSARCOMA

Sarcomas are malignant connective tissue tumours which are classified according to their differentiation, i.e. fibrosarcoma, osteogenic sarcoma, myosarcoma, et cetera (1, 2, 16). Fibrosarcomas occur at any age, with peaks in early infancy and late adulthood (2, 4). In children a slight male predominance is reported (4, 17). Fibrosarcomas grow infiltratively into the surrounding tissues, and recurrence after local surgical excision is common (2, 4). The degree of fibrosarcoma differentiation is relevant for their growth pattern and clinical behaviour (17). Relatively well differentiated tumours may show extensive collagen production, and are firm and fibrous. Poorly differentiated fibrosarcomas are usually soft and friable and may contain large areas of necrosis. While infrequent in the low-grade fibrosarcomas, metastasis, especially pulmonary, may be frequent in high-grade tumours. In children the low-grade, highly differentiated fibrosarcomas predominate, associated with a generally higher survival rate (4, 17, 18).

Sarcoma occurrence in the central nervous system is rare (1, 14, 15, 16), the work of Bailey in 1929 being one of the first publications contributing to the present knowledge of this subject (3). Subsequent investigative attempts and literature studies have attempted to deal with the problems of brain sarcoma description (1, 14, 16), and attention has been given to the problems of classification, such as their distinction from meningeal neoplasms or from variants of tumours of glial origin (16).

Macroscopically, brain sarcomas do not differ from sarcomas found elsewhere in the body. Those situated in the meninges are described as somewhat firmer than sarcomas situated more deeply within the brain itself (16). There is no site of predeliction within the central nervous system (1, 14, 16). The occurrence of multiple primary brain sarcomas has been reported (5, 10), and sarcomas have been found to occur in association with other tumour types (13, 14, 19). Fibrosarcomas occurring in the brain are generally primary in origin, although reports of metastatic occurrence have been made (9, 12, 20).

Estimates of sarcoma incidence have been cited ranging from 0.5% to 3% of all primary intracranial tumours (11, 13, 14). (One exceptionally high incidence of 7% cited by Distelmaier (6) is probably inflated by the inclusion of lympho-reticular malignancies and other neoplasm types within his category of primary brain sarcomas.) Rubinstein, after correction for the inclusion of controversial

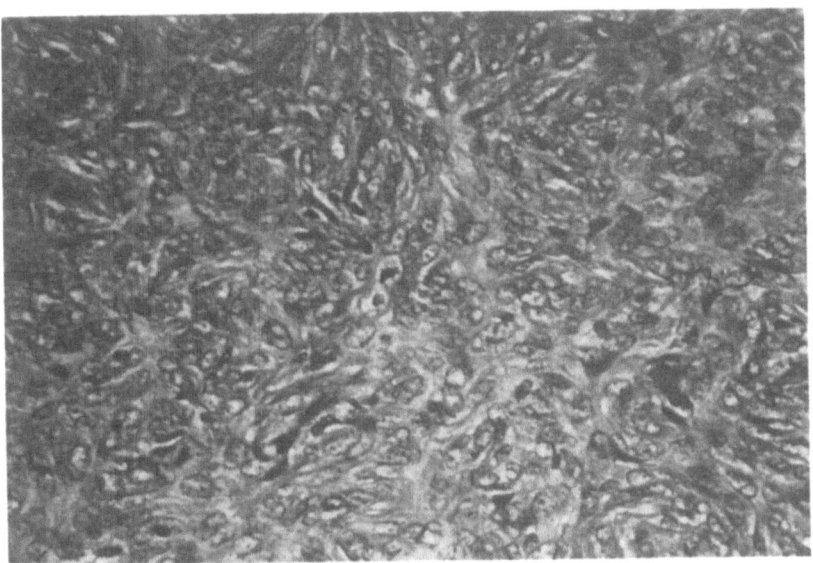

Fig. 1. Microscopic appearance of a cerebral fibrosarcoma
HE, 250x

tumour types cites an incidence of 1.2% (16). The percentage of fibrosarcoma of
all primary brain sarcomas varies from 12% in some series (6) to 25% in reviews
of the literature (1), with percentages as high as 66% in reports of small series
(14). The reported cases of cerebral fibrosarcoma were found occurring predominantly in adult life, the total age range of the patients being 17 months to 69
years (1, 6, 14). While a difference in sex incidence in the occurrence of brain
sarcomas in general has not been established (14, 16), at least one report of
male predominance in the occurrence of fibrosarcoma of the brain has been made
(6).

Cerebral fibrosarcomas do not demonstrate a distinctive clinical picture (16),
the symptomatology depending on the location and rate of growth of the neoplasm
(1, 14), the degree of malignancy being determined by the characteristics of the
neoplasm, some of the more differentiated fibrosarcomas possibly demonstrating
little aggressive growth (16).

Previous radiation therapy has been implicated in the etiology of cerebral
sarcomas, the latency period being approximately 5 to 10 years (15, 16) within
a range of 2 to 20 years (16).

FAMILIAL ASPECTS OF CEREBRAL FIBROSARCOMA

Insufficient reports of the familial occurrence of cerebral fibrosarcomas
have been made to warrant definite conclusions as to the role of hereditary
factors in the etiology of these neoplasms.

Gainer et al. (8) report the familial occurrence of fibrosarcomas in two
families, describing a 73-year-old man who was operated upon for a fibrosarcoma
of the right occipital lobe, and his 59-year-old daughter who died of two
separate cerebral fibrosarcomas, one of the left inferior frontal gyrus, the
other in the left precentral and postcentral gyri. In the case of the daughter
the problem of tumour differentiation again appears, as while the diagnosis of
multiple fibrosarcomas is made, the possibility of 'gliosarcomas' is not
excluded (V.C.1.1). In their second family two sisters are reported demonstrating
cerebral fibrosarcomas. The youngest, 64 years of age, was operated upon for a
fibrosarcoma *involving the inferior frontal and medial temporal lobes*. Her sister
at 69 years demonstrated a tumour of the right temporal area. The diagnosis of
fibrosarcoma was made with, in parentheses, the qualification *meningeal sarcoma,
malignant meningioma* (V.B.1.1). The authors speculate on the possibility of
malignant degeneration of previously benign meningiomas as a possible etiological
factor in the occurrence of these 4 cases. They also report the remarkable similarity in tumour cells of the neoplasms occurring in the two sisters, noting that
histological similarity in familially occurring tumours has been encountered
previously.

Distelmaier (6) refers to the occurrence of a cerebral fibrosarcoma in a
patient whose father and whose child had previously died as the result of brain
tumours. Unfortunately no other information regarding this report is cited, so
that the character of the neoplasms in the first and third generations remain
unspecified. As a question of choice this report has been categorized within the
section on discordant tumours (V.C.2.1).

Although no other reports of the familial occurrence of cerebral fibrosarcomas
are presently available, the familial occurrence of fibrosarcomas outside of the
central nervous system has been reported. Epstein et al. (7) report osteogenic
sarcomas occurring in direct familial lineage, and summarize a number of reports
of familial sarcoma occurrence. They speculate on the etiological influence of
hereditary susceptibility to possible carcinogens. As studies reviewing infantile

fibrosarcomas report incidences of 32% (17) to 37% (4) of the cases occurring at birth, congenital influences may also be considered in the discussion of such etiological factors.

REFERENCES

1. ABBOTT KH, KERNOHAN JW 1943
   Primary sarcomas of the brain. Review of the literature and report of twelve cases.
   Arch Neurol Psychiatr 50:43-66
2. ANDERSON WAD, SCOTTI TM 1968
   Synopsis of Pathology 7th ed.
   The CV Mosby Co, St Louis
3. BAILEY P 1929
   Intracranial sarcomatous tumors of leptomeningeal origin.
   Arch Surg 18:1359-1402
4. CHUNG EB, ENZINGER FM 1976
   Infantile fibrosarcoma.
   Cancer 38:729-739
5. COTTRELL L 1939
   Primary fibrosarcoma of the brain.
   Arch Pathol 27:895-901
6. DISTELMAIER P 1977
   Klinik, Differentialdiagnose und radiologisches Bild der primären Hirnsarkome.
   Nervenarzt 48:405-418
7. EPSTEIN LI, BIXLER D, BENNET JE 1970
   An incident of familial cancer. Including 3 cases of osteogenic sarcoma.
   Cancer 25:889-891
8. GAINER Jr JV, CHOU SM, CHADDUCK WM 1975
   Familial cerebral sarcomas.
   Arch Neurol 32:665-668
9. HO KL 1979
   Sarcoma metastatic to the central nervous system. Report of three cases and review of the literature.
   Neurosurgery 5:44-48
10. HOULTON TL 1926
    Report of a case of multiple sarcoma of the brain.
    Nebr Med J 11:169-174
11. KERNOHAN JW, UIHLEIN A 1962
    Sarcomas of the brain.
    Charles C Thomas, Springfield, Ill
12. MATA GONZALEZ PR, ESTADES VENTURA A, VAZQUEZ HERRERO C, RUIZ-OCANA C 1978
    Dermatofibrosarcoma con metástasis en el cerebro. A propósito de un caso poco frecuente.
    Rev Clin Esp 149:307-308
13. MENA H, GARCIA JH 1978
    Primary brain sarcomas. Light and electron microscopic features.
    Cancer 42:1298-1307

14. NICHOLS Jr P, WAGNER JA   1952
    Primary intracranial sarcoma. Report of nine cases with suggested
    classification.
    J Neuropathol Exp Neurol 11:215-234
15. NOETZLI M, MALAMUD N   1962
    Postirradiation fibrosarcoma of the brain.
    Cancer 15:617-622
16. RUBINSTEIN LJ   1972
    Tumours of the central nervous system.
    In: Atlas of Tumor Pathology. 2nd series, Fasc 6.
    Armed Forces Inst of Pathol, Washington DC p 190-204
17. SOULE EH, PRITCHARD DJ   1977
    Fibrosarcoma in infants and children. A review of 110 cases.
    Cancer 40:1711-1721
18. STOUT AP   1962
    Fibrosarcoma in infants and children.
    Cancer 15:1028-1040
19. WHITCOMB BB, TENNANT R   1966
    Brain tumors of diverse germinal origin arising in juxtaposition.
    Report of three cases.
    J Neurosurg 25:194-198
20. ZUCKER DK, KATZ R, KOTO A, HOROUPIAN DS   1978
    Sarcomas metastatic to the brain. Case report of a metastatic fibro-
    sarcoma, and review of literature.
    Surg Neurol 9:177-180

Chapter VI

FAMILIAL PINEALOMA

CASE REPORTS

CLASSIFICATION

A. *TWINS*

    1. Monozygotic twins with concordant tumour

    2. Monozygotic twins with discordant tumour

    3. Monozygotic twins, one demonstrating pinealoma

    4. Dizygotic twins

B. *SIBLINGS*

    1. Siblings with concordant tumour

    2. Siblings with discordant tumour

C. *OTHER GENERATIONS AND DISTANT RELATIVES*

    1. Other generations and distant relatives with concordant tumour

    2. Other generations and distant relatives with discordant tumour

TABLES

VI.A.   *TWINS*

VI.A.1.   MONOZYGOTIC TWINS WITH CONCORDANT TUMOUR

VI.A.1.1. <u>Waldbaur et al. 1976 - Erlangen, Germany</u> (25)

Monozygotic twins. Female. German.

Two monozygotic twin sisters are described, 5 and 16 months of age, having
respectively a medulloblastoma of the cerebellum and a pineoblastoma. These
tumours are considered to be concordant by the authors of the article.
This article has been reported and is described further in the chapter on
familial medulloblastoma (II.A.1.2).

VI.A.2.   MONOZYGOTIC TWINS WITH DISCORDANT TUMOUR

The twins described in case VI.A.1.1. (and II.A.1.2) might possibly have
been considered as having discordant tumours, depending on ones interpretation
of the differences in diagnosis between pineoblastoma and medulloblastoma.
The choice has been made here to register this case under the condordant
tumours.

VI.A.3. MONOZYGOTIC TWINS, ONE DEMONSTRATING PINEALOMA

Reports of pinealoma occurrence in one member of monozygotic twins have not been available in the literature.

VI.A.4. DIZYGOTIC TWINS

Reports of pinealoma occurrence in dizygotic twins have not been available in the literature.

VI.B.   *SIBLINGS*

VI.B.1.   SIBLINGS WITH CONCORDANT TUMOUR

VI.B.1.1. Mendenhall 1950 - Fort Wayne, U.S.A. (9)

Two sisters and a brother. American.

Case 1 (proband)

History: The medical history of this girl included an early dentition beginning with the appearance of the first tooth at the age of two months. At 6 months of age a sarcoma of the left ovary was removed. At 3 years she demonstrated polydipsia and polyuria, and sugar was found in the urine. These symptoms disappeared with regular diet. At 5 years she had measles and whooping cough, and at 6 years a tonsillectomy, without complications. At the age of 8 years she demonstrated small abscesses near the rectum and on her legs. *For some time she had been complaining of headache and drowsiness.* As her blood sugar was high she was admitted to hospital for examination (1934). Diet and insulin could not influence her hyperglycaemia, and she was discharged after approximately 5 1/2 weeks. A definite diagnosis had not been established by examination. Ten weeks later she was readmitted to hospital for 3 days. Approximately 7 months later she died of an acute pneumonia.

Autopsy: revealed a bronchial pneumonia, early involution of the thymus, atypical Graafian follicle development, a pituitary cyst, congenital right kidney abnormality, fibrosis of the islands of Langerhans of the pancreas, and a tumour of the pineal gland.

Microscopic study (of the pineal): Pinealoma.

Diagnosis: Pinealoma.

Case 2

History: This male child was first examined at the age of 4 years as he *had the physical characteristics of his older sister.* No abnormalities were then found. At 7 years of age sugar was found in his urine. His blood sugar was found to remain high despite diet or insulin treatment.

In December 1939 the child was hospitalized because of bronchitis. He died shortly thereafter.

Autopsy: revealed a haemangioma of the brain, vascular hyperaemia of the pituitary, hypertrophy with signs of fibrotic changes in the pancreas islands of Langerhans, and a pinealoma measuring 2 x 2 x 1 cm.

Microscopic study (of the pineal): Pinealoma.

Diagnosis: Pinealoma.

Case 3

History: This girl was carefully observed from birth *because her appearance was identical with the other two abnormal children*. Dentition initiated at the age of three months. She had a *potbelly* and precocious hair development. At 2 1/2 to 3 years of age her skin began to wrinkle and become pigmented, her face began to look *older*, and her nails became abnormally hard. There was precocious development of the labia majora and minora, and of the clitoris. She had whooping cough and chicken-pox at the ages four to five. At 5 1/2 years *she entered school and was a very bright pupil* .... In September, 1946, sugar was found in the urine. *She began to complain of headaches about this time.* She was hospitalized for several days. Treatment was found to have little effect on her hyperglycaemia.

In October, 1947, *she developed pyelonephritis and died from septicemia.*

Autopsy: Severe fibrosis and hypertrophy of the pancreas, simple cyst of the pituitary, kidney abscesses, bilateral perinephric abscess, and hyperplasia of the pineal gland (3 x 2 x 1 cm).

Microscopic study (of the pineal): Pinealoma.

Diagnosis: Pinealoma.

Family: The parents of these children were white Americans. There were seven children. The first-born child was a normal female, who later gave birth to two normal daughters. The second-born child is described in case 1. The third child was a normal female, who later gave birth to a normal son. The fourth-born is described in case 2. The fifth child in this family died at the age of six months as the result of an intussusception. No other abnormality was found at autopsy, but brain examination did not take place. This child is said to have had *the same physical characteristics* as the children in the described cases, but as this child was the first of the children to die no special attention was aroused by this observation. *The sixth child was born an anencephalic and died a few days after birth.* The seventh child is described in case 3.

The author notes that the patients' *maternal grandmother had diabetes and died of pulmonary tuberculosis.* The mother and the normal daughters (first and third born children) demonstrated a *slightly increased amount of hair on their arms and legs.*

No other family members with pathology were known.

196

1 = case 1

2 = case 2

3 = case 3

4   died a few days
    after birth
    anencephalic

5   died at 6 m of
    intussusception

6   diabetes; died
    of tuberculosis

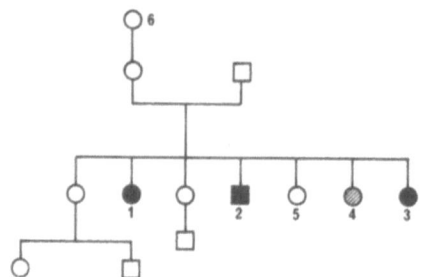

<u>COMMENT</u>

Three out of seven siblings are reported demonstrating abnormalities of the
pituitary, pancreas and pineal glands, with a clinical syndrome demonstrating
high insulin resistance. The exact age at death in the three cases is not
reported.

The gender of the fifth and sixth child in this family is not reported.

The syndrome which was not originally apparent by the first death in the
family (of the fifth-born child) may be summarized by: an old appearance of
the face, hirsutism, pigmented skin, protruding abdomen, hardened finger nails,
early dentition, enlarged external genitalia, therapy resistant hyperglycaemia,
and death by concomitant cause or disease.

VI.B.1.2. Kjellin et al. 1960 - Stockholm, Sweden (7)

Two half-brothers. Swedish.

Case 1

History: This 11-year-old male was admitted to hospital, having suffered from *headaches, diplopia, and vomiting for 2 weeks* ....

On examination *neck rigidity, bilateral papilledema, left abducens and right trochlear paralysis, positional nystagmus, impairment of gait, and slight clumsiness in both arms* were found.

Operation revealed *a dense, rather well-defined reddish-gray tumor* ..., *apparently originating from the pineal region.*

The patient died four months after the operation, approximately 4½ months after the onset of the disease.

Autopsy: Was not performed.

Microscopic study (of the biopsy): *showed a cellular tumor without any mitoses. The cells had a fairly large, dark, rounded or elongated nuclei surrounded by a sparse rim of cytoplasm, and were frequently arranged in small groups separated by septa* .... *Nowhere was the usual two-cell pattern of pinealoma encountered.*

Diagnosis: *Adult type* tumour of the pineal region.

Case 2

History: This 14-year-old male was admitted to hospital with a medical history of *tonic fits, vomiting, and headache for 1 year, and increasing impairment of vision for 2 months.*

On admission *he was stuporous, had bilateral papilledema, extensor plantar reflexes, and was clumsy in arms and legs. He was unable to elevate his eyes, there was impairment of conjugate depression, and the pupils were fixed to light.*

At operation an approximately walnut sized well-defined soft, vascularized, reddish-gray tumour was found *between the corpus callosum, cerebellum and both internal veins* ..., compressing the quadrigeminal plate.

The patient died 11 hours after the operation ....

Autopsy: revealed a large haematoma at the tumour site, extending into the fourth and part of the third ventricle.

Microscopic study: showed *a cellular tumor without mitoses. The cells had large, rounded, dark, rather monomorphic nuclei surrounded by sparse cytoplasm and were arranged in some places in groups separated by glia fibers* ....

198

Diagnosis: Tumour in the pineal region of *adult type*.

Family: These two half-brothers were members of a family of nine children. No other information concerning family members is given.

COMMENT

According to the authors the microscopic diagnosis in these cases was made upon the basis of the classification of Ringertz, Nordenstam and Flyger (12).

VI.B.1.3. <u>Wakai et al. 1980 - Tokyo/Chiba, Japan</u> (24)

Two brothers. Japanese.

<u>Case 1</u> (proband)

<u>History</u>: Born at full term after normal pregnancy. No developmental abnor-malities. At the age of 13 years this boy was admitted to hospital *with a 7-month history of polydipsia, polyuria, and loss of appetite.*
On admission he showed bitemporal hemianopsia, upward gaze palsy, horizontal nystagmus with lateral gaze, and ataxic gait. Pneumoventriculography showed only *moderately dilated lateral ventricles.* Angiograms were not indicative of pineal neoplasms.
He was treated for hydrocephalus by placement of a ventriculoperitoneal shunt, and improved gradually until a month after operation, his condition then dete-riorating. A second pneumoventriculogram performed approximately five months after operation *disclosed a small mass in the pineal region.*
He was treated with radiation therapy, but died after approximately nine weeks, nine months and one week after admission.
<u>Autopsy</u>: revealed a *tumor with a small cyst, 0.8 cm in diameter,* in the pineal region invading the wall of the third and lateral ventricles.
<u>Microscopic study</u>: ... *the tumor was composed of keratinized squamous epi-thelium, sebaceous glands, fat tissues, and columnar epithelium, with goblet and Paneth cells indicating intestinal structures .... In addition to these three germinal components, the tumor contained germinomatous elements, which infiltrated into the parenchyma of the surrounding brain ....*
<u>Diagnosis</u>: *Pineal teratoma with some germinomatous components.*

<u>Case 2</u>

<u>History</u>: Born at full term after normal pregnancy. *At 11 years of age, a plain skull film showed abnormal intracranial calcification.* At 17 years of age this boy was admitted to hospital *because of a progressive right-sided hemiparesis with a 2-year history of diplopia.*
On examination *upward gaze palsy and horizontal nystagmus with lateral gaze* were found. *There was a spastic hemiparesis and a hemihypesthesia with extensor plantar response on the right side. Computerized tomography (CT) revealed a large mass, with calcification in the pineal region, that encroached upon the posterior portion of the third ventricle. There was a low-density area in the left frontal horn .... angiograms showed a mass in the posterior third ventricle and a diffuse vascular shadow in the left posterior portion of the*

200

lateral ventricle .... Titer of alpha-fetoprotein and human chorionic gonado-
tropin in both serum and cerebrospinal fluid were within normal range.
Craniotomy revealed a mass in the *posterior part of the third ventricle and*
the pineal region consisting of white cheese-like material, hair, and finger-
tip sized bone .... The left half of the mass was quite vascular in nature,
infiltrating the left thalamus and posterior limb of the internal capsule. As
the histological diagnosis of this part during operation was found to be a
germinoma, radical resection was not attempted. A ventriculoperitoneal shunt
was placed 16 days later, and the patient received a course of radiation therapy.
He remains bedridden.

Microscopic study: *The tumor consisted of germinal elements, including skin*
with sebaceous glands, smooth muscle, bone, and intestine .... A germinoma-like
structure that had cells with relatively large nuclei intermingled with small
lymphoid cells was present in the specimen taken from the left half of the
tumor ....

Diagnosis: *Pineal teratoma with some germinomatous components.*

Family: The patients reported here were the eldest (case 1) and second-born
(case 2) of three siblings. Their younger sister was reported examined by
computer tomography, but no abnormality was found. Her age is not reported.
The parents of these children were healthy, without consanguinity.

COMMENT

The authors state that to their knowledge this is the first report of pineal
teratoma occurrence in siblings, and that lack of such reports, and the authors'
low calculation of their occurrence rate, *support the role of intrauterine*
factors in the pathogenesis of this tumor.

VI.C.   *OTHER GENERATIONS AND DISTANT RELATIVES*

VI.C.1.   OTHER GENERATIONS AND DISTANT RELATIVES WITH CONCORDANT TUMOUR

Reports of concordant pineal neoplasm occurrence in more than one generation or in distant relatives have not been available in the literature.

VI.C.2.   OTHER GENERATIONS AND DISTANT RELATIVES WITH DISCORDANT TUMOUR

Reports of discordant pineal neoplasm occurrence in more than one generation or in distant relatives have not been available in the literature.

TABLE 1 - SIBLINGS WITH CONCORDANT TUMOUR (VI.B.1)

	case	gender	relationship	number of unaffected siblings	race or nationality	age at symptom occurrence	age at death	location of the tumour
VI.B.1.1. Mendenhall 1950	1	f	s	4	white Amer.	2 m	estimated approx. 9 y	pineal gland
	2	m	br	4	white Amer.	7 y	estimated approx. 7 y	pineal gland
	3	f	s	4	white Amer.	3 m	estimated approx. 7 y	pineal gland
VI.B.1.2. Kjellin 1960	1	m	half br	7	Swed.	11 y	11 y	pineal region
	2	m	half br	7	Swed.	13 y	14 y	pineal region
VI.B.1.3. Wakai 1980	1	m	br	1	Japan.	13 y	approx. 13 y	pineal region
	2	m	br	1	Japan.	17 y	-	pineal region

diagnosis	biopsy	autopsy	associated physical or mental conditions	family	comment
Pinealoma	-	+	Pituitary, pancreas, kidney, thymus, ovary abnormalities; hyperglycaemia; pneumonia	Maternal grand-mother: diabetes, TBC. 2 normal sisters. 1 sib died of intussusception at 6 m; 1 sib died a few days after birth, anencephalic	Syndrome described involving physio-gnomy, hair, skin, abdomen, nails, dentition, and external genitalia
Pinealoma	-	+	Pituitary, pancreas abnormalities; brain haemangioma; hyperglycaemia		
Pinealoma	-	+	Pituitary, pancreas, kidney abnormali-ties; perinephric abscess; hyper-glycaemia		
Adult type tumour of pineal region	+	-	-	Family of 9 children. No additional in-formation given	
Adult type tumour of pineal region	+	+	Haematoma at tumour site		
Pineal teratoma with some germinomatous components	-	+	Gaze palsy, nystag-mus, ataxic gait; hydrocephalus	Parents healthy. 1 normal younger sister	
Pineal teratoma with some germinomatous components	+	-	Abnormal intracra-nial calcification at 11 y; diplopia for 2 y prior to hospital admission at age 17. Right-sided hemiparesis, gaze palsy, nystag-mus		

GENERAL ASPECTS OF PINEALOMA

The term pinealoma was first introduced into the literature by Krabbe in 1916; in the Anglo-Saxon literature in 1923. Evaluation of the following literature has often presented difficulties, many of the different tumour types occurring in the pineal region sometimes being referred to as pinealomas. As the knowledge concerning pineal neoplasms increased these tumours were generally classified into 'pinealomas', teratomas, and gliomatous lesions (1, 12, 13, 21). This classification has recently benefited from the recognition of the distinction between pineal neoplasms composed of parenchymal cell derivatives and those of germ cell origin.

Tumours of germ cell origin arising from primitive cells and differentiating into various tissue components are the most frequently occurring neoplasms in the pineal region (15, 21, 23). They are mostly immature germ cell tumours and are called germinomas. Macroscopically germinomas are soft, pinkish-gray and of

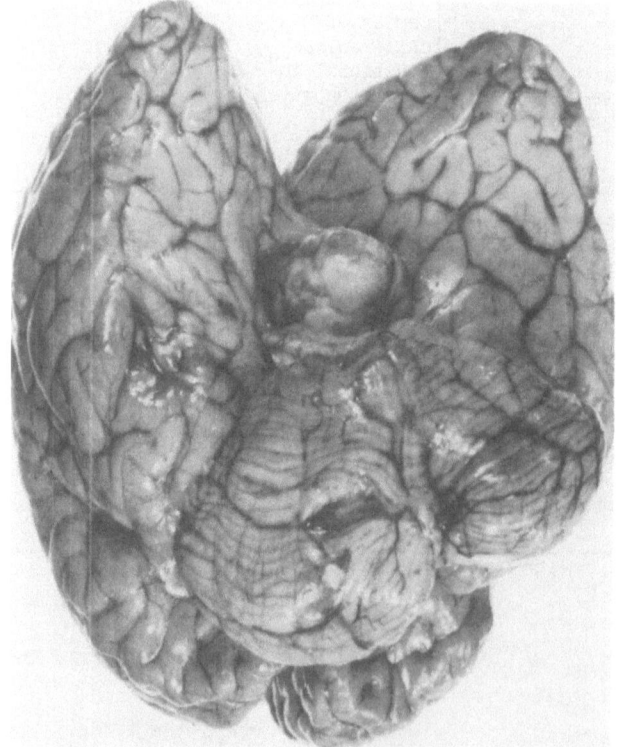

Fig. 1

Macroscopic appearance
of a germinoma of the
pineal gland.

granular consistency. Microscopically two cell types dominate: large cells with conspicuous central nuclei, and groups of small, darkly staining cells resembling lymphocytes (15, 21). Foci of differentiation into other tissue components are indicative of their teratomatous character (15), and they have synonymously been called atypical teratomas. When occurring in the midline hypothalamic region these tumours have been designated by the term suprasellar germinoma. Germinomas show infiltration into the surrounding tissues (22) and metastasis outside the CNS has been reported (14, 15). These tumours are regarded as being highly radiosensitive (15, 23).

Germ cell tumours with a high degree of differentiation into various tissue elements are called (typical) teratomas. They do not differ essentially from teratomas arising elsewhere in the body. They are circumscribed and of relatively benign behaviour, and may often contain less differentiated areas such as those characteristic of the germinoma (15).

Highly malignant variants of such germ cell neoplasms as choriocarcinoma and embryonal carcinoma, as well as mixed forms, are infrequently described (15, 17).

The term pinealoma itself can best be reserved for tumours arising from pineal parenchymal cells (10, 15, 21). Traditionally two types of neoplasm are

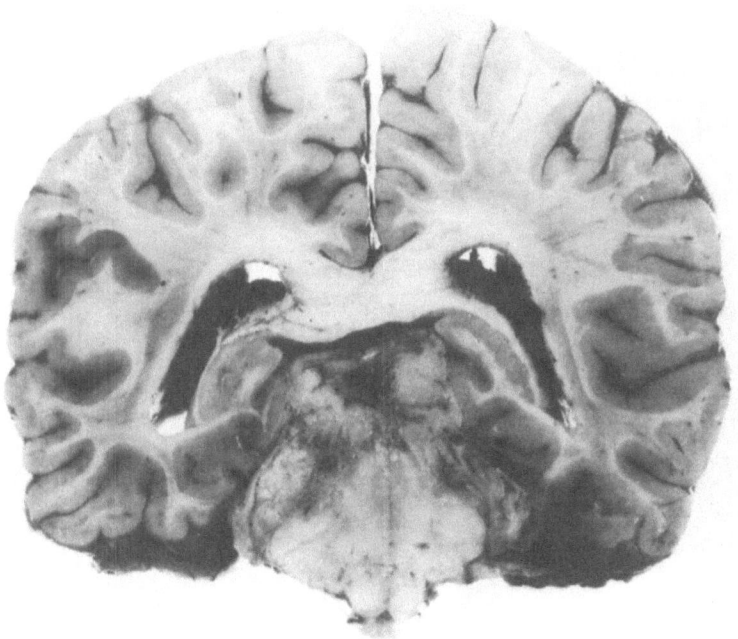

Fig. 2. Cross-section of a tumour of the pineal gland

distinguished: a primitive form, the highly malignant pineoblastoma, composed of immature cells with an ill-defined cytoplasm, which strongly resembles the medulloblastoma both histologically and in behaviour (3, 15, 17), and the pineocytoma, composed of relatively mature pineal parenchymal cells and resembling the normal pineal gland (10, 15, 16). Pineocytomas may demonstrate a slow, noninvasive growth (3, 15), but a more aggressive growth pattern also occurs. It seems from recent investigations (16, 17) that the more benign behaviour is found in those tumours in which cells show neuronal, or neuronal and astrocytic differentiation.

Sporadically other neoplasm types occur in the pineal region, including glial forms and cysts (15, 21). Metastasis to the pineal from tumours elsewhere is uncommon, but has been known to occur (21).

The clinical manifestations of pineal region neoplasms are determined by their type, dimensions and location. Generally, the presenting complaint is the result of acute or chronically increased intracranial pressure (3, 4, 5, 11, 12, 20, 21). Headache, and visual or motor symptoms may occur, as well as disturbances in endocrine and hypothalamic function, resulting in such symptoms as diabetes insipidus or pubertas praecox (4, 15, 20, 21, 22).

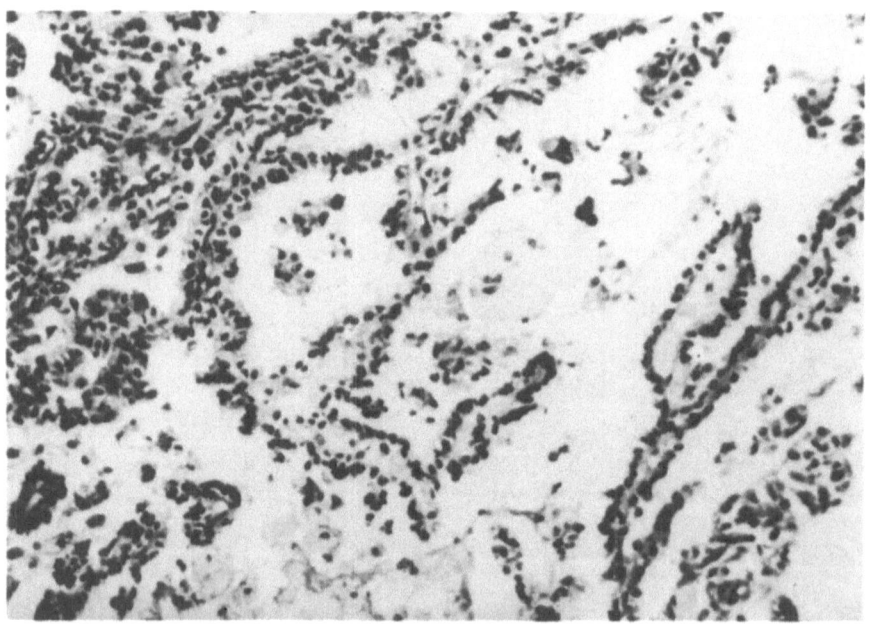

Fig. 3. CT-scan of a tumour of the pineal gland (not enhanced)

Various estimations of the occurrence of pineal neoplasms have been cited, and variation in geographical distribution has been demonstrated. The general incidence has been estimated at 0.4 to 1 or 2% of all brain tumours (2, 15, 21). The exception is Japan, where incidences varying from 2.1 to approximately 10% have been cited (2, 8, 11, 18).

Atypical (and typical) teratomas form the majority of the pineal region neoplasms (8, 15, 18, 21, 23), but establishment of their relative occurrence within the group of pineal tumours is unclear due to the lack of a consequently used classification.

In the pineal region a male preponderance is reported (6, 8, 12, 18, 19, 21, 23), but sex difference seems absent in tumours of the suprasellar region (15, 17, 18, 22).

Germinomas and teratomas are found occurring mainly in the first three decades of life, with a peak in the second (3, 15, 17, 18, 21, 22). Pineoblastomas occur mainly in children and young adults (3, 15, 17). Pineocytomas appear to occur at any age (15, 17).

FAMILIAL ASPECTS OF PINEALOMA

Reports concerning the familial occurrence of pineal region tumours have been
extremely infrequent. Waldbaur et al. (VI.A.1.1; II.A.1.2) reported two monozygotic twin sisters, 5 and 16 months of age, demonstrating respectively a
medulloblastoma of the cerebellum and a pineoblastoma. The histological indis-
tinguishability of these tumour types has been noted, and the authors of this
report have considered these tumours to be concordant. Other reports of twins
demonstrating pinealomas are not available in the literature.

Three reports have been made of pineal neoplasm occurrence in siblings.
Mendenhall (VI.B.1.1) reported two sisters and a brother demonstrating pineal
gland tumours in the first life decade. One of these sisters had been operated
upon for an ovarial sarcoma at the age of six months. The brother showed a brain
haemangioma at autopsy. All three children demonstrated pituitary, pancreas, and
kidney abnormalities, and a syndrome including precocious external genital development and therapy-resistant hyperglycaemia. A fourth child in this family was
said to have had the same physical characteristics as the children in the described
cases, but as this child was the first in the family to die (of intussusception),
no attention was aroused by this observation.
Kjellin et al. (VI.B.1.2) reported two half-brothers, aged 11 and 14 years,
demonstrating histologically similar tumours of the pineal region.
Wakai et al. (VI.B.1.3) reported two brothers having pineal teratomas at respectively 13 and 17 years of age. The 13-year-old died approximately nine months
after hospital admission. The other brother was alive at the time of article
completion.
Further reports of familial pineal neoplasm occurrence are not encountered in the
literature.

All the cases reported were found occurring in children. There was no sexual
predominance of occurrence in these cases.

The etiology of pineal neoplasms remains obscure. The lack of reports, as well
as specificity in terminology use in the designation of these neoplasms, makes
the interpretation of the role of familial or hereditary factors in their etiology
unclear. The geographical variation noted in their occurrence may be indicative
of genetic or environmental factors.

REFERENCES

1. ANDERSON WAD, SCOTTI TM 1968
   Synopsis of Pathology
   CV Mosby Co, St. Louis
2. BEHREND RC 1974
   Epidemiology of brain tumours.
   In: Vinken PJ, Bruyn GW (eds) Handbook of Clinical Neurology.
   North-Holland Publ Co, Amsterdam vol 16:56-88
3. BORIT A, BLACKWOOD W, MAIR WGP 1980
   The separation of pineocytoma from pineoblastoma.
   Cancer 45:1408-1418
4. BUEHLER BA 1979
   The clinical diagnosis of pinealoma.
   Ann Clin Lab Sci 9:243-246
5. DELONG GR, ADAMS RD 1975
   Clinical aspects of tumors of the posterior fossa in childhood.
   In: Vinken PJ, Bruyn GW (eds) Handbook of Clinical Neurology.
   North-Holland Publ Co, Amsterdam vol 18:387-411
6. FAHLBUSCH R, MARGUTH F 1974
   Endocrine disorderd associated with intracranial tumours.
   In: Vinken PJ, Bruyn GW (eds) Handbook of Clinical Neurology.
   North-Holland Publ Co, Amsterdam vol 16:341-359
7. KJELLIN K, MÜLLER R, ASTRÖM KE 1960
   The occurrence of brain tumors in several members of a family.
   J Neuropathol Exp Neurol 19:528-537
8. KOIDE O, WATANABE Y, SATO K 1980
   A pathological survey of intracranial germinoma and pinealoma in
   Japan.
   Cancer 45:2119-2130
9. MENDENHALL EM 1950
   Tumor of the pineal body with high insulin resistance.
   J Indiana State Med Assoc 43:32-36
10. NEUWELT EA, GLASBERG M, FRENKEL E, CLARK WK 1979
    Malignant pineal region tumors; a clinico-pathological study.
    J Neurosurg 51:597-607
11. ONOYAMA Y, ONO K, NAKAJIMA T, HIRAOKA M, ABE M 1979
    Radiation therapy of pineal tumors.
    Radiology 130:757-760
12. RINGERTS N, NORDENSTAM H, FLYGER G 1954
    Tumors of the pineal region.
    J Neuropathol Exp Neurol 13:540-561
13. ROBBINS SL 1974
    Pathologic basis of disease.
    WB Saunders Co, Philadelphia p 1370-1371
14. RUBERY ED, WHEELER TK 1980
    Metastases outside the central nervous system from a presumed
    pineal germinoma. Case report.
    J Neurosurg 53:562-565

210

15. RUBINSTEIN LJ   1972
    Tumors of the central nervous system.
    In: Atlas of Tumor Pathology. 2nd series, Fasc 6.
    Armed Forces Inst of Pathol, Washington DC p 269-284
16. RUBINSTEIN LJ   1979
    Cytogenesis and differentiation of pineal neoplasms.
    Lakartidningen 76:4374-4377
17. RUBINSTEIN LJ   1981
    Cytogenesis and differentiation of pineal neoplasms.
    Hum Pathol 12:441-448
18. SANO K, MATSUTANI M   1981
    Pinealoma (Germinoma) treated by direct surgery and postoperative
    irradiation. A long-term follow up.
    Child's Brain 8:81-97
19. SAYK J   1974
    The cerebrospinal fluid in brain tumours.
    In: Vinken PJ, Bruyn GW (eds) Handbook of Clinical Neurology.
    North-Holland Publ Co, Amsterdam vol 16:360-417
20. SLOOFF ACJ, SLOOFF JL   1975
    Supratentorial tumours in children.
    In: Vinken PJ, Bruyn GW (eds) Handbook of Clinical Neurology.
    North-Holland Publ Co, Amsterdam vol 18:305-386
21. SMITH RA, ESTRIDGE MN   1974
    Pineal tumors.
    In: Vinken PJ, Bruyn GW (eds) Handbook of Clinical Neurology.
    North-Holland Publ Co, Amsterdam vol 17:648-665
22. SUNG DII, HARISLADIS L, CHANG CH   1978
    Midline pineal tumors and suprasellar germinomas: highly curable by
    irradiation.
    Radiology 128:745-751
23. VALK J   1975
    The radiotherapy of brain tumours.
    In: Vinken PJ, Bruyn GW (eds) Handbook of Clinical Neurology.
    North-Holland Publ Co, Amsterdam vol 18:481-516
24. WAKAI S, SEGAWA H, KITAHARA S, ASANO T, SANO K, OGIHARA R, TOMITA S
    1980
    Teratoma in the pineal region in two brothers. Case reports.
    J Neurosurg 53:239-243
25. WALDBAUR H, GOTTSCHALDT M, SCHMIDT H, NEUHÄUSER G   1976
    Medulloblastom des Kleinhirns und Pineoblastom bei eineiigen
    Zwillingen.
    Klin Pädiat 188:366-371

Chapter VII

FAMILIAL GLIOMA

(excluding medulloblastoma, choroid plexus papilloma,
pinealoma, neuroblastoma, optic glioma)

CASE REPORTS

CLASSIFICATION

A. *TWINS*

　　1. Monozygotic twins with concordant tumour

　　2. Monozygotic twins with discordant tumour

　　3. Monozygotic twins, one demonstrating glioma

　　4. Dizygotic twins

B. *SIBLINGS*

　　1. Siblings with concordant tumour

　　2. Siblings with discordant tumour

C. *OTHER GENERATIONS AND DISTANT RELATIVES*

　　1. Other generations and distant relatives with concordant tumour

　　2. Other generations and distant relatives with discordant tumour

TABLES

VII.A.   *TWINS*

VII.A.1.   MONOZYGOTIC TWINS WITH CONCORDANT TUMOUR

VII.A.1.1.   Joughin 1928 - U.S.A. (112)

Identical twins. Female. Jewish.

Case 1

   History: The patient was the second born twin. At the age of 32 years she
was admitted to hospital because of *occipital headache for six months, pro-*
gressively growing worse. Other complaints were *weakness of the left extremi-*
ties for three months, numbness of the left hand and foot and an annoying
'drawing sensation' through the left side of the trunk for three months,
transitory intermittent diplopia on looking to the right for two months, and
diminution of vision for two or three months.
On neurological examination *a left hemiparesis of moderate degree was ...*
demonstrated, with slight hypertonia of the left leg. On the left all tendon
reflexes were increased, and all cutaneous reflexes decreased. All non-
equilibratory coordination tests were definitely poorly performed on the left.
Left hemihypesthesia and hemihypalgesia, affecting all modalities of super-
ficial sensibility, was present. Muscle, joint and tendon sense was deficient
on the left, especially in the feet. Stereognostic sense was deficient in the
left hand. Investigation of the cranial nerves showed an *anisocoria, the left*
pupil the larger, papilledema of 4 diopters in each eye and a *complete left*
homonymous hemianopia.
The diagnosis of intracerebral neoplasm was suspected and a right craniotomy
performed. At operation *the brain was under great pressure. The ventricles*
were aspirated, and ... yellowish fluid with abundant cholesterol crystals,
was withdrawn.
The patient failed to rally and died twelve hours after the operation.
   Autopsy: *a large fungating tumor mass was seen on the base of the brain,*
probably originating from the right hippocampal gyrus, compressing and
distorting the optic chiasm. This mass extended upward into the third ven-
tricle, occluded the right foramen of Monro and produced a marked dilatation
of the right lateral ventricle .... The brain tissue was firm, translucent
and grayish white and showed signs of repeated abundant old and recent
haemorrhages.

<u>Microscopic study</u>: The histological diagnosis was glioma.

<u>Diagnosis</u>: Right temporal glioma.

Case 2

<u>History</u>: This was the first born twin, who preceded her sister by an interval of five minutes. At the age of 34 years she complained of *'spells' of seven years' duration. These 'spells' consisted of a tingling feeling in the right foot,* followed by a loss of strength of the right leg. These 'spells' were at first confined to the right leg, but later also involved the left. First neurological examination did not reveal abnormalities. A few months later she complained of recurring occipital headaches that progressively grew worse. She also had tinnitus.

Neurological examination at that time revealed a *beginning choked disk ..., slight right facial weakness, slight weakness of the right arm and right leg,* and *tendon reflexes increased on the right ....*

A cerebral tumour was suspected and a left craniotomy performed. At operation a huge subcortical tumour was partially removed from the left hemisphere. *The tumor mass extended into the left ventricle and beneath the falx into the right hemisphere.*

The patient rallied well and went home. Six months later she succumbed from shock shortly after a second surgical operation.

<u>Autopsy</u>: Not mentioned.

<u>Microscopic study</u>: The histological diagnosis was glioma.

<u>Diagnosis</u>: Left subcortical glioma.

<u>Family</u>: The family history of the patients was traced for three generations, but information of genetical interest could not be discovered. The maternal aunt gave birth to male twins who died at an advanced age, one of diabetes, the other of pneumonia.

COMMENT

The twins were assumed to be identical, as they were of the same sex, had eyes and hair of the same colour, were of the same weight until adult life, and were of the same general mental and emotional make-up. The authors state in their article that until that time no brain tumours have been reported in twins, identical or nonidentical. Unfortunately the histological nature of the glioma is not recorded in the article.

VII.A.1.2. Kjellin et al. 1960 - Stockholm, Sweden (123)

Identical twins. Male. Swedish.

Case 1

History: The patient was admitted to hospital at the age of 33 years. One week before admission he had an epileptic fit, which subsequently developed into continuous convulsions in the left half of the face.
On examination he was found to have bilateral papilledema and left-sided hemiplegia including the left side of the face.
At operation a tough tumor with the appearance of an astrocytoma was found in the anterior part of the right temporal lobe. A piece was removed for histologic examination. The subsequent course was rather uneventful until the patient died approximately 5 years after the operation ....

Autopsy: Not performed.

Microscopic study: the biopsy specimen showed a rather acellular tumor with slight pleomorphism and no mitoses. Most cells had the appearance of large astrocytes; in addition, there were a number of gemistocytes. There were no vascular abnormalities and no necroses.

Diagnosis: Right temporal astrocytoma grade I.

Case 2

History: This patient was admitted to hospital at the age of 50 years. He had uncinate fits about 1 year before admission ....
Examination revealed slight left-sided facial paresis of central type.
At operation a gelatinous, gray-red, partly soft tumor with the appearance of an astrocytoma was partially removed from the anterior part of the right temporal lobe.
The patient died 3 months after the operation ....

Autopsy: showed a whitish, rather tough, solid tumor in the anterior part of the right temporal lobe.

Microscopic study: biopsy specimens showed a rather acellular and mono-morphic tumor composed of astrocyte-like cells and without mitoses. The blood vessels were normal, and there were no necroses. The tumor was somewhat more cellular, polymorphic and rich in gemistocytic forms in sections from autopsy specimens.

Diagnosis: Right temporal astrocytoma grade I-II.

Family: The twin brothers came from a family of 6 children. No further
data are mentioned in the article.

COMMENT

That the brothers were uniovular twins was not confirmed. They were reported
as having a very similar appearance.

VII.A.1.3. <u>Fairburn and Urich 1971</u> - Romford/London, England (66)

Identical twins. Male. English.

The twin boys were born after a normal delivery and were said to have a common placenta. The pregnancy had been normal and there was no exposure to X-rays or any significant illness.

Case 1

<u>History</u>: At the age of 2 years and 11 months this boy developed progressive unsteadiness of gait. *He was also noticed to have difficulty in controlling the use of his left hand. Ten days before his admission to hospital ..., he began to vomit in the mornings.*

On examination *his fundi showed bilateral early papilloedema. He had ataxia of the left limbs and bilateral extensor plantar responses. Skull radiography showed suture diastasis. Ventriculography ... showed marked hydrocephalus due to the presence of a left cerebellar tumour.*

After a Torkildsen's operation a *suboccipital exploration with partial removal of an infiltrating tumour, occupying the vermis and the left cerebellar hemisphere, was carried out.* Biopsy of the tumour showed a malignant neoplasm which at first was erroneously diagnosed as a medulloblastoma and he was given a course of radiotherapy. On discharge six months later *he was speaking a few words and walking with assistance.*

He was readmitted two months later *with a two weeks' history of recurrence of ataxia, vomiting, and irritability.*

His condition rapidly deteriorated, and he died in coma one week later.

<u>Autopsy</u>: showed a tumour ... *occupying the white matter of the left cerebellar hemisphere ventral to the dentate nucleus, the adjacent brachium pontis, the restiform body, and the dorsolateral part of the medulla. The cut surface of the tumour was soft, pinkish-grey, and mottled with haemorrhages in its upper part. ... towards the lower end it was firm, white and homogeneous.*

<u>Microscopic study</u>: *the tumour consisted of two distinct parts.* The part corresponding to the soft, greyish-pink areas had the appearances of a malignant oligodendroglioma. The white, solid part was probably astrocytic in origin. *The boundary between the two types of tumour was not clear-cut and both types of cell intermingled freely in a broad transition zone.*

<u>Diagnosis</u>: Mixed glioma with oligodendroglial and astrocytic elements in the left cerebellar hemisphere and brain stem.

Case 2

<u>History</u>: At the age of 7 1/2 years this boy was admitted to hospital.

... *he complained of intermittent headaches and had two focal epileptic*
attacks affecting the right arm in the previous month. Once this was followed
by a generalized convulsion.

On examination he showed no abnormal signs. *Electroencephalogram, brain scan,*
and left carotid angiography suggested the presence of a small left parietal
tumour. ... *no surgical treatment was advised at that time and he was dis-*
charged home on anti-convulsant drugs.

One month later he was readmitted *with a week's history of weakness of the*
right hand and dragging of the right leg.

On examination he was drowsy and had *severe bilateral papilloedema and a mild*
right hemiparesis. A left carotid angiogram was repeated and showed a very
large left parietal tumour. A left parietal burr-hole was made and *at a depth*
of 3 cm a cystic cavity was entered from which 20 ml. of clear yellow fluid
was aspirated. A needle biopsy of solid tumour deep to the cyst was obtained
at the same time.

... *his condition improved temporarily* .... *no surgical or radiotherapeutic*
treatment was undertaken. The patient remained well until two months later
when *he went rapidly downhill in the course of a few days and died in a coma*
a few days later.

Autopsy: *revealed a large tumour* ... *occupying the white matter of the*
posterior end of the third frontal convolution and most of the parietal lobe.
The cut surface of the tumour showed a variegated appearance, the anterior
end being white and homogeneous, the centre necrotic and haemorrhagic, the
posterior end soft, greyish and stippled with small haemorrhages.

Microscopic study: *This tumour* ... *consisted of an oligodendroglial and an*
astrocytic part, the former comprising the bulk of the tumour, the latter
forming its anterior end. The demarcation of the two parts was more abrupt
than in the first twin.

Diagnosis: Mixed glioma with oligodengroglial and astrocytic elements
left fronto-parietal.

Family: The father was aged 27 and the mother 26 years. There were no
other children. The parents had been healthy and there was no consanguinity.

COMMENT

The boys were very alike both in appearance and personality and were
regarded as identical twins.

VII.A.1.4. <u>Clarenbach et al. 1979 - Freiburg, Germany</u> (46)

Identical twins. Male. German.

The twins were born after a normal pregnancy, labour and delivery. Two placen-
tae and three allantoic membranes were found. Uniovularity was confirmed by
serological data.

Case 1

<u>History</u>: The patient was admitted to hospital at the age of 22 years. He
complained of *early vomiting, disturbances of balance, and pulsating headaches*.

On examination he showed only minimal papilloedema. *The retinal fundus had a
particularly red appearance* .... The pupillary light reflex was reduced, but
there were prompt contractions on convergence. Investigation of the vestibulo-
oculomotor system revealed *approximately symmetrical impairment of fixation,
suppression of vestibulo-ocular reflexes, horizontal gaze nystagmus, cog-
wheeled smooth pursuit, impaired optokinetic nystagmus, and central positional
nystagmus*. Cerebellar ataxia of posture and gait were present. ... *angiography
and computerized tomography scan showed a tumor in the posterior fossa extending from the midline into the right cerebellar hemisphere, and a pronounced
occlusive hydrocephalus. Ventriculography indicated an intraventricular growth
in the fourth ventricle* ....

At operation *a midline tumor of the posterior fossa reached down to the C-2
vertebra, infiltrating the right corpus restiforme, the cerebral peduncles,
and at several separate points in the medullo oblongata. A subtotal resection
was performed, followed by placement of atrioventricular shunts*.

Postoperatively there was an *improvement of smooth pursuit, of optokinetic
nystagmus, and of horizontal gaze nystagmus*. Cerebellar ataxia also improved.
A CT-scan 10 months later showed no increase in size of the residual tumour.

<u>Microscopic study</u>: ... *led to the diagnosis of subependymoma* ....
... *there was a clear demarcation of the tumor from adjacent brain tissue*.

<u>Diagnosis</u>: Subependymoma of the fourth ventricle.

Case 2

<u>History</u>: The patient was admitted to hospital at the age of 22 years with
a history of early vomiting, disturbances of balance, and pulsating headaches.
On examination he *displayed papilledema of about 3 diopters in both eyes, his
visual acuity was reduced to 0.7 and 0.6 respectively, and his visual field
showed impairment of the inferior segments with enlargement of the blind spot*.

He showed reduced pupillary light reflexes, but prompt contractions on conver-
gence. The retinal fundus had a particularly red appearance .... The vestibulo-
oculomotor system showed the same disturbances as in case 1. *In addition, he*
showed spontaneous nystagmus to the left and directional preponderance to the
left at rotation. Cerebellar ataxia of posture and gait were present.

... angiography and computerized tomography scan showed a tumor in the poste-
rior fossa extending from the midline into the right cerebellar hemisphere,
and a pronounced occlusive hydrocephalus. Ventriculography indicated an intra-
ventricular growth in the fourth ventricle ....
At operation *a midline tumor was found ... : caudally it reached the upper*
edge of the C-2 vertebra. It was well demarcated from the medulla oblongata ....
The cerebellar tonsils, the corpus restiforme of the brain stem, and the floor
of the fourth ventricle were infiltrated on the right side. A subtotal resection
was performed, followed by placement of atrioventricular shunts.
Postoperatively *the papilledema disappeared and there was gradual improvement*
of visual acuity and visual fields. The eye movement disorders and cerebellar
ataxia also improved. A CT-scan 10 months later showed no increase in size of
the residual tumour.

Microscopic study: *... led to the diagnosis of subependymoma ....*
... there was a clear demarcation of the tumor from adjacent brain tissue.

Diagnosis: Subependymoma of the fourth ventricle.

Family: *The family history revealed no parental consanguinity.* Their mother
(66 years old) showed no neurological symptoms and their father died of myo-
cardial infarction at the age of 40 years. *... no neoplastic disorders have*
occurred in the older brother or in the two older sisters.

COMMENT

These identical twins with subependymomas were also reported by Voigt and
Marquardt in 1979. They describe the angiographic diagnostic features of the
concordant tumours in these monozygotic twins. They mention that there was
no growth of the residual tumours in the 3 years after operation, as investigated by regular CT-scan control (273).

VII.A.2.   MONOZYGOTIC TWINS WITH DISCORDANT TUMOUR

VII.A.2.1.   <u>Hoppe 1952 - Berlin, Germany</u> (104)

Identical twins. Male. German.

One twin (case 1) had a meningioma, the other (case 2) had a glioblastoma.
These cases have been described in the chapter on meningioma (III.A.2.1).

VII.A.2.2. <u>Koch et al. 1957 - Münster, Germany</u> (130)

Identical twins. Male. German.

Case 1

<u>History</u>: This 48-year-old teacher was hospitalized because of tonic-clonic seizures and mental disturbances of three month duration.

On examination the patient was unconscious with irregular breathing, and funduscopy showed papilloedema on both sides. Right carotid angiography revealed a tumour in the temporal lobe.

At operation a mandarin size infiltrating tumour in the right temporal lobe was removed.

The patient died eleven months after the operation.

<u>Autopsy</u>: Not performed.

<u>Microscopic study</u>: showed a glioblastoma multiforme.

A small cyst of the septum pellucidum was also found.

<u>Diagnosis</u>: Right temporal glioblastoma multiforme.

Septum pellucidum cyst.

Case 2

<u>History</u>: This government inspector had a first tonic-clonic generalized seizure at the age of 35 years and a second left-sided partial seizure at the age of 42 years for which he was admitted to hospital.

On examination a slight spasm of the left arm, a left-sided positive Babinski sign, a dysdiadochokinesis of the left hand and a right abducens paresis were found. Angiography was indicative of a basomedially situated process on the right side.

At operation a strongly elevated intracranial pressure because of brain oedema was found and as the tumour was considered inoperable no tissue was removed.

At the age of 45 years ventriculography was performed, which showed a displacement of both lateral ventricles. A diagnosis of septum pellucidum cyst was made.

The patient died two years later in coma with extensor spasms of all extremities.

<u>Autopsy</u>: Not performed.

<u>Microscopic study</u>: Not performed.

<u>Diagnosis</u>: Septum pellucidum cyst.

Family: The twins were the fourth and fifth of seven children. The father died at the age of 85 years and the mother at the age of 80. The eldest brother died in a traffic accident. An older sister died at the age of 50 years of liver cirrhosis; another sister of lung tuberculosis. The two other sisters were healthy. No occurrences of neurological or mental diseases or deformities were known of in the family.

COMMENT

Diagnosis of case 2 was made on clinical grounds, no histological verification could be performed.

VII.A.3.   MONOZYGOTIC TWINS, ONE DEMONSTRATING GLIOMA

The reports on monozygotic twins with one of the twins demonstrating a glioma are too numerous for separate description. These cases are frequently mentioned in the framework of an extensive investigation of brain tumours in twins or families (92, 127, 272), and details are often lacking in these reports. Such investigations will be discussed under the heading of familial aspects of glioma.

VII.A.4.   DIZYGOTIC TWINS

No reports on concordant glioma in dizygotic twins are presently available in the literature.

VII.B.   *SIBLINGS*

VII.B.1.   SIBLINGS WITH CONCORDANT TUMOUR

VII.B.1.1.   <u>Besold 1896 - Erlangen, Germany</u> (22)

Two sisters. German.

Case 1

<u>History</u>: At the age of 17 years this patient was admitted to hospital with
a 10-month history of headaches, vomiting, and seizures. She also complained
of blurred vision, diplopia and difficulty in walking.
On examination she had a right facial paresis and impaired vision. Funduscopy
showed an atrophy of the optical nerve. Her speech was remarkably slow. There
was abasia and astasia. The deep tendon reflexes were somewhat brisk. Hearing
was diminished.
In the following months the patient's condition gradually declined: she became
apathetic, incontinent and suffered from progressive headache and vomiting.
The epileptic seizures became more frequent and worse.
She died 11 months after admission.

<u>Autopsy</u>: revealed a greyish-red, rough, lobulated tumour mass in the region
of the corpora quadrigemina and third ventricle, originating from the region
of the left thalamus opticus and accompanied by an enormous chronic internal
hydrocephalus.
Other autopsy findings were an open foramen ovale, cysts in the thyroid gland,
pancreatic haemorrhages, and a double left-sided ureter.

<u>Microscopic study</u>: The histological diagnosis of 'medullar sarcoma probably
of ependymal origin' was made.

<u>Diagnosis</u>: Sarcomatous tumour of ependymal origin of the third ventricle,
originating in the region of the left thalamus opticus.

Case 2

<u>History</u>: At the age of 12 years this female was admitted to hospital with
a 16-month history of progressive headache, vomiting and seizures. She also
complained of disturbances of vision and difficulting in walking.
On examination the patient was somewhat apathetic and bradyfrenic. She was
totally blind. Funduscopy showed bilateral atrophic papillae. Impaired hearing
on both sides was discovered. Her speech was very slow and monotone. She was

incontinent of urine. There was a paraparesis.

During the stay in the hospital her condition gradually deteriorated; she had progressive seizures and disturbances of consciousness.

She died in the hospital at the age of 14 years, 22 months after admission.

Autopsy: A tumour mass was found in the third ventricle originating from the region of the left thalamus opticus and incorporating the pineal gland, corpora quadrigemina, posterior part of the left corpus striatum, and the right thalamus opticus. An enormous internal hydrocephalus was present.

Microscopic study: revealed an angiosarcomatous tumour of ependymal origin.

Diagnosis: Sarcomatous tumour of ependymal origin of the third ventricle originating in the region of the left thalamus opticus.

Family: The parents of the two sisters were healthy. The grandmother died of a 'brain suppuration'. Nothing was known about the other members of the family.

COMMENT

According to the histological description in the article both tumours must be classified as ependymal tumours of the anaplastic type in modern nomenclature.

VII.B.1.2. Böhmig 1918 - Dresden, Germany (32)

A brother and a sister. German.

Case 1 (brother)

History: The patient was admitted to hospital at the age of 24 years. He had a one-year history of progressive headaches, vomiting and convulsions. His medical history noted severe convulsions at the age of 3 months with residual strabismus and a right foot paresis.
Shortly after admission he died subsequent to a severe convulsion.

Autopsy: revealed a 4 cm rather soft tumour in the left frontal lobe with a cyst in the parietal lobe. The left hemisphere was very oedematous.

Diagnosis: Left fronto-parietal tumour cerebri (glioma).

Case 2 (sister)

History: The patient died at the age of 38 years after a 'convulsion'. She had a one-year history of progressive intermittent headaches with vomiting and flickering of the eyes, and drop attacks. She also had paraesthesia of the arms and legs.
On repeated neurological examination, also performed during an attack, no abnormalities were found except for slight papilloedema on both sides, on the right more than the left.

Autopsy: revealed a 8 x 5 x 4 cm partly white, partly red-grayish tumour in the right frontal lobe.

Microscopic study: Oedematous glioma.

Diagnosis: Right frontal glioma.

Family: The father died of a 'paralysis'. No further data are available. There were no hereditary diseases in the family.

COMMENT

It is not mentioned in the article whether the histological diagnosis in case 1 was confirmed by microscopic study.

VII.B.1.3. Hoffmann 1919 - Tübingen, Germany (102)

Two brothers. German.

Case 1

History: At the age of 30 years this patient began to complain of headaches and started to have generalized convulsions. Subsequently his mental condition declined. A few years later he also showed disturbances of speech and noticed a loss of strength in his right arm and leg. He began to complain of blurring of vision and had disturbances of gait. A few weeks before admission at the age of 33 years he became apathetic and drowsy.
On examination the patient was somnolent, disoriented in time, and bradyfrenic. Examination revealed a slight right facial paresis and a spastic hemiparesis of the right arm and leg with elevated deep tendon reflexes. A slight anisocoria was present. Vision was diminished and funduscopy showed papilloedema on both sides. There were disturbances of gait.
After admission his condition gradually declined and he died a few months later after a rise of temperature.
Autopsy: showed a somewhat lobulated, firm tumour of the left gyrus hippo-campi and gyrus occipito-temporalis, extending into half of the temporal lobe.
Microscopic study: revealed a cell-rich glioma without further particulari-ties.
Diagnosis: Glioma of the left gyrus hippocampi and gyrus occipito-temporalis.

Case 2

History: At the age of 48 years the patient was admitted to hospital with a history of vomiting and vertigo since a few months.
On examination the patient was disoriented, somnolent, and somewhat bradyfrenic. He also complained of headaches. Examination revealed a first degree nystagmus, a doubtful left-sided hemianopsia and disturbances of gait with a tendency to fall to the right. Ophthalmological examination showed beginning left papill-oedema.
Because of the continuing vomiting and decline of mental condition a palliative trepanation on both sides was performed under local anaesthesia.
Two days later the patient died.
Autopsy: A soft tumour mass was found in the right hippocampus and gyrus hippocampi.
Microscopic study: revealed a cell-rich glioma without particularities.
Diagnosis: Glioma of the right hippocampus and gyrus hippocampi.

230

Family:

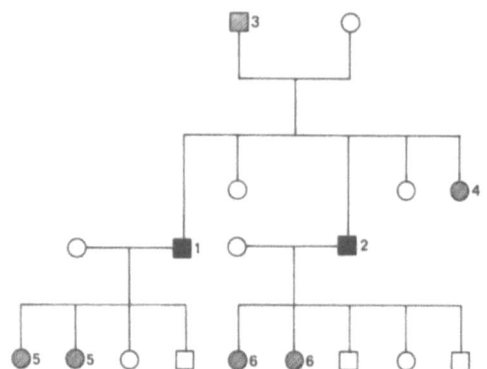

1 = case 1
2 = case 2
3 = convulsions
4 = feeble-minded
5 + 6 = died very young

The father died at the age of 74 years of a cerebrovascular accident. The
last years before his death he suffered from convulsions (3). The mother
died at the age of 61 years of 'Wassersucht'. A sister of the two probands
was strange and feeble-minded (4). She suffered now and then from convulsions,
probably of hysterical nature. The other sisters were healthy.
Both probands had two children who died very young (5 and 6). The other
children were healthy in their second and third decade of life.

VII.B.1.4. Bender and Panse 1932 - Berlin, Germany (21)

Hallervorden 1936 - Landsberg-Warthe, Germany (87)

Three brothers. German.

Case 1

History: The patient was admitted to hospital at the age of 58 years
because of a tentamen suicide. He had been drinking alcohol excessively for
many years and was impotent since his 47th year. Two years prior to admission
he had also made a suicide attempt. Since that time he complained of headaches
and loss of memory.

On examination he was disoriented in time. He had a lipoma near the left
trochanter, scattered naevi and pes caves on both sides. Neurological examination was normal, but the Pandy reaction of the cerebrospinal fluid was elevated.
The following months his condition, in particular mentally, declined and a few
months later he also had neurological disorders: a left facial paresis, hypertonia of the extremities, more on the right than on the left, and a positive
Babinski sign on the right. At funduscopy papilloedema on both sides was found.
There was a tendency to fall backwards.

A few weeks later the patient demonstrated a convulsive state and died a few
days later.

Autopsy: A highly vascular, soft tumour mass was found in the lateral and
third ventricles, infiltrating great parts of the central brain structures.

Microscopic study: showed a non-mature, cell-rich glioma with polymorphic,
dysplastic and partly mitotic cell forms with considerable cell dystopia in
the hemispheres and partly in the cerebellum. The histological diagnosis was
spongioblastoma.

Diagnosis: Spongioblastoma of the central region.

Case 2

History: The patient had been an alcoholic since the age of 34 years. At
the age of 40 he became depressive and a year later he attempted to commit
suicide.

On examination he had a right frontal subcutaneous firm tumour as large as a
cherry, a naevus of the cheek, and little skin tumours of the neck. On both
sides pes caves were found. Neurological examination showed a slight facial
paresis and a tongue paresis on the left.

A few months later he suffered a loss of consciousness followed by periods of
agitation. He then also had difficulties in finding words and his speech was

somewhat dysarthric.

The next year choreiform movements of the head and extremities were discovered, especially of the left arm. The attacks of unconsciousness recurred. A repeated neurological examination showed no abnormalities.. The patient was in an obviously psychotic state with acoustic hallucinations. Once he had a general-ized convulsion. Finally he became blind and apathetic.

He died at the age of 46 years.

Autopsy: A large, greyish-red, cystic tumour was found in the right temporal lobe infiltrating the hippocampus.

Microscopic study: The tumour consisted of undifferentiated small glia cells with stark proliferating capacity. These cells extended into the whole brain, also in the brain stem and cerebellum, without sharp limitation. A histological diagnosis of diffuse glioblastomatosis with local accumulation in the temporal lobe was made.

Diagnosis: Diffuse glioblastomatosis with local accumulation in the right temporal lobe.

Case 3

History: At the age of 47 years the patient began complaining of progressive headaches and vomiting.

On examination seven months later he was disoriented and slow minded. There was a striking rigidity of the extremities and a bilateral ptosis. The cerebro-spinal fluid pressure was elevated and he had bilateral papilloedema. He had two naevi on the shoulder and pes caves on both sides. After a temporary improvement his condition declined and he became incontinent of urine and faeces. He died at the age of 47 years after a few hour period of vomiting.

Autopsy: Was not performed.

Diagnosis: A clinical diagnosis of brain tumour was made.

Family: Fifty-four other members of the family in five generations were investigated. Among these relatives no brain tumour was found. Four persons were oligofrenic, among them two sisters of the probands. One person had epi-lepsy, two had pes caves (one sister) and five had naevi (one brother, one sister).

COMMENT

In case 3 a clinical diagnosis of brain tumour was made, but no autopsy or microscopic study was performed. The three brothers were first reported by Bender and Panse in 1932. At that time the brother of case 2 was still alive and a brain tumour was suspected on clinical grounds. The autopsy, microscopic study and histological diagnosis of this case were reported 4 years later by Hallervorden in 1936.

Stigmata of the neurofibromatosis complex are present in the probands and their relatives, which suggests a relationship with this disease entity.

VII.B.1.5. <u>Glauberman 1936</u> (83)

(cited by Manuelidis 1972) (322)

Two brothers.

Glauberman reported two brothers, 56 and 51 years of age, each having spongioblastoma multiforme located in the same site of the brain, the left temporal
lobe.

<u>COMMENT</u>

The occurrence is cited by Manuelidis 1972. No further data are mentioned
concerning these cases. It was not possible to obtain the original article.

VII.B.1.6. <u>Pass 1938 - Hamburg, Germany</u> (197)

Two half-sisters. German.

<u>Case 1</u> (proband)
This patient died of a histologically verified glioma of the frontal lobe at
the age of 49 years.

<u>Case 2</u>
This patient died at the age of 46 years of a histologically verified glioma
of the temporal lobe.

<u>Family:</u>

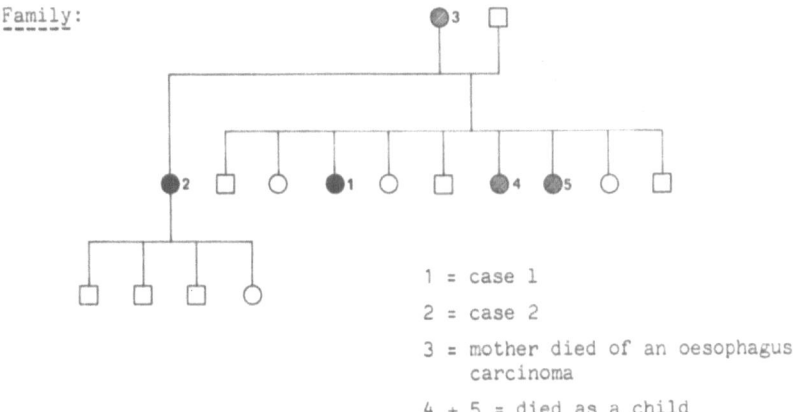

1 = case 1
2 = case 2
3 = mother died of an oesophagus
    carcinoma
4 + 5 = died as a child

<u>COMMENT</u>
In his study the author investigated 30 families of patients with brain
tumours (glioblastoma, astrocytoma, meningioma). This was the only case of
familial occurrence of brain tumours in his material.

VII.B.1.7. Geyer and Pedersen 1939 - Berlin-Buch, Germany (81)

A brother and sister. German.

Case 1 (brother)
This patient died of a histologically verified glioblastoma multiforme of the frontal lobe at the age of 43 years.

Case 2 (sister)
This patient died at the age of 44 years of a glioblastoma multiforme of the frontal lobe. The diagnosis could only be made macroscopically at autopsy.

COMMENT
No further data are mentioned in the article.

VII.B.1.8. Halpern 1943 - Israel (88)
(cited by Peyser and Beller 1951 (202) and Manuelidis 1972 (322))

Two brothers.

Halpern described two brothers, 42 and 43 years of age. One brother had an astroblastoma located in the left peduncle, the other an astroblastoma in the left temporal lobe.

COMMENT
This report was cited by Peyser and Beller (202) and Manuelidis (322). No further data are mentioned concerning the cases. It was not possible to obtain the original report.

VII.B.1.9. Riese et al. 1944 - Richmond, U.S.A. (218)

A brother and a sister. American.

Case 1 (brother)

History: This white male was admitted to hospital at the age of 50 years. Two months prior to admission he fell while at work. *Following this fall he began complaining of headaches, dizziness, and felt that his 'mind and vision were crossed'*. He gradually developed *mental symptoms of forgetfulness, seclusiveness, agitation, and depression. There was incontinence of urine and feces*.

Neurological examination on admission revealed *generalized hyperactive deep reflexes, slight ataxia, and equilibratory incoordination which necessitated walking on a broad base*. Investigation of the spinal fluid was normal. Mental examination showed *considerable memory defect for both recent and remote events*. Three weeks after admission the patient was found in a stuporous state, which was followed by frequent vomiting and a series of convulsive seizures. Neurological examination revealed *mild choking of the optic discs*. There was progressive elevation of temperature with evidence of bronchopneumonia and he died a few days later.

Autopsy: ... *a rather extensive growth could be seen, situated in the right cerebral hemisphere, involving the basal ganglia in the central portion of the growth, especially the striopallidum and thalamus, and spreading to the hypothalamic region and to the opposite side. This growth has definite hemorrhagic aspect* .... *The tumor extends from the posterior region of the frontal lobe to the parietal lobe* ....

Microscopic study: A histological diagnosis of glioblastoma multiforme was made.

Diagnosis: Right fronto-parietal glioblastoma multiforme.

Case 2 (sister)

History: This female was admitted to hospital at the age of 39 years. Two months before admission she developed left-sided convulsions.

On examination *she was moderately drowsy. She did not talk at all spontaneously* .... *There was moderate choking of the disks bilaterally* .... *Moderate weakness of the left arm and leg, especially the latter, could be demonstrated* .... *There was a positive Babinski sign of the left side* .... *A careful lumbar puncture* showed a spinal fluid pressure of 35 cm H_2O; the investigation of the fluid was normal. Ventriculography showed *marked displacement of the entire*

*ventricular system to the left side by a presumed right-sided temporo-parietal
tumor ....*

At operation *a diffuse infiltrating tumor was found on the cortex, extending
... subcortically as well. The tumor was subtotally removed.*

Postoperatively the patient's condition was of a steady down-hill course and
she died four days after operation.

Autopsy: *Gross diagnoses were: (1) primary bronchiogenic carcinoma of the
left lung with miliary metastases throughout the left lung. (2) malignant
right temporal lobe ... tumor .... Hemorrhage was seen into the basal ganglia
between the external and internal capsules in both ... hemispheres. (3) Leiomyomata uteri ....*

Microscopic study (operative specimen): *revealed a neoplasm having the
characteristic features of glioblastoma multiforme.*

Diagnosis: Right temporal glioblastoma multiforme.

Family: The father was murdered at 30 years of age. The mother died of
asthma at the age of 59 years. No further data concerning the relatives are
mentioned in the article.

COMMENT

Some doubt may exist as to the subclassification of the tumour in case 1.
Another brain tumour specialist was *inclined to classify it with the
astroblastomata.*

VII.B.1.10. Lange-Cosack 1949
                (cited by Van der Wiel 1959) (286)

Two sisters.

This case is cited by Van der Wiel (286) in his table on familial incidence
of gliomas. It concerns two sisters with glioma cerebri in both. No further
information is given about the cases. No reference was mentioned in the
thesis or could be obtained from the author.

VII.B.1.11. Zülch 1951 (297)
                (cited by Koch 1954) (127)

Two brothers.

Two brothers having glioblastoma of the parieto-occipital region are reported.
One died at the age of 54 years, the other at the age of 61 years. No further
details are mentioned.

COMMENT
This case is cited by Koch (127) and also mentioned by Zülch (299) in his
Handbook. The original report was not available.

VII.B.1.12. Almeida Lima - 1954
                (personal communication in Koch 1954) (127)

Two brothers.

This case is cited by Koch in 1954 as a personal communication. It concerns
two brothers with astrocytoma. No further information concerning the cases
is given in the article.

VII.B.1.13. <u>Koch 1954 - Münster, Germany</u> (127)

A sister and brother. German.

<u>Case 1</u> (sister)
This female had an anatomically diagnosed ependymoma of the posterior part of the right lateral ventricle at the age of 47 years. She suffered from epilepsy.

<u>Case 2</u> (brother)
At the age of 53 years this male had a cystic glioma of the right fronto-temporal lobe (anatomical diagnosis).

<u>Family:</u>

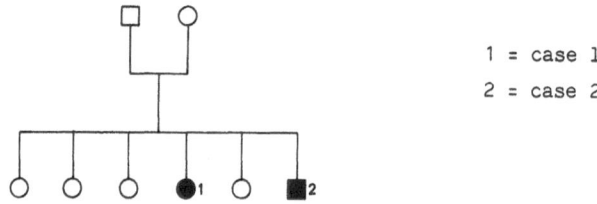

1 = case 1
2 = case 2

<u>COMMENT</u>
This case was mentioned in an extensive study of 350 female patients with CNS tumour. No further data about the patients are given in the article.

VII.B.1.14. <u>Appelman 1956 - The Netherlands</u>
            (personal communication in Van der Wiel 1959) (286)

Two brothers with glioblastoma.
No further details are known concerning these cases.
Personal communication cited by van der Wiel, 1959.

VII.B.1.15. Noetzel 1959 - Freiburg, Germany (186)

A brother and sister. German.

Case 1 (brother)
   History: This carpenter was admitted to hospital at the age of 43 years.
The day before admission he had a head injury and the following day he suffered
from headaches, vertigo and temporary dullness of the senses.
On examination the patient at first showed no neurological disorders. Three
days later his pulse became slow. Examination then revealed an anisocoria
greater on the right than on the left, a positive Babinski sign, and ankle
clonus on the left. There was a progressive loss of consciousness the following
days and a bilateral trepanation was performed on suspicion of a subdural
haematoma.
The patient died three days later of central respiratory paralysis.
   Autopsy: A tumour was found in the left parieto-occipital region with hydrocephalus of the lateral and third ventricles.
Other organs showed a partly cystical nodular goiter, persisting foetal 'Lappung'
of the kidneys and adenoma of the prostate.
   Microscopic study: Glioblastoma multiforme.
   Diagnosis: Left parieto-occipital glioblastoma multiforme.

Case 2 (sister)
   History: At the age of 32 years this housemaid was acutely admitted to
hospital because of sudden onset of severe headache during her work. She had
a history of headaches and depression during the previous four year period.
On examination a bilateral myosis was found and a rapidly progressive loss of
consciousness.
She died a few hours later of central respiratory paralysis.
   Autopsy: revealed a tumour of the right frontal lobe extending into the
corpus callosum and the midbrain. The other organs showed no abnormalities.
   Microscopic study: Glioblastoma fusiforme.
   Diagnosis: Right frontal glioblastoma fusiforme.

   Family: The parents were healthy. No further data are available.

VII.B.1.16. Noetzel 1959 - Freiburg, Germany (186)

Two brothers. German.

Case 1

History: This shoemaker was admitted to hospital at the age of 48 years.
At the age of 40 his right eye was enucleated because of a shell splinter
injury. Since that time he complained of headaches. At the age of 49 he had
a focal seizure of the right arm and leg. Focal seizures became more frequent
during the following months.
On examination he had a left facial paresis and a positive Babinski sign on
the left. He was disoriented and sleepy. Electroencephalogram and angiography
indicated a large inoperable tumour in the right temporal region.
He died four weeks after admission of central respiratory paralysis.
Autopsy: showed a diffuse growing glioma, extending over the corpus
callosum and the fornix into both occipital lobes. The other organs were
normal.
Microscopic study: Glioblastoma consisting of small cells.
Diagnosis: Glioblastoma of the posterior corpus callosum.

Case 2

History: This cashier was admitted to hospital at the age of 59 years.
Three months prior to admission he had bumped his head (frontal, right) and
two days later he suffered from headache. Five weeks thereafter he complained
of nausea, vomiting, vertigo, calculation and concentration disturbances, and
temporary dullness.
On examination he had bilateral papilloedema, left facial paresis, amnestic
aphasia and acalculia. During electroencephalography the patient had a
generalized convulsion. Ventriculography showed a slight displacement of the
ventricle system to the right.
At operation a tumour in the left parieto-occipital region was subtotally
removed.
Postoperative course was good. The patient died one year later.
Autopsy: Not performed.
Microscopic study: Glioblastoma fusiforme.
Diagnosis: Left parieto-occipital glioblastoma fusiforme.

Family: The mother died of tuberculosis, the father of heart failure.
Seven siblings were alive and well.

VII.B.1.17. <u>Grosz and Plaschkes 1960 - Tel-Aviv, Israel</u> (86)

A brother and sister.

Case 1 (brother)

<u>History</u>: This man was a musical prodigy and was very young when he had established himself as a concert violonist and a teacher at the conservatory of music. At the age of 29 years he became withdrawn and reclusive. The family noticed musical deterioration and he lost social contact. At the age of 50 years *he began to show attacks of twitching at the right corner of his mouth and developed impairment of speech.*
On examination *there was a slight paresis of the buccal portion of the facial nerve on the right, of the right palatal arc and a slight deviation of the outstretched tongue to the left.* His speech difficulty was *not of an aphasic nature but consisted rather of a certain bradylalia and indistinctness of speech. His skull was of a pointed shape.* Electroencephalogram and pneumence-phalogram were indicative of a cerebral tumour. *On ventriculography, the tumor was located in the posterior part of the left temporal lobe.*
At craniotomy *the tumor was found in the posterior part of the left temporal lobe* and partially removed.
Postoperatively there was a complete hemiplegia on the right. The patient was given roentgen irradiation and died two months later.

    <u>Autopsy</u>: Was not performed.
    <u>Microscopic study</u>: Glioblastoma multiforme.
    <u>Diagnosis</u>: Left temporal glioblastoma multiforme.

Case 2 (sister)

<u>History</u>: At the age of 32 years this female, *who had always been healthy physically as well as mentally,* had started complaining of headaches, vomiting and impairment of speech.
On examination she showed aphasia.
After a long period of observation a craniotomy was performed ... and a *cerebral tumor was found* ....
Postoperatively there was hemiplegia and aphasia.
She died a few months later in Vienna, 22 years prior to the death of her brother.

    <u>Microscopic study</u>: The tumour was histologically diagnosed as a glioma.
    <u>Diagnosis</u>: Left temporal glioma.

Family: Both patients came from a well-known family of musicians. The
father was a professional violinist and his father also had been a musician.
The brothers of the mother also had been musicians. All five children of
this family were highly talented musicians from their earliest youth.

COMMENT

No further details on the histological structure of the tumour of case 2 are
available in the article. The sister had died 22 years earlier than the
brother in Vienna in a private sanatorium. She had been under the observation
of one of the authors at that time and he recalled the information concerning
this case.

VII.B.1.18. Symonds 1960 - London, England (259)

A brother and sister. English.

Case 1 (brother)

History: This man was admitted to hospital at the age of 35 years. He was
a scientific worker of high intelligence with no previous evidence of mental
abnormality. In the fortnight before his admission he had *several attacks of*
an epileptic character. During this period he had also developed symptoms
which, on admission, were indistinguishable from those of a schizophrenic
psychosis.
On examination he showed *incongruity of thought ar.d affect, thought disorder,*
and bizarre delusional ideas ... without ... any clouding of consciousness.
Subsequently he became drowsy, with signs suggesting a left frontal tumour,
and he died a fortnight after his admission to hospital after ventriculography
and biopsy.
Autopsy: *a tumour was found involving the corpus callosum and extending*
forward into the left frontal lobe.
Microscopic study: Glioblastoma.
Diagnosis: Glioblastoma of the corpus callosum and left frontal lobe.

Case 2 (sister)

History: This female was a school-teacher with no mental abnormality. At
the age of 34 years she came under medical care *on account of occasional epi-*
leptic seizures. In the course of time physical signs developed, leading to
the diagnosis of a left posterior frontal tumour, and five years after the
first symptom an exploratory craniotomy ... revealed an infiltrating glioma
in this situation.
After the operation she rapidly developed symptoms of mental disorder, and
was transferred to a mental hospital .... The mental disorders were *typical*
of a schizophrenic psychosis.
Microscopic study: Oligodendroglioma.
Diagnosis: Left posterior frontal oligodendroglioma.

Family: No information regarding the family is reported.

VII.B.1.19. <u>Koch and Middendorf 1960 - Münster, Germany</u> (131)

Three sisters. German.

Case 1

<u>History</u>: At the age of 54 years this housewife was admitted to hospital. She complained of headaches for ten weeks, forgetfulness for 2 weeks, and temporary confusion. Two weeks before admission she started vomiting and suffered a collapse.

On examination she was disoriented. There was an obvious adjusting nystagmus with rotatory component. Funduscopy revealed papilloedema, more on the right than on the left. A right facial paresis and slight spastic paresis of the right arm and leg with high tendon reflexes were found. Gordon and Oppenheim signs were positive and there was a dysdiadochokinesis on the right. An electroencephalogram showed moderate diffuse disturbances, and focal dys-rhythmia right temporo-parietal. A right carotid angiography indicated a deep tumour in the posterior part of the frontal and the parietal lobe with infil-tration into the posterior third of the corpus callosum.

The following days the patient deteriorated progressively and died six days after admission.

<u>Autopsy</u>: Not performed.

<u>Diagnosis</u>: Infiltrating tumour on the dorsal part of the right frontal and parietal lobe (probably a glioblastoma multiforme).

Case 2

<u>History</u>: At the age of 51 years this housewife was admitted to hospital because of sudden illness followed by loss of consciousness.

On examination she was unconscious and had tonic-clonic spasms. The pupils were wide and did not respond to light or convergence. There was a positive Babinski sign on the left. The next weeks the patient made a good recovery and was discharged home. Ten days later she complained of sudden headaches and nausea, and was readmitted.

On examination she had obvious bilateral papilloedema, positive Babinski sign on the right, and deviation of gait to the right. A sleep EEG showed irritative potentials praecentral and frontal. Ventriculography and angiography revealed an intracerebral tumour deep in the right temporal lobe.

A right temporal trepanation was performed and a tumour was found extending to the sphenoidal wing and medially to the basal ganglia. The tumour was partially removed.

The patient died one day after operation from elevated intracranial pressure.

Autopsy: Not performed.

Microscopic study: Glioblastoma multiforme.

Diagnosis: Right temporal glioblastoma multiforme.

Case 3

History: This charwoman was admitted to hospital at the age of 50 years. At school she had been a feeble-minded pupil. She started complaining of progressive headaches a day before admission and the next day suddenly vomited and later lost consciousness. A few weeks earlier she had been somewhat confused for some days.

On examination she was unconscious and had a conjugate gaze to the left. She recovered but a few days later the same symptoms recurred. There was papilloedema on both sides and a slight anisocoria, left greater than right. The deep tendon reflexes were elevated on the right. Coordination on the right was slightly disturbed. Orientation was impaired and the patient was apathetic.

An electroencephalogram showed focal left temporal disturbances. Left carotid angiography showed the anterior cerebral artery pushed over the median line and the middle cerebral artery displaced upwards.

At operation a large, soft, cystical tumour was found in the left temporal lobe and also infiltrating into parts of the brain stem.

Postoperatively the patient gradually deteriorated, and died a few days thereafter.

Autopsy: Not performed.

Microscopic study: Glioblastoma multiforme.

Diagnosis: Left temporal glioblastoma multiforme.

Family: At the time of the report the mother was still alive (78 years) and had suffered from diabetes at older age. The father died at the age of 79 years of severe arteriosclerosis cerebri. Neurological or mental disturbances could not be discovered in the family. Two brothers had died at the age of 2 years of unmentioned cause. The first sister had 2 healthy children, the second sister four. The third sister was not married and had no children.

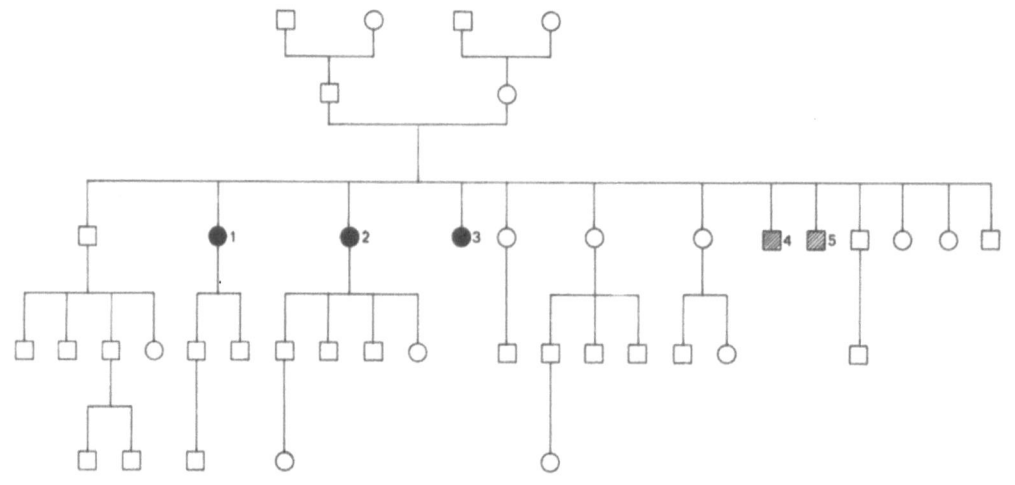

1 = case 1

2 = case 2

3 = case 3

4 + 5 = died at the age
        of 2 years

COMMENT

The diagnosis of the tumour in case 1 was not histologically verified.
The disease began in all three sisters in the beginning or shortly after
the beginning of the menopause.

VII.B.1.20. <u>Parkinson and Hall 1962 - Winnipeg, Canada</u> (195)

Two brothers. Canadian.

<u>Case 1</u>

<u>History</u>: This farmer was admitted to hospital at the age of 39 years. He *had been having grand mal seizures for approximately 6 years. For 2 weeks he had been complaining of severe headaches and his relatives noted a progressive decrease in his level of consciousness.*
On examination *there was no response to voice but the patient responded briskly to light painful stimuli and equally so from either side of the body. There were no lateralizing signs* .... Radiographs of his skull were normal. *An electroencephalogram gave abnormally slow waves from both hemispheres but more pronounced from the left than the right. Left carotid angiography revealed ... displacement of the anterior cerebral artery ....*
At operation *neoplastic tissue was disclosed along the surface adjacent to the falx ... and beneath the tumor was a cyst containing ... dark yellow fluid ....* *All visible neoplastic tissue was removed ....*
The patient made a good recovery and was dismissed from the hospital in a symptom free condition.
<u>Microscopic study</u>: Histological diagnosis was oligodendroglioma.
<u>Diagnosis</u>: Left frontal oligodendroglioma.

<u>Case 2</u>

<u>History</u>: This 35-year old labourer was admitted to hospital in coma. His history indicated that he had been examined five years earlier in another hospital *because of grand mal seizures with an aura of a peculiar feeling of well being which was followed closely by a feeling of faintness. Lately he had complained of progressive headache and blurring of vision and his associates noted increasing drowsiness and frequent vomiting.*
On examination the patient was *stuporous, responding to spoken voice only if aroused with painful stimuli previously. He had bilateral acute papilledema with multiple hemorrhages. Films of the skull revealed calcification above, in front, and to the left of the tuberculum sellae. Left carotid angiography suggested a space-occupying lesion on the left and ventriculography localized a mass near the mid-line in the left frontal lobe.*
At operation *neoplastic tissue was disclosed between the left carotid artery and the chiasm.* There was extension of the tumour into the third and lateral ventricles. The tumour was removed widely but *it was felt that a complete*

removal was not obtained.

Postoperatively the patient made a gradual recovery. *He was given deep roentgen-ray therapy* .... At the time of the report he had *poor memory for distant and recent events* but was caring for himself although at that time *not earning a living.*

Microscopic study: Histological diagnosis was oligodendroglioma. Some areas showed *more activity indistinguishable from that of highly malignant gliomas of the astrocytic series.*

Diagnosis: Subfrontal oligodendroglioma extending in third and lateral ventricles.

Family: No information concerning the family is given in the article.

VII.B.1.21. Metzel 1963 - Freiburg, Germany (170)

Two brothers. German.

Case 1

History: This boy was hospitalized with symptoms of acute elevated intracranial pressure, and died shortly thereafter.

Autopsy: A tumour was found in the right hemisphere occluding Monroe's
foramen.

Microscopic study: A histological diagnosis of ependymoma was made.

Diagnosis: Ependymoma of the right hemisphere.

Case 2

History: This 9-year-old boy was admitted to hospital because of vomiting
and frontal headaches of a year duration. Two days prior to admission he
suffered from short extension spasms, and a disturbance of gait was noticed.
On examination the child was restless and dazed, and there was a deviation of
the head to the left. A left-sided hemisyndrome with pyramidal tract signs was
found.
A right-sided ventricle drain was placed, improving the level of consciousness.
Ventriculography showed an internal hydrocephalus with a large tumour mass in
the right ventricle, extending over the midline.
Definitive atrio-ventricular drainage was made, which some time later became
obstructed.
The patient died with signs of an elevated intracranial pressure.

Autopsy: Was not permitted.

Microscopic study: The cytological examination of the cerebrospinal fluid
was compatible with a diagnosis of ependymoma.

Diagnosis: Ependymoma of the right ventricle.

Family: The mother suffered from seizures until her first pregnancy. The
grandmother (mother's side) was said to be mentally deteriorated.

COMMENT

The diagnosis of case 2 was based on the cytological examination of the
cerebrospinal fluid, which gives no definite proof of the histological
diagnosis. According to the authors in their discussion, the age of the boy
of case 1 must have been approximately the same as his brother of case 2.

VII.B.1.22. <u>Metzel 1964 - Freiburg, Germany</u> (171)

A brother and sister. German.

In this article the author describes a patient with an arachnoidal cyst in
the cisterna magna who was operated upon at the age of 19 years. His mother
died at the age of 28 years of a histologically verified ependymoma of the
fourth ventricle. Her brother was operated upon in the same year as the son
because of a glioblastoma.
No further information is mentioned in the article concerning these two cases.

The author made a study of 393 patients with brain tumours of the glioma
group - also containing 21 medulloblastomas - and found familial occurrence
in siblings in three cases. Apart from the above mentioned case two pairs of
brothers with astrocytomas and ependymomas were also discovered. No further
data are given concerning these cases, for which reason they are not registered
in the table separately.

VII.B.1.23. <u>Armstrong and Hanson 1969 - Toronto, Canada</u> (10)

Two brothers and a sister. Canadian.

Case 1 (brother)

History: This man was admitted to hospital at the age of 64 years. *As board chairman of a manufacturing concern, he had, for several months, noted difficulty with recall of names and business information* ... and *he had felt 'fatigued'.*

On examination the patient was *inattentive and had obvious difficulty with simple tests of memory and in following instruction* .... *Right ptosis was present and had been noted by the patient for many years. There was weakness of the left lower face and the left tendon jerks were brisker than the right. The left leg was weak.*

Roentgenograms of the skull were normal. *The EEG showed disorganization of normal activity over the right hemisphere and slowing over the right posterior and midtemporal region. Pertechnetate brain scan and angiography demonstrated a mass lesion in the right temporal lobe.*

At operation *a large amount of tumor mass was removed from the right temporal lobe.*

The patient died at home several months later.

Autopsy: Not performed.

Microscopic study: The tumour was interpreted as a malignant astrocytoma grade II to III.

Diagnosis: Right temporal astrocytoma grade II to III.

Case 2 (brother)

History: This man was admitted to hospital at the age of 50 years, *following the sudden onset of a right hemiplegia.*

On examination *he was stuporous and aphasic.* Roentgenograms of the skull were normal. *Pneumoencephalogram demonstrated a left-sided mass lesion.*

At operation a tumour was found in the left posterior temporal lobe.

Following operation the patient deteriorated, and died a few months later.

Autopsy: Not performed.

Microscopic study: Astrocytoma grade II to III.

Diagnosis: Left temporal astrocytoma grade II to III.

Case 3 (sister)

History: This woman was admitted to hospital at the age of 57 years. *She had complained of headache for a week prior to admission. The day of admission*

254

she had an episode of dizziness, vomiting and syncope.

Roentgenograms of the skull were normal. *Arteriography demonstrated a mass lesion of the right hemisphere.*

At craniotomy a biopsy was taken from the right temporal lobe.

The patient died shortly after surgery.

    Autopsy: Not performed.

    Microscopic study: Astrocytoma grade II to III.

    Diagnosis: Right temporal astrocytoma grade II to III.

    Family: There were six other siblings who were alive and in good health. The family history is unremarkable.

VII.B.1.24. Baughman et al. 1969 - Grand Rapids, Mich., U.S.A. (18)

Two brothers and two sisters. American.

Case 1 (sister)

History: This 12-year-old girl was admitted to hospital *2 weeks after a seizure involving the right arm and leg. She also complained of frontal headache and diarrhea.*
On examination *there was a single café-au-lait spot on the back and a pigmented nevus on the right leg. There was bilateral papilledema but no other neurologic abnormalities. An electroencephalogram was diffusely abnormal.* Ventriculography at first showed only slight dilatation of the lateral and third ventricles, but two months later ventriculography *delineated left temporo-thalamic and right thalamic mass lesions.*
Bilateral subtemporal decompression and biopsy was followed by cobalt therapy.
Diarrhea persisted and a sigmoidoscopy disclosed *2 polyps in the rectal ampulla and a villus adenoma located 10 cm above the anal ring.*
The patient died two years after operation.

Autopsy: *There were no additional bowel lesions. The larger polyp showed both villus hyperplasia and clusters of atypical cells invading the muscularis mucosa. Brain sections revealed a well circumscribed, infiltrating tumor of the white matter of both hemispheres.*

Microscopic study: *The histological diagnosis was glioblastoma multiforme. There was also an increased population of hyperchromatic glial cells in the medulla and in sections from the dorsal spinal cord. The tumor seemed multicentric.*

Diagnosis: Glioblastoma multiforme of the white matter of both hemispheres; polyposis of the colon.

Case 2 (brother)

History: This 25-year-old man was admitted to hospital because of *seizures and a progressive right hemiparesis. Five years previously he had undergone surgery for carcinoma of the colon.*
On examination *pigmented nevi were abundant over the back and abdomen. There was a mild right hemiparesis and dysphasia. ... chromosome analysis from leukocyte culture was within normal limits. The brain scan and left carotid arteriogram delineated a tumor of the left temporal lobe.*
The patient died approximately one year later.

Autopsy: *showed approximately 2 dozen polyps ... in the colon and rectum.*

Brain sections disclosed an infiltrating tumor beginning at the level of the head of the caudate nucleus and spreading through the isthmus of the temporal lobe into the white matter of the temporal lobe proper.

Microscopic study: Two polyps were examined. *One showed polypoid hyperplasia, and the other malignant change, with a formation of signet cells invading the stump.* The histologic diagnosis of the brain tumour was glioblastoma multiforme.

Diagnosis: Left temporal glioblastoma multiforme;
polyposis of the colon.

Case 3 (brother)

History: This 12-year-old boy was admitted to hospital because of *convulsions, headaches with vomiting and diplopia.*
On examination *four café-au-lait spots were noted. He had bilateral papilledema and a mild right hemiparesis and dysphasia. X-ray study showed separation of suture lines; ventriculography demonstrated a left fronto-parietal mass.*
At craniotomy a *subcortical, grayish-red cystic tumor* was found.
He died 3 months later at home.

Autopsy: Not performed.
Microscopic study: *The histologic diagnosis was glioblastoma multiforme.*
Diagnosis: Left fronto-parietal subcortical glioblastoma multiforme.

Case 4 (sister)

History: This 21-year-old woman was admitted to hospital *after 2 generalized seizures.*
An electroencephalogram showed slow and sharp activity from the left hemisphere, but a brain scan, pneumoencephalography, spinal-fluid analysis, barium-enema study and sigmoidoscopy were negative.
Four months later she was readmitted and examination then showed bilateral papilloedema. *A brain scan and left carotid arteriogram indicated a left posterior frontal tumor ....*
At operation this tumour was partially resected.
Sigmoidoscopic examination revealed *'2 tiny polyps, benign appearing, sessile ... 13 cm from the anal verge'.*

Microscopic study: The histologic diagnosis of the brain tissue was glioblastoma multiforme.

Diagnosis: Left frontal glioblastoma multiforme;
two polyps of the colon.

Family: The medical histories of 76 family members of five generations were investigated. One additional case of brain tumour was ascertained. This was a posterior-fossa ependymoma in a three-year-old girl, a maternal second cousin of the siblings. There were no additional cases of polyposis and no occurrence of neurofibromatosis.

The father and mother and two sisters were in good health and there was no consanguinity.

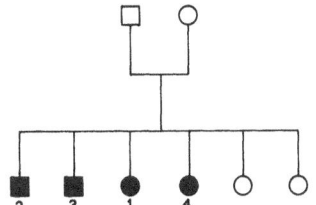

1 = case 1
2 = case 2
3 = case 3
4 = case 4

COMMENT

This family manifests the so-called glioma-polyposis syndrome, a disease with a possible autosomal recessive mode of transmission (see discussion of familial aspects). Three of the siblings had café-au-lait spots and pigmented naevi, suggesting a relationship with central neurofibromatosis. Remarkably, glioblastoma was found occurring in all four siblings at an early age.

VII.B.1.25. Blaauw and Schenk 1971 - Rotterdam, The Netherlands (27)

Two brothers. Dutch.

Case 1

History: This 21-year-old male was admitted to hospital *because of fever and a tender neck*. He was known to have a factor VIII-deficiency and *had 6 previous admissions for bleeding episodes from the mouth and retroperitoneally, and for haemarthrosis and haematuria. Six years prior to this admission he was treated with bedrest for pain and stiffness of the neck.*
On examination *there was a Horner's syndrome on the left side. The abdominal reflexes were diminished on the left side. The left knee and ankle jerks were increased and the left plantar response was extensor. In the next 5 days he developed a partial transverse cord lesion at the lower cervical level. Lumbar puncture yielded yellow CSF containing no cells, protein 243 mg/100 ml. Ascending myelography revealed a total block of the contrast medium at T_1.*
At operation *the spinal cord protruded markedly. Its diameter was much increased and it was greenish-blue. Upon puncture in the midline a few drops of viscous blood were obtained.*
Postoperatively the spinal cord lesion showed no improvement. *A second and fatal haemorrhage occurred on the 13th postoperative day.*

Autopsy: *The cord was swollen and this swelling ended inferiorly far below the site of operation.* The brain was *exceptionally large and heavy ....*

Microscopic study:

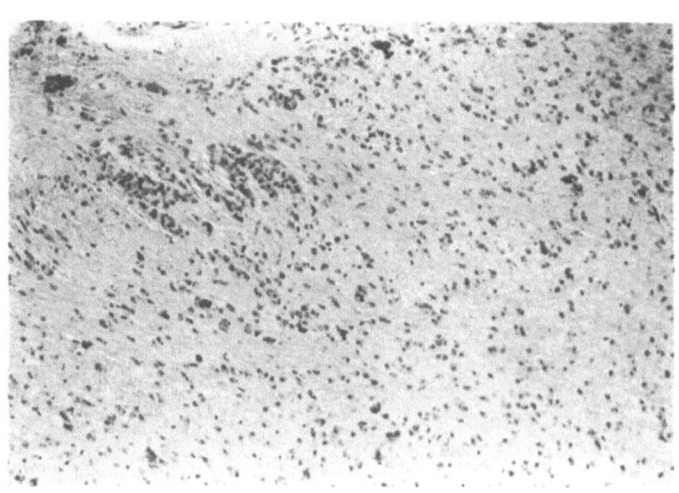

Fig. 1.
Microscopic
appearance
of tumour of
case 1.
FE.

*Sagittal section showed an uninterrupted haemorrhage, extending into the
lumbar cord .... In the superior cervical cord the central canal was very wide.
It was surrounded by a glial mantle .... In the lower cervical segments gliomatous tissue surrounded the central canal.* At the site of operation a large
blood clot filled a wide cavity which was ruptured dorsally. The clot continued
caudal until L_1. *In the lumbar cord a central core of gliomatous tissue was
found with irregular features of ependyma. The brain revealed an occasional
punctate haemorrhage, and oedematous swelling of the intercellular material.*

Diagnosis: Cervical subependymoma. Syringomyelia. Factor VIII-deficiency
(haemophilia).

Case 2

History: This male was admitted to hospital at the age of 18 years. *He
awoke ... with a tender neck and shoulders. Approximately 11 hr later he
experienced burning pain in the back of the neck, which was quickly followed
by progressive weakness of arms and legs. He had noted some weakness of the
left hands for a few months.* The patient was known to have a factor VIII-
deficiency and had four prior admissions for haemarthrosis, retroperitoneal
bleeding, and haematuria.
On examination *there was flaccid quadriplegia. He had diaphragmatic respiration.
The reflexes from the trunk and extremities could not be elicited. There was
priapism and retention of urine. Lumbar puncture yielded colourless CSF
containing no cells, protein 195 mg/100 ml. Ascending myelography showed a
total block of the contrast medium at T_1.*
At operation *the canal seemed to be very wide, giving the impression of a
chronic process. ... a swollen cord was found with appearances of intramedullary
tumour. A biopsy was taken.*
Postoperatively there was no improvement of the transverse cord lesion and the
patient died in shock from a massive intestinal haemorrhage on the 19th postoperative day.

Autopsy: *the spinal cord was extremely swollen* and *in some parts there were
fresh haemorrhages.*

Microscopic study: *In the mid-cervical region there was a tumour in the
posterior parts of the cord. It consisted of spindle-shaped cells and cells
resembling ependyma. Some gial cells were seen. A syringomyelic cyst was not
seen.*

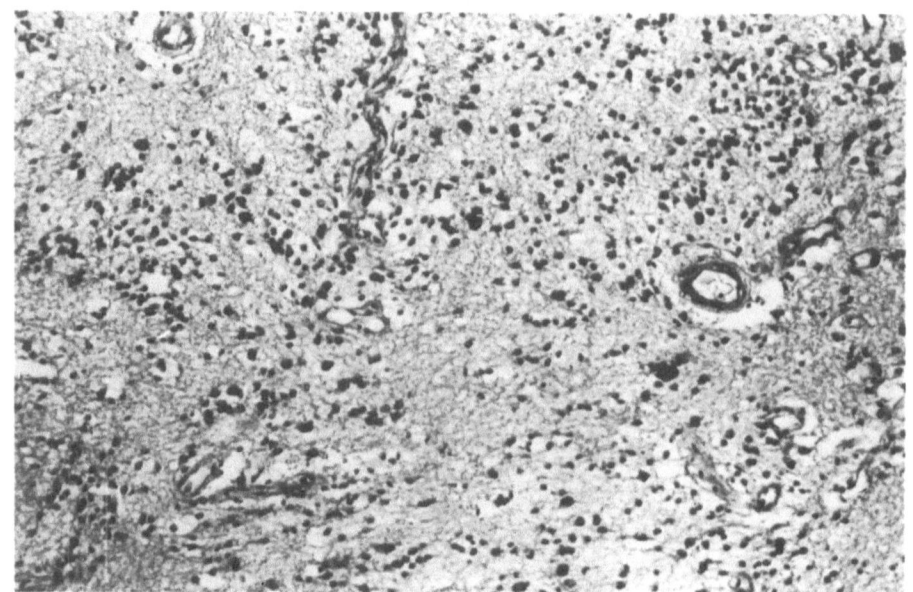

Fig. 2. Microscopic appearance of tumour of case 2.
HE.
(Blaauw G, Schenk VWD 1971 (27))

Diagnosis: Mid-cervical subependymoma. Factor VIII-deficiency (haemophilia).

Family: There were other relatives with haemophilia in the family.

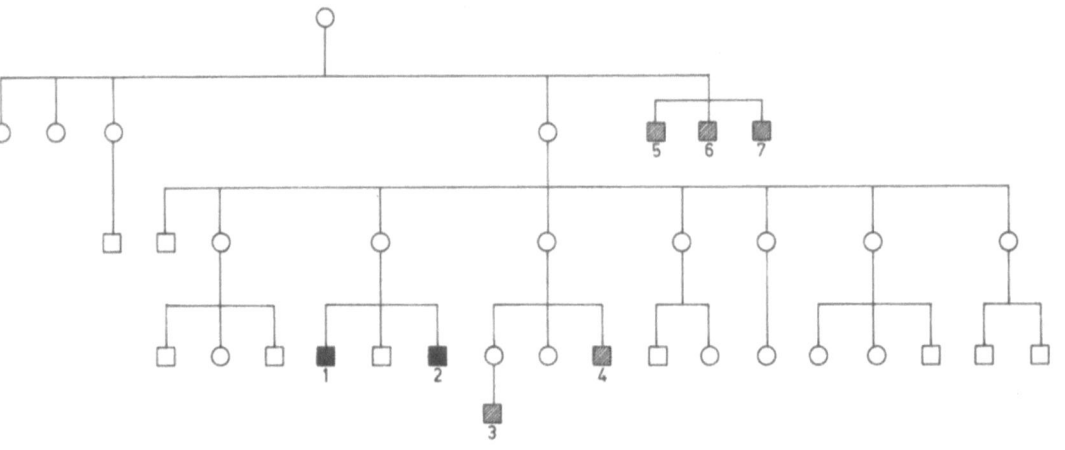

1 = case 1;   2 = case 2;   3 - 7 = haemophiliacs

COMMENT

In both cases the presence of a cord tumour was not suspected prior to operation. In these cases there is a coincidence of familial occurrence of subependymoma with another familial disease (haemophilia).

VII.B.1.26. Kaufman and Brisman 1972 - New York, U.S.A. (116)

Two brothers. American.

Case 1

History: This 38-year-old man was hospitalized because of *difficulty with speech and right-sided weakness.*
Examination suggested a deep left cerebral mass lesion which was confirmed by pneumoencephalography and arteriography.
The patient was treated with radiotherapy and cytostatic drugs with transient improvement.
He died 9 months later.

Autopsy: A tumour was found involving structures from the left thalamus to the brain stem.

Microscopic study: Cystic glioblastoma multiforme.

Diagnosis: Glioblastoma multiforme from left thalamus to the brain stem.

Case 2

History: This 50-year-old man was hospitalized *with a history of right cerebellar and cranial nerve symptoms and signs which were confirmed on examination.*
Arteriography and ventriculography suggested a mass in the right cerebellar hemisphere.
Suboccipital craniectomy revealed a tumour in the right cerebellar hemisphere. The patient died 3 weeks postoperatively.

Autopsy: A tumour was found in the right cerebellar hemisphere involving the brain stem.

Microscopic study: Glioblastoma multiforme with histological characteristics comparable with those of case 1.

Diagnosis: Cerebellar glioblastoma multiforme.

Family: A detailed family pedigree was obtained (see figure).
The mother of the siblings had diabetes mellitus and died at the age of 76 years. The father had emphysema and died at 69 years. There were three other siblings. One brother had diabetes, the other had gout. The sister suffered from migraine.

262

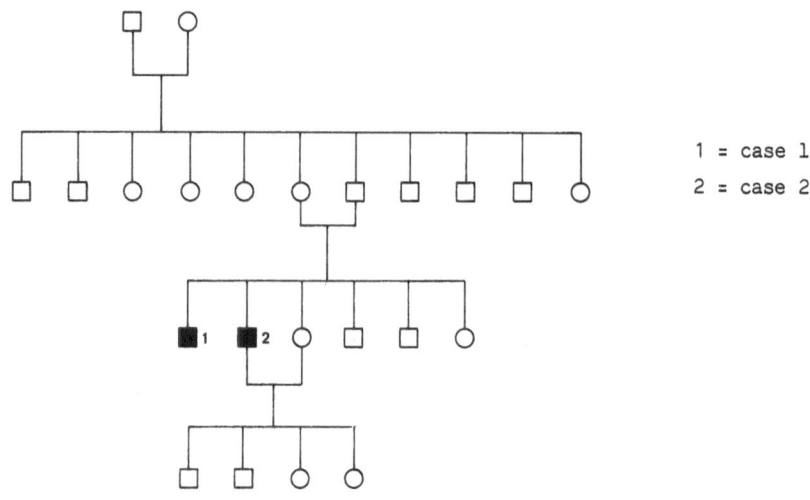

1 = case 1
2 = case 2

COMMENT

The article also mentions two first cousins with brain tumour. One had a
malignant astrocytoma of the lower brain stem, the other a relatively benign
cystic cerebellar astrocytoma (see other generations and distant relatives).

VII.B.1.27. <u>Isamat et al. 1974 - Barcelona, Spain</u> (109)

Two sisters. Spanish.

Case 1

<u>History</u>: The onset of symptoms occurred at a similar age in both sisters.
The patient had blood-group A. No further details are described.
She was operated on in the anterior part of the third ventricle at the age
of 55 years.

<u>Microscopic study</u>: Astrocytoma.

<u>Diagnosis</u>: Astrocytoma of anterior third ventricle.

Case 2

<u>History</u>: This patient had blood-group A.
She was operated on a postfrontal tumour at the age of 57 years.

<u>Microscopic study</u>: Astrocytoma grade III.

<u>Diagnosis</u>: Postfrontal astrocytoma grade III.

<u>Family</u>: No information is given concerning the family.

COMMENT

These two siblings are described in a report on six families with intracranial gliomas. The age at death was not mentioned in the article.

VII.B.1.28. <u>Isamat et al. 1974 - Barcelona, Spain</u> (109)

Two brothers. Spanish.

<u>Case 1</u>

<u>History</u>: This patient had blood-group A. The onset of symptoms occurred at a similar age as his brother.

He was operated on a bifrontal corpus callosum tumour at the age of 49 years. No further information is given in the article.

<u>Microscopic study</u>: Astrocytoma grade IV.

<u>Diagnosis</u>: Bifrontal astrocytoma grade IV of the corpus callosum.

<u>Case 2</u>

<u>History</u>: This brother also had blood-group A.

He was operated on a temporal brain tumour at the age of 48 years.

<u>Microscopic study</u>: Astrocytoma grade IV.

<u>Diagnosis</u>: Temporal astrocytoma grade IV.

<u>Family</u>: A nephew of the affected siblings *had an aqueductal stenosis, presumably due to gliosis*.

<u>COMMENT</u>

These two brothers are mentioned in a report on six families with intracranial gliomas. The age at death was not mentioned in the article.

VII.B.1.29. Schoenberg et al. 1975 - Rochester (Minn.), U.S.A. (327)

A brother and two sisters. American.

Case 1 (brother)

    History: This 12-year-old boy was admitted to hospital because of *frontal headaches and intermittent diplopia for six weeks and nausea and vomiting for three days* ....

On examination a *paresis of the left superior oblique muscle and bilateral papilledema* was found. A ventriculogram showed *features of a tumor on the dorsal surface of the aqueduct of Sylvius. A biopsy was not done because of the location of the mass.*

A bilateral Torkelson ventriculocisternostomy relieved his symptoms for several months, but progressive neurologic deterioration then ensued.

He died 1 1/2 years after the onset of symptoms.

    Autopsy: Not performed.

    Diagnosis: Brain tumour on the dorsal surface of the aqueduct of Sylvius.

Case 2 (sister)

    History: This 6-year-old girl was admitted to hospital because of *a generalized tonic-clonic seizure with focal onset involving the left lower extremity.* She *had a history of a generalized convulsion at the age of two years* ....

On examination bilateral early papilloedema was found and electroencephalography *showed slowing in the right temporoparietal area.*

At craniotomy a tumour was removed with excision of a large portion of the right parietal and posterior temporal lobes. *The patient did not receive radiation therapy.*

On discharge her only neurological defect was a left homonymous visual field defect.

At the age of 21 years *she had intermittent diplopia and a generalized seizure.* Neurological examination was normal except for the visual field defect. Computerized tomography and angiography showed a mass in the right temporo-parietal area.

At craniotomy *subtotal removal of a cystic tumor was performed. The cystic element extended into the right lateral ventricle and the ventricular wall was studded with tumor nodules.*

The patient received radiation therapy and was doing well three months later.

    Microscopic study: The tumour from the first operation was diagnosed as a grade II astrocytoma and that of the second operation as a grade III astrocytoma.

    Diagnosis: Right temporo-parietal astrocytoma, grade II and III.

266

Case 3 (sister)

History: This 12-year-old girl was hospitalized because of progressive occipital headaches, and nausea and vomiting. She had previously *undergone excision of a presacral lipoma at the age of six years* ....
On examination papilloedema was found. *A left carotid angiogram revealed a left frontal lobe mass.*
At craniotomy the tumour was partially excised.
She received radiation therapy, but died a few months later.

Autopsy: Not performed.
Microscopic study: Grade III astrocytoma.
Diagnosis: Left frontal astrocytoma grade III.

Family: A fourth sibling, a brother, was operated upon because of a mediastinal cystic hydroma at the age of 9 years. The paternal grandfather died at the age of 68 years of *prostatic cancer* and the paternal grandmother died at the age of 36 years of *pneumonia and kidney disease*.
There was no known history of brain tumors in any other family members, nor was there any evidence suggestive of neurofibromatosis.

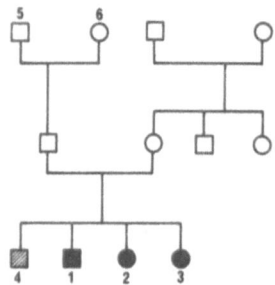

1 = case 1
2 = case
3 = case 3
4 = mediastinal cystic hydroma
5 = prostatic cancer
6 = kidney disease

VII.B.1.30. Li et al. 1977 - New Haven, U.S.A. (145)

Two brothers. White. American.
Unremarkable pregnancy and delivery at term.

Case 1

History: This 6-year-old Caucasian boy was admitted to hospital *for evaluation of headaches, vomiting, ataxia, and right abducens nerve palsy. History revealed prior excision of a 2 cm x 1 cm congenital nevoid scalp lesion, a meningocoele with vascular malformation ....*
Examination of peripheral blood and spinal fluid showed no leukemia or tumor cells. Ventriculogram demonstrated agenesis of the corpus callosum.
Craniotomy revealed at the floor of the fourth ventricle a tumor that could not be biopsied or resected. Glioma was diagnosed and brain irradiation initiated.
Two months postoperatively the patient developed *fever, anemia, abdominal masses, and skin nodules. Studies of the peripheral blood and bone marrow showed acute leukemia of a poorly differentiated cell-type.*
The patient died suddenly four days later.

Autopsy: Not performed.
Diagnosis: Glioma of the floor of the fourth ventricle;
          acute leukaemia.

Case 2

History: This 11-year-old Caucasian boy was hospitalized *because of an anterior mediastinal mass.*
Examination revealed a *cafe-au-lait spot on the right cheek, and several punctate flat pigmented nevi on the face and trunk. Peripheral blood and bone marrow ... were normal. Thoracotomy showed a diffuse, poorly differentiated lymphocytic lymphoma ....* Radiotherapy and chemotherapy were administered.
Four months later *while in clinical remission of lymphoma, the patient developed headache, vomiting, and bilateral abducens nerve palsies. Cerebral arteriogram showed a large frontal lobe mass* for which the patient was operated upon and a biopsy taken.
Postoperatively the patient was treated with radiotherapy and chemotherapy. He died eight months later with recurrent brain tumour.

Autopsy: Not performed.
Microscopic study: Glioblastoma multiforme.
Diagnosis: Glioblastoma multiforme of the frontal lobe;
          lymphocytic lymphoma.

Family: A 35-month-old brother of the two siblings (3) suffered from meylogenous leukaemia. He had *a small haemangioma on the right arm, and multiple yellowish raised skin lesions diagnosed by ... biopsy as nevoxanthoendothelioma.* He died *with cardiac failure, pulmonary infiltrates, and focal seizures with left hemiparesis.* No autopsy study was performed.

Another brother (4) died in the eleventh week of life *with cardiac malformations: dextroversion, anomalous pulmonary venous return with obstruction, and atrial septal defect. He may have been exposed to rubella in the second trimester of gestation. Soon after birth a ... squamous papilloma was excised from his abdomen.*

Both parents were in good health except for recurrent herpetic stomatitis in the mother, and infectious mononucleosis and polio during adolescence in the father. The parents showed absence of congenital malformations and skin lesions other than several raised moles in the mother. *The father had an uncle who died with myelofibrosis at age 59 years, and several distant relatives who reportedly had cancer. There was no parental consanguinity.*

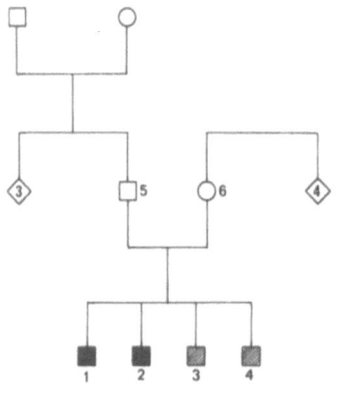

1 = case 1 (glioma, acute leukaemia meningocoele)

2 = case 2 (glioblastoma multiforme, lymphocytic lymphoma, café-au-lait spots and pigmented naevi)

3 = brother with cardiac malformations and squamous papilloma

4 = brother with myelogenous leukaemia multiple nevoxanthoendotheliomata

5 = father had infectious mononucleosis and polio during adolescence

6 = mother had recurrent herpetic stomatitis and several small raised moles

COMMENT

The proband (case 2) and his parents showed no diagnostic laboratory character-istics of a familial syndrome with susceptibility to cancer. Chromosome analysis of the peripheral blood of each parent revealed isolated abnormalities: fragments, breaks, and aneuploidy. The mother had elevated nerve-growth stimu-lating activity which raised the possibility of Von Recklinghausen's neuro-fibromatosis, but she had no clinical evidence of the disease. The serologic

reactivity to cultured allogeneic human astrocytoma cells was increased in the
father, and SV-40 viral T-antigen expression in cultured skin fibroblasts of
both parents was increased. However, no definite oncogenic role could be
assigned to these findings. The parents showed no immunologic defects.
The familial tendency of childhood brain tumour aggregated with leukaemia or
lymphoma is suggested by this and also several other published reports.
Unfortunately, no histological verification of the tumour in case 1 was made
and diagnosis of glioma was made macroscopically at operation.
Perhaps this report on familial occurrence of multiple primary malignancies,
cardiac malformations and disorders of the skin must be regarded as a form of
Von Recklinghausen's neurofibromatosis or another underlying inherited
family cancer syndrome.

VII.B.1.31. Pelgrom von Motz et al. 1977 - The Hague, The Netherlands
             (200)

Three sisters. Dutch.

Case 1

   History: This 69-year-old woman was hospitalized *with complaints of general*
feebleness, right-sided headaches, and drowsiness.
On examination *consciousness was variably clouded. Slight left-sided facial*
paresis was present. There was weakness of the left arm and leg .... *The*
plantar response was extensor on the left. Dysdiadochokinesia and slight
dysmetria were present on the left. Skull X-rays were normal. *Electroencephalo-*
graphy, brain scan, and right carotid angiography revealed a voluminous fronto-
parietal lesion ....
The patient died 3 months later.

   Autopsy: *A voluminous tumor was found in the insular region of the right*
hemisphere, growing into the central nuclei ....

   Microscopic study: The appearance of the tumour was consistent with
astrocytoma grade III.

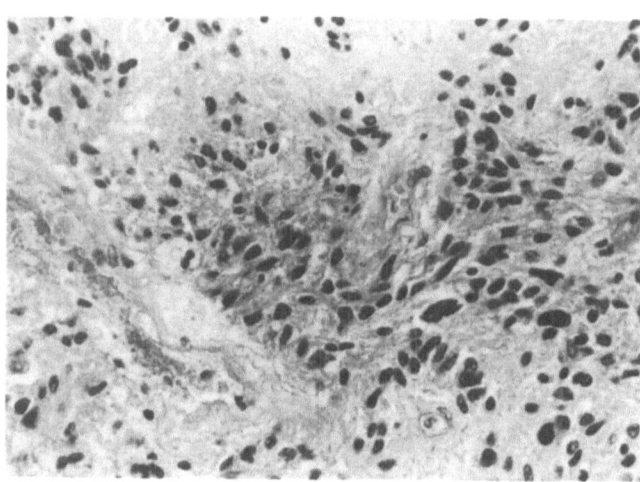

Fig. 1.
Microscopic appearance
of tumour of case 1.
HE.
(Pelgrom von Motz I,
Bots GTAM, Endtz LJ
1977 (200))

   Diagnosis: Astrocytoma grade III in the right insular region.

Case 2

   History: This nurse was admitted to hospital at the age of 53 years. *She*
complained of headache, nausea, and disturbances in the right visual field,

and had difficulty in picking up objects with the right hand. ... a gradual
psychic alteration had been noted for 1 or 2 years.
On examination no abnormalities were found *apart from slight dysdiadocho-*
kinesia on the right and some alteration of the position-sense of the right
foot. Skull radiography showed decalcification of the dorsum sellae. Electro-
encephalography, brain scan, and left carotid angiography showed a left-sided
mass in the parieto-occipital region on which she was operated.
Postoperatively the patient received radiotherapy.
Her condition deteriorated and she died a few months later.
Autopsy: Not performed.
Microscopic study: The general appearance was that of astrocytoma grade III.

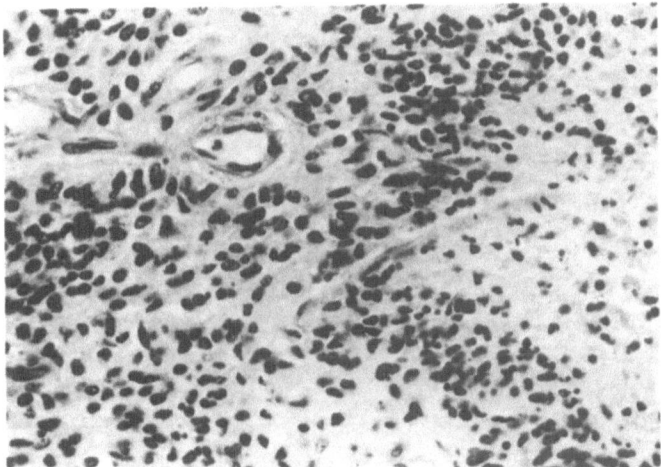

Fig. 2.
Microscopic appearance
of tumour of case 2.
HE.
(Pelgrom von Motz I,
Bots GTAM, Endtz LJ
1977 (200))

Diagnosis: Left parieto-occipital astrocytoma grade III.

Case 3

Diagnosis: This 73-year-old nurse was hospitalized because of a month long
difficulty in walking. *Six months previously she had been admitted to the*
same hospital for acute weakness of the right leg and arm and aphasia. She
recovered within a few days, and was discharged with the tentative diagnosis
of stroke.
On examination *orientation was defective. Slight right-sided facial paresis*
was present. Electroencephalography, brain scan, and bilateral carotid angio-
graphy revealed a voluminous left frontoparietal lesion and suggested another
mass in the right temporoparietal region.
The patient's condition rapidly deteriorated and she died one month later.

Autopsy: Two tumours were found, one in the right frontal region and the other in the left parietal region. *There was no direct connection between these two tumors.* No other abnormalities were found, apart from hyperplasia of the left adrenal.

Microscopic study: Both tumours were microscopically identical. The general appearance was consistent with astrocytoma grade III.

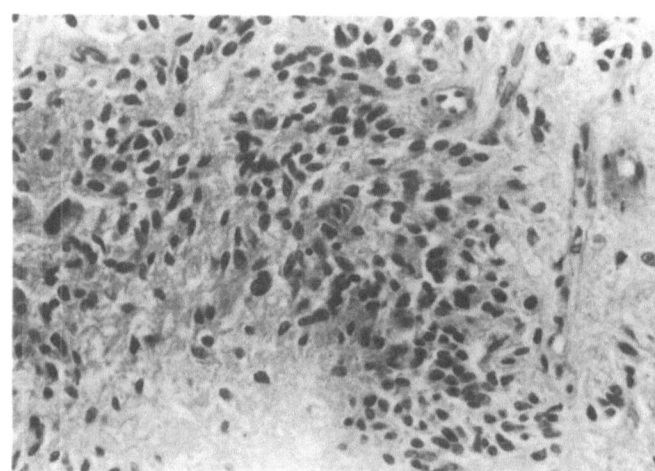

Fig. 3.
Microscopic appearance
of tumour of case 3.
HE.
(Pelgrom von Motz I,
Bots GTAM, Endtz LJ
1977 (200))

Diagnosis: Astrocytoma grade III, right frontal and left parietal.

Family: *Three brothers and three sisters, all older than 65, and the three children of case 1 were alive and in good health .... The two other affected sisters were childless. Malignancy seems to be over-represented in the family, but no other cases of brain tumor were known to the relatives.*
Two sisters of the father, in a family of eight siblings, had died of malignant diseases (carcinoma of the breast in one and carcinoma of the uterus in the other). Two of the 19 children of three brothers and one sister of the father had also died of malignant diseases (carcinoma of the lung and carcinoma of the breast). The grandfather had died of carcinoma of the stomach. The mother, one of three siblings, had died of esophageal carcinoma, and one of her brothers died of carcinoma of the stomach. The two brothers of the mother had seven children; one of these also had died of carcinoma of the stomach.
There was no consanguinity between the parents or grandparents, who did not stem from known isolated regions.

VII.B.1.32. De Tribolet et al. 1979 - Lausanne, Switzerland (265)

Two brothers. Swiss.

Case 1

History: This 50-year-old man was hospitalized after a two month period of speech difficulties, followed by right-sided weakness.

On examination *he presented with right sided hemiparesis, right homonymous hemianopia and motor aphasia. A left carotid angiogram revealed a left temporal mass.*

At operation the tumour was partially excised.

Postoperative course was complicated by brain oedema and the patient died two days later.

Autopsy: showed a tumour involving *the left temporal lobe, the thalamus, the mesencephalon and the pons.*

Microscopic study: the tumour consisted of *glial cells with considerable variations in size. Mitotic figures were abundant. Some areas contained gemistocytic astrocytes with single or multiple nuclei. There were extensive areas of necrosis.* A histological diagnosis of glioblastoma (glioma grade IV) was made.

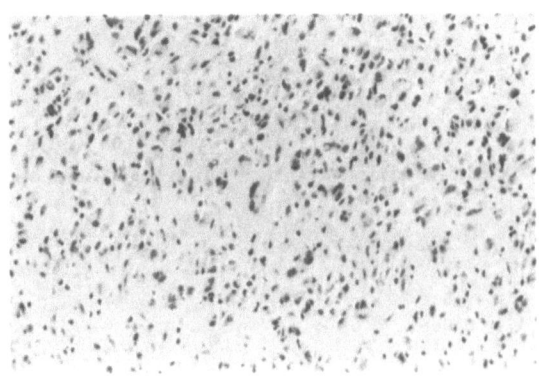

Fig. 1
Microscopic appearance
of tumour in case 1.
HE.
(De Tribolet N, Deruaz JP,
Zander E 1979
Neurochirurgia 22:225-228
Georg Thieme Verlag
Stuttgart)

Diagnosis: Left temporal glioblastoma.

Case 2

History: This man was hospitalized at the age of 69 years. He became *hemiparetic on the left side three weeks prior to admission.*

On examination he had a *left spastic hemiparesis with decreased sensation to pin-prick on the same side.* He was *somnolent and there was bilateral papill-oedema. Radioisotopic brain scan and bilateral carotid angiography showed a right temporal hypervascularized tumour.*

At operation this tumour was subtotally excised.

The patient died of pulmonary embolism 3 weeks later ....

Autopsy: *revealed involvement of the right temporal lobe ....*

Microscopic study: *the tissue was highly cellular with mitotic figures,* areas of necrosis and new vessel formation Gemistocytic astrocytes predomi-nated in some areas. The histological diagnosis was glioblastoma (glioma grade IV).

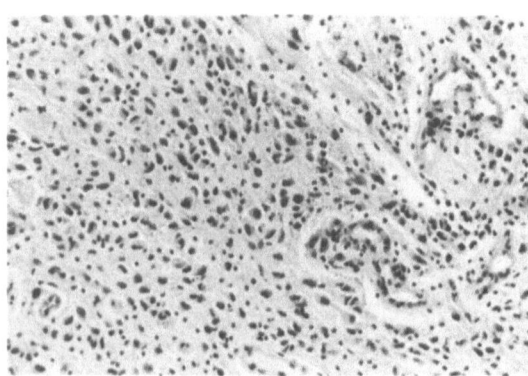

Fig. 2
Microscopic appearance
of tumour in case 2.
HE.
(De Tribolet N, Deruaz JP,
Zander E 1979
Neurochirurgia 22:225-228
Georg Thieme Verlag
Stuttgart)

Diagnosis: Right temporal glioblastoma.

Family: No information concerning the relatives is given in the article.

VII.B.1.33. Sulla et al. 1979 - Kosice, Czechoslovakia (257)

Two brothers. Czech.

Case 1

History: This electrical engineer was admitted to hospital at the age of
61 years. He had complained of progressive headaches and personality changes
during the previous month. Shortly after admission he had an epileptic seizure.
On examination a left hemiparesis was found. Carotid angiography revealed a
tumour mass with pathological vascularity in the right temporal lobe.
At craniotomy an infiltrating tumour found in the right temporal lobe was
partially resected.
The patient was discharged home, and died 6 weeks postoperatively.
    Autopsy: Not performed.
    Microscopic study: Astrocytoma grade II.
    Diagnosis: Right temporal astrocytoma grade II.

Case 2

History: This forest labourer was hospitalized at the age of 59 years. He
had complained of progressive headaches accompanied by psychic disturbances
for several months.
Carotid angiography revealed a tumour mass in the rostral part of the right
frontal lobe.
At craniotomy an infiltrating tumour in the right frontal lobe was partially
removed.
The patient died 3 weeks postoperatively.
    Autopsy: Not performed.
    Microscopic study: Astrocytoma grade III.
    Diagnosis: Right frontal astrocytoma grade III.

Family: The two brothers had 6 other siblings, all of whom were healthy.
Their father had died of pneumonia, their mother was healthy and alive (82
years). Both patients had four healthy children. No reports of relatives with
brain tumour or phacomatosis had been made.

COMMENT
Both patients had an AB, Rhesus positive blood-group.

276

VII.B.1.34. Schouwink 1980 - Arnhem, The Netherlands
             (personal communication)

Two brothers. Dutch.

Case 1

   History: This man was admitted to hospital at the age of 59 years. He
complained of attacks of abdominal pain and of pain in the right arm and leg,
accompanied by palpitations, perspiration and fear. His medical history showed
a luetic infection at the age of 22 and two admissions in a psychiatric hospital because of 'pre-tabes' symptoms that were treated with penicillin.
On examination narrow, irregular pupils were found that did not respond to
light. There was a slightly disturbed Romberg test, a dysarthric speech and
emotional unstableness. A beginning dementia was present. Deep tendon reflexes
were symmetrically low on both sides. The luetic reactions were positive.
Cerebrospinal fluid showed no other abnormalities than a slightly elevated
protein content and positive luetic reactions. The patient again received
antibiotic therapy.
In the course of a few months he gradually deteriorated an became apathetic
without developing other neurological symptoms.
He died a short time later of bronchopneumonia.
   Autopsy: A 4 centimetre in diameter, greyish tumour was found in the right
frontal lobe. No signs of tabo-paralysis were found.
   Microscopic study: A histological diagnosis of astrocytoma was made.
   Diagnosis: Right frontal astrocytoma.

Case 2

   History: This patient was admitted to hospital at the age of 51 years. He
had become unwell at his work and the diagnosis of apoplexia was made by a
consulting physician. In the weeks prior to admission he had become inactive
and irritable, and he had complained of headaches for two weeks.
On examination the patient was drowsy and confused, his speech was dysarthric.
There was slight ptosis, left more than right. The pupils were small and
responded slowly to light. There was a tetraparesis, more on the left than on
the right. Deep tendon reflexes were symmetrical. The electroencephalogram
showed a disturbance of the left frontal region. Angiography revealed a large
left frontal process.
Surgical therapy was decided upon, but the patient suddenly deteriorated with
high fever, and died a few days later.

<u>Autopsy</u>: A necrotic tumour was found in the left frontal lobe.

<u>Microscopic study</u>: Histological diagnosis was astrocytoma.

<u>Diagnosis</u>: Left frontal astrocytoma.

<u>Family</u>: A third brother died at a young age supposedly of a brain tumour, but no further data are known concerning this case.

A fourth brother complained of disturbances of balance and headaches for years, but on examination no disorder could be found.

No further information concerning relatives is available.

VII.B.1.35. Spit and Hoff 1980 - The Netherlands
             (personal communication)

A brother and sister. Dutch.

Case 1 (sister)

   History: This 64-year-old woman was admitted to hospital with a history of
acute left hemiparesis. She also complained of a tendency to fall to the left.
Her medical history revealed a chronic hypertension.
On examination she had a left hemiparesis and a left hemihypaesthesia. Deep
tendon reflexes were higher on the left than on the right. An electroencephalogram showed disturbances of both hemispheres, more on the right than on the left.
Carotid angiography revealed an obstruction of the right external carotid and no
further abnormalities. On computerized tomography a tumour was discovered in the
right thalamus and basal ganglia with extension into the temporal lobe.
At operation a tumour found in the right temporal lobe was totally removed.
Postoperatively the patient remained very apathetic, and died a short time
thereafter.
   Autopsy: Not performed.
   Microscopic study: Astrocytoma grade III to IV.
   Diagnosis: Right temporal astrocytoma grade III to IV.

Case 2 (brother)

   History: This 61-year-old man was hospitalized because of a left hemiparesis.
A brain tumour was diagnosed.
At operation a right frontal tumour was found and a subtotal right frontal
lobectomy was performed.
Postoperatively the patient received radiotherapy.
His condition gradually deteriorated in the following months and he died five
months postoperatively.
   Autopsy: No information is available.
   Microscopic study: Astrocytoma grade III.
   Diagnosis: Right frontal astrocytoma grade III.

   Family: No information concerning the family members is available.

VII.B.1.36. <u>Todd et al. 1981 - Fargo, U.S.A.</u> (263)

Two brothers and a sister. American.

<u>Case 1</u> (sister)

    <u>History</u>: *This 17-year-old girl ... presented with a glioblastoma multiforme in the left frontal lobe. Following surgery the patient initially did well and enrolled in college but then died at the age of 19 years ....*
There was no history or documentation of gastrointestinal problems.

    <u>Autopsy</u>: Not performed.

    <u>Microscopic study</u>: Glioblastoma multiforme.

    <u>Diagnosis</u>: Left frontal glioblastoma multiforme.

<u>Case 2</u> (brother)

    <u>History</u>: *This child ... presented at the age of 10 years with a two-month history of headaches and vomiting.*
Neurological examination and subsequent surgery revealed a cystic grade III astrocytoma of the right temporooccipital area.
One year later a partial colectomy was performed and *examination of the cecum and terminal ileum showed Hodgkin's disease. Another solitary lesion of the cecum was shown to be a true adenomatous polyp.*
The patient's neurological status gradually worsened, and he died at the age of 12 years.

    <u>Autopsy</u>: showed an extensive right temporo-parietal tumour with extension into the brain stem. *Several adenomatous polyps were present in the remaining portion of the ileum.*

    <u>Microscopic study</u>: Astrocytoma grade III.

    <u>Diagnosis</u>: Right temporo-parieto-occipital astrocytoma grade III.
                  Hodgkin's disease. Polyposis coli.

<u>Case 3</u> (brother)

    <u>History</u>: *This 18-year-old boy ... presented with a left cerebral glioblastoma multiforme.*
Postoperatively he received radiation therapy as well as CCNU.
One year later multiple benign adenomatous polyps of the colon were found.
... because of a carcinomatous change in one lesion, a right hemicolectomy was performed that revealed a mucinous adenocarcinoma of the ascending colon as well as multiple benign polyps.
At the age of 23 years the patient developed recurrent episodes of pneumonia and died.

<u>Autopsy</u>: *showed recurrent glioma in the left frontal lobe, multiple polyps in the ascending colon, and a chronic granulomatous pneumonia ....*

<u>Microscopic study</u>: Glioblastoma multiforme.

<u>Diagnosis</u>: Left frontal glioblastoma multiforme.

Polyposis coli.

<u>Family</u>: There were three siblings; case 1 was the eldest child, case 2 the second-born and case 3 the youngest. *The family history is negative for similar disease*. The father died of myocardial infarction, the mother was living and well. The siblings of the father and mother had no gastrointestinal or cerebral problems. The maternal grandfather died at 80 years of age of myocardial infarction, and at autopsy an incidental carcinoma of the stomach was discovered.

<u>COMMENT</u>

This family manifests the Turcot syndrome, i.e. the occurrence of polyposis coli with glioma or medulloblastoma (see also VII.B.1.24 and II.B.2.1). The authors state that the genetic pattern of this syndrome is uncertain. *An autosomal recessive trait is most probable but a dominant trait with variable expression cannot be excluded* (see also discussion on familial aspects).

VII.B.2.   SIBLINGS WITH DISCORDANT TUMOUR

VII.B.2.1.   Oehler 1936 - Münster, Germany (189)

Two brothers. German.

Case 1

   History: This left-handed man was admitted to hospital at the age of 29
years. He suffered from epileptic seizures for three years. For two years he
had also complained of vertigo, nausea, disturbances of gait and smell,
diminished vision and clumsiness.
On examination he had multiple pigmented naevi, and a papilloma on his tongue.
A right facial paresis and a slight right ptosis were present. There was
ataxia of the right arm and leg and a tendency to fall. Deep tendon reflexes
were brisker on the right. Ophthalmological examination showed bilateral
papilloedema and a second grade nystagmus. Cerebrospinal fluid showed no
abnormalities apart from a somewhat elevated protein content. Ventriculography
was indicative of a left frontal and temporal tumour mass.
At operation under local anaesthesia a soft greyish-red tumour found in the
left temporal and frontal lobe was partially removed.
The patient died two days postoperatively.
   Autopsy: Remnants were found of a diffuse brain tumour of the left frontal
and temporal lobe.
   Microscopic study: A histological diagnosis of glioblastoma multiforme was
made.
   Diagnosis: Left fronto-temporal glioblastoma multiforme.

Case 2

   History: This man was hospitalized four times between the age of 35 and 36
years. He had suffered from epileptic seizures, progressive headaches and
impaired vision for three years. He also complained of memory impairment and
disturbances of concentration.
On examination there was a left facial paresis. A Babinski sign was positive
on the left, and there was anosmia. Papilloedema was apparent on both sides,
more on the right than on the left. Cerebrospinal fluid showed an elevated
pressure but no further abnormalities. Radiographs of the sella turcica
revealed a diffuse enlargement the size of a cherry.
A clinical diagnosis of hypophysis tumour was made and the patient was discharged.

He died at home at the age of 38 years.

Autopsy: Not performed.

Microscopic study: Not performed.

Diagnosis: A clinical diagnosis of tumour of the hypophysis was made.

Family: The mother died at the age of 52 years of cancer of the uterus. The father was alive and healthy. A brother of the father suffered from depressions and had committed suicide.

There were eight brothers and sisters. One sister suffered from vertigo and headaches and one brother had stomach complaints. The other siblings were alive and healthy.

COMMENT

No histological diagnosis of the tumour of case 2 was made.

VII.B.2.2. <u>Hallervorden 1936 - Landsberg-Warthe, Germany</u> (87)

A brother and a sister. German.

<u>Case 1</u> (brother)

<u>History</u>: This man was hospitalized at the age of 44 years. At the age of 42 years he had suffered a brain injury and subsequently was subject to seizures. A few days prior to admission a 'Jackson attack' was seen by his doctor. On examination a fibroma was discovered on his back but no neurological symptoms were apparent.
The epileptic seizures were progressive and he died after an attack at the age of 47 years.

<u>Autopsy</u>: Diffuse neoplastic tissue was found in the right and left hemisphere and brain stem. This tissue was especially seen in the basal ganglia, gyrus cinguli, thalamus, tectum and the pons.

<u>Microscopic study</u>: The neoplastic tissue consisted of blastomatous glial cells.

<u>Diagnosis</u>: Diffuse glioblastomatosis.

<u>Case 2</u> (sister)

<u>History</u>: This sister died at the age of 42 years of a brain tumour. Only a clinical diagnosis was made and no autopsy performed.

<u>Diagnosis</u>: Brain tumour.

<u>Family</u>: Two other sisters were healthy. The father died at the age of 50 years of a cerebrovascular accident. The mother died of intestinal cancer at the age of 70 years. The patient of case 1 had three healthy children.

VII.B.2.3. <u>Peyser and Beller 1951 - Jerusalem, Israel</u> (202)

Two brothers. Israeli.

One brother had a choroid plexus papilloma of the right cerebral hemisphere, the other a glioblastoma multiforme of the left frontal horn (see IV.B.2.2).

VII.B.2.4. Koch 1954 - Münster, Germany (127)

A brother and a sister. German.

Case 1 (brother)
   History: This man died of a right temporal glioma (anatomical diagnosis)
at the age of 45 years.
   Diagnosis: Right temporal glioma.

Case 2 (sister)
   History: This woman died at the age of 57 years of a left frontal brain
tumour.
   Microscopic study: No histological diagnosis was made.
   Diagnosis: Left frontal brain tumour.

   Family: A brother (3) died of a liver carcinoma.

         1 = case 1
         2 = case 2
         3 = liver carcinoma

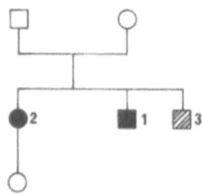

COMMENT
The tumour in case 1 was anatomically diagnosed. Apparently some form of
histological examination was made, but no further details are given.
This case was mentioned in an extensive study on 350 female patients with
CNS tumours.

VII.B.2.5. Henschen 1955 (96)
          (cited by Kemper 1964) (117)

A brother and sister.

A 55-year-old male with a temporal glioblastoma and his 42-year-old sister
having a clinically diagnosed brain tumour are reported.

COMMENT
This case is cited by Kemper (117). No additional information is given. It
was not possible to obtain the original report.

VII.B.2.6. Turcot et al. 1959 - Quebec, Canada (267)

A sister and brother. Canadian.

The sister had a glioblastoma of the left frontal lobe, the brother a medulloblastoma of the spinal cord.
Both siblings also had polyposis of the colon. This family is a manifestation
of the glioma-polyposis or Turcot syndrome (see II.B.2.1 and discussion on
familial aspects of glioma).

VII.B.2.7. <u>Hauge and Harvald 1960 - Copenhagen, Denmark</u> (92)

Two sisters and two brothers. Danish.

<u>Case 1</u> (sister)

<u>History</u>: This female died at the age of 55 years of a tumour in the right temporal lobe.

<u>Microscopic study</u>: Fibrillary astrocytoma.

<u>Diagnosis</u>: Right temporal astrocytoma.

<u>Case 2</u> (brother)

<u>History</u>: This male *died at the age of 45 years from cerebral tumour (hospital diagnosis).*

<u>Case 3</u> (brother)

<u>History</u>: This male *died at the age of 46 years from cerebral gliomatosis (hospital diagnosis).*

<u>Case 4</u> (sister)

<u>History</u>: This female *died at the age of 49 years from cerebral tumour (hospital diagnosis).*

<u>Family</u>: The father committed suicide at the age of 59 years. The mother died at the age of 83 years from cardial asthma. There were 8 other siblings, all male. One died in infancy from unknown causes. One brother died at the age of 59 years from malaria and possible cerebral abscess. One brother died at the age of 37 years from tuberculosis and another brother at the age of 37 years from cardiac disease. One brother died at the age of 81 years from myocardial degeneration accompanied by right-sided hemiplegia. Another died at the age of 71 years suffering from severe bilateral nephrolithiasis, pyonephritis and previous lues.

<u>COMMENT</u>

As no further information is given in the article it is not clear whether the diagnosis in case 3 has been confirmed by microscopic study. If this was the case, this report should be registered among siblings with concordant tumour.

VII.B.2.8. Kjellin et al. 1960 - Stockholm, Sweden (123)

A brother and sister. Swedish.

Case 1

History: This 11-year-old boy was admitted to hospital because of *headache of 3 months duration, and loss of vision in the right eye and diplopia for one month....*

On examination the patient was *stuporous and had right-sided palsy of the oculomotor and facial nerves, homonymous hemianopsia on the left side, and bilateral papilledema.*

At operation *the right occipital lobe, which contained a deep-seated tumor of gliomatous appearance, was removed.*

The patient died one and a half years after operation.

Autopsy: Not performed.

Microscopic study: Malignant glioma of the astrocytoma-group.

Diagnosis: Right occipital astrocytoma.

Case 2

History: This 25-year-old woman was admitted to hospital because of *increasing symptoms of fatigue, headache, dizziness, and impaired vision over a period of 4 months. In addition, she reported diplopia for 2 months, and fits of generalized convulsions in increasing frequency during the last month before admission....*

On examination *she was found to have neck rigidity, bilateral anosmia, papilledema, and paralysis of ocular muscles. Ventriculography revealed a centrally located expanding process, which appeared to be situated mainly in the basal ganglia on the left side.*

A craniotomy was performed but no brain tissue was removed.

The patient died 5 months after the operation.

Autopsy: Not performed.

Microscopic study: No material available.

Diagnosis: Brain tumour in the left basal ganglia.

Family: No information is available in the article.

COMMENT

Unfortunately a histological diagnosis is lacking in case 2. The signs and symptoms, the findings at ventriculography and operation and the rapid progress of symptoms suggest a diagnosis of glioma.

VII.B.2.9. <u>Metzel 1963 - Freiburg, Germany</u> (170)

Two brothers. German.

Case 1

<u>History</u>: This male patient was hospitalized at the age of 42 years. He had suffered from temporal seizures with a visceral aura. His history revealed word-finding difficulties and a slight clumsiness of the right arm and leg which had existed for several months.

On examination a slight papilloedema, a right facial paresis and a paresis of the right arm were found. He had difficulties in finding words. His mental condition was depressive. An electroencephalogram showed a delta focus in the left temporal region, and left carotid angiography revealed a temporo-medial tumour mass, the presence of which was confirmed at operation.

The patient died 10 days postoperatively of a lung embolus.

<u>Autopsy</u>: Showed a bloody cavity and tumour in the left temporal lobe, with tumour growth into the basal ganglia.

<u>Microscopic study</u>: Astrocytoma.

<u>Diagnosis</u>: Left temporal astrocytoma.

Case 2

<u>History</u>: This male died at the age of 55 years of a clinically diagnosed brain tumour of the left temporal lobe. The diagnosis was confirmed by angiography.

Operation or autopsy was not performed.

<u>Diagnosis</u>: Left temporal brain tumour.

<u>Family</u>: No information is available in the article.

COMMENT

Based on the angiography and the rapidly progressive course of the disease, a diagnosis of gliomatous tumour in case 2 has been suggested by the author.

VII.B.2.10. <u>Kemper 1964 - Münster, Germany</u> (117)

Two sisters. German.

Case 1
   <u>History</u>: This female was hospitalized at the age of 64 years. She had
complained of severe headaches and difficulties in finding words for several
months. A few weeks prior to admission she had suffered a loss of strength on
the right side and impairment of vision.
On examination a right central facial paresis and a hypotonic right-sided
hemiparesis were found. There was an expressive, and partly receptive, aphasia.
A positive Babinski sign was present on the right. On both sides papilloedema
was present. Her mental condition was unstable. An encephalogram was indicative
of a left-sided tumour.
One day later the patient died suddenly of central respiratory failure.
   <u>Autopsy</u>: Revealed a partly necrotic, haemorrhagic tumour in the left
occipital lobe. A fresh haemorrhage around the tumour had burst into the
lateral ventricle.
   <u>Microscopic study</u>: Showed a glioblastoma multiforme.
   <u>Diagnosis</u>: Left occipital glioblastoma multiforme.

Case 2
   <u>History</u>: This female died during the war of a brain tumour. She is said to
have presented symptoms similar to those of her sister in case 1, such as
disturbances of speech. Further information is not available.
   <u>Diagnosis</u>: Brain tumour.

   <u>Family</u>:

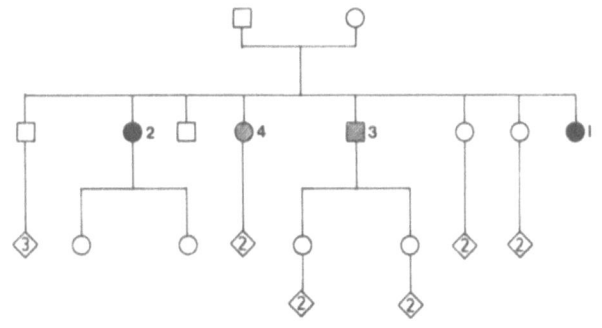

1 = case 1
2 = case 2
3 = died of carcinoma
    of the stomach
4 = operated because
    of tumour of the
    face

A brother of these two sisters died of a carcinoma of the stomach at the age of 38 years. A sister had been operated upon because of a tumour of the face. She died later of cardiac failure and cachexia.

No further information concerning other relatives was available.

COMMENT

This case was reported in an extensive study of 254 male and 199 female patients with brain tumours. No medical history was available in case 2.

VII.B.2.11. Colafranceschi and Mennonna 1970 - Florence, Italy (50)

Two brothers. Italian.

Case 1

History: This 50-year-old male labourer was hospitalized with a 3-month medical history of mental change, speech disturbance and loss of strength on the right side.

On examination a right central facial paresis and a right hemiparesis were present. The patient also had expressive aphasic disorders (paraphasia). His blood-group was O, Rhesus negative. An electroencephalogram showed disturbances in the left fronto-temporal region and left carotid angiography revealed an expansive process in the left temporal area.

At operation a cystic tumour in the left temporal lobe was partially removed. Postoperatively the patient made a good recovery and was discharged.

He died 11 months thereafter.

Autopsy: Not performed

Microscopic study: A diagnosis of glioblastoma multiforme was made

Diagnosis: Left temporal glioblastoma multiforme.

Case 2

History: This 57-year-old male labourer was admitted to hospital because of headaches, loss of strength on the left side of the body and disturbances of consciousness.

On examination beginning papilloedema and a left central facial paresis was found. A left hemiparesis and a positive Babinski sign were present. His blood-group was O, Rhesus negative. An electroencephalogram showed disturbances of the right temporal region, and right carotid angiography demonstrated a pathological process in the right posterior frontal area indicative of a glioma.

The patient refused operation and was treated with radiotherapy.

He died a few months later.

Autopsy: Not performed.

Diagnosis: Right frontal brain tumour.

Family: These two brothers had 3 sisters and 3 other brothers. The mother had 9 siblings and the father 7. None of the other family members died of a brain tumour. A brother of the mother, a brother of the father, and a nephew on the father's side died of cancer of the stomach. Another brother of the father died of leukemia.

292

COMMENT

Unfortunately no histological diagnosis could be made of the tumour in case 2. The examination findings and clinical course are suggestive of a glioma. As this diagnosis was not corroborated this case has been registered within the discordant group.

VII.B.2.12. Chen et al. 1970 - Rochester, Minn., U.S.A. (42)

Two sisters and two brothers. Guamanian.

History: The authors investigated the clinical and genetic patterns of
neurological diseases on Guam. They discovered a family demonstrating 4
patients (2 male and 2 female) with brain tumours and 2 with acute myelogenous leukaemia in a sibship of 14. The brain tumours were diagnosed from
material collected at autopsy and included 2 medulloblastomas, 1 glioblastoma
and 1 paraventricular haemangioma. The two patients with medulloblastomas were
sisters who died at the ages of 7 and 13 years. One sister had black naevi on
the back and hypoplasia of the corpus callosum, the other had several café-
au-lait spots and haemangiomata on the right leg and also in the spleen. One
brother had a glioblastoma in the left hemisphere and died at the age of 5
years. He also had café-au-lait spots on the back. The other brother having
a paraventricular haemangioma, who died at the age of 5 years of a rupture,
also had a haemangioma in the right hemisphere.

Family:

1 = case 1
2 = case 2
3 = case 3
4 = case 4
5 = acute myelogenous leukaemia
6 = acute myelogenous leukaemia
7 = hepatoma
8 = hepatoma
9 = laryngeal cancer

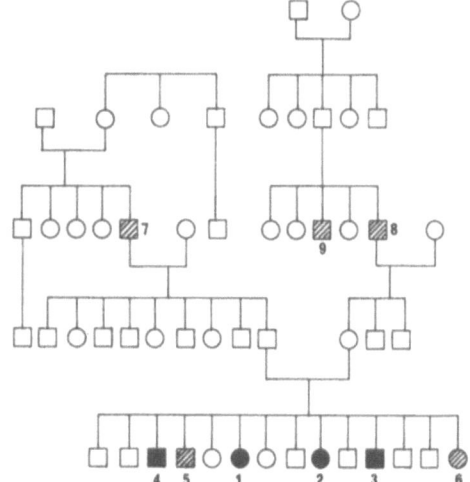

Both paternal (7) and maternal (8) grandfathers died of a primary hepatoma,
and a maternal great-uncle died of laryngeal cancer (9). Amyotrophic lateral
sclerosis had been diagnosed in a great-uncle of the patients and in his son.
Other members of the sibship had clinical features associated with the phacomatosis complex, such as café-au-lait spots and black neavi. *There was no*

roentgenographic evidence of jaw cyst or forking ribs.

COMMENT

The association of the brain tumours with stigmata of phacomatosis, such as café-au-lait spots and black naevi (neurofibromatosis), and haemangiomata (Hippel-Lindau) makes a relationship very likely. Considering the occurrence of leukaemia and other forms of cancer (hepatoma, laryngeal cancer), a manifestation of the family cancer syndrome (SBLA syndrome) also cannot be excluded.

This report has also been registered among the concordant familial medulloblastoma (II.B.1.5).

VII.B.2.13. De Tribolet et al. 1979 - Lausanne, Switzerland (265)

A brother and sister. Swiss.

Case 1 (brother)

History: This male was admitted to hospital at the age of 21 years. He
started complaining of severe bifrontal headache and vomiting one month prior
to admission.
On examination *there was marked bilateral papilloedema and a discrete left*
hemiparesis. Radioisotopic brain-scan and arteriography showed a right frontal
mass.
At operation the tumour was totally excised.
Postoperatively the patient received radiotherapy and *two and a half years*
later the patient has no neurological deficit and works full time.

Microscopic study: Glioblastoma multiforme.
Diagnosis: Right frontal glioblastoma multiforme.

Case 2 (sister)

History: This female was hospitalized at the age of 15 years. She *noticed*
slight weakness and numbnes on the left side of her body 2 weeks prior to
admission.
On examination a paresis of her left leg with diminished vibration sense was
found. *A right carotid angiogram revealed a right thalamic mass, hypervascu-*
larized and with numerous arteriovenous shunts.
The patient was not treated and she died one month later.

Autopsy: Not performed.
Diagnosis: Right thalamic brain tumour.

Family: No further information is given in the article.

COMMENT
The tumour of case 2 was felt by the authors to be most compatible with the
diagnosis of glioblastoma multiforme, but this was not histologically verified.

296

VII.B.2.14. Blattner et al. 1979 - Miami, U.S.A. (29)

Two brothers. American.

Case 1

History: This male was hospitalized at the age of 37 years. His early development had been normal, *although the left testicle did not descend into the scrotal sac until age 13 years.* At the age of 33 years he *experienced psychomotor seizures ...,* which increased in frequency in the years preceding admission.
An EEG showed a right temporal lobe focus, and computerized tomography *disclosed a right temporal lobe lesion ...,* for which the patient was operated upon.

Microscopic study: Low-grade astrocytoma.
Diagnosis: Right temporal low-grade astrocytoma.

Case 2

History: This 2-year-old male was admitted to hospital as he had *experienced a stiff back, anorexia, weight loss, drowsiness, and projectile vomiting during a two-month period ....*
A clinical diagnosis of tuberculous meningitis was made, but autopsy showed a tumour *originating in the wall of the fourth ventricle.*

Microscopic study: Medulloblastoma.
Diagnosis: Medulloblastoma of the fourth ventricle.

Family: A sister had a single grand mal seizure at the age of 27 years, but cerebral CAT was normal. A distant relative was hospitalized at 27 years of age with headache, visual problems, vertigo, mental confusion and vomiting. *A midline cerebellar tumor was excised. It was a highly cellular papillary, rosette-forming tumor possibly of choroid epithelial origin; it may have been metastatic, but no other primary tumor was found.* A comprehensive family study showed a constellation of tumours in the family - a total of 16 cases of cancer - including bony and soft tissue sarcomas, neural tumours, brain tumours, leukaemia and breast carcinoma.

COMMENT

The tumours in this family are a manifestation of the so-called SBLA cancer syndrome, a dominantly inherited predisposition to certain kinds of cancer (see also discussion on familial aspects).

VII.C.   *OTHER GENERATIONS AND DISTANT RELATIVES*

VII.C.1.   OTHER GENERATIONS AND DISTANT RELATIVES WITH CONCORDANT TUMOUR

VII.C.1.1.   Ostertag 1948 - Germany
            (personal communication in Koch 1949) (126)

A mother and daughter. German.

History: The mother had a glioblastomatosis in the parieto-occipital region
at the age of 23 years. She had a premature still-born daughter with a glioblastomatosis of the same region. Both tumours were histologically verified.
No further information concerning the patients or the family is given in the
article.

COMMENT
This was the first reported case of histologically verified glioma in two
generations. It is mentioned by Koch (1949) as a personal communication.

VII.C.1.2. <u>Koch 1949 - Tübingen, Germany</u> (126)

A mother, daughter and son. German.

<u>Case 1</u> (mother)

<u>History</u>: This 51-year-old female was admitted to hospital with a one month
history of speech disturbance, headache and vomiting. Two days prior to admission she suddenly noticed a loss of strength on the right side. Her medical
history revealed an abdominal occlusion for which she was operated upon at
the age of 38 years.
On examination an amnestic aphasia, slight anisocoria, a right hypotonic hemiparesis, disturbed sensibility on the right and a positive Babinski sign on
the right were found. Roentgenograms of the skull were normal.
The neurological condition gradually deteriorated with papilloedema developing
on both sides and she died 18 days after admission.

<u>Autopsy</u>: A greyish-red tumour was found in the parietal lobe extending into
the posterior horn of the lateral ventricle and the occipital lobe. Autopsy of
the body showed no remarkable disorders.

<u>Microscopic study</u>: Not mentioned in the article.

<u>Diagnosis</u>: Left parieto-occipital glioma.

<u>Case 2</u> (daughter)

<u>History</u>: This 23-year-old teacher was admitted to hospital with a four
month history of numbness and strange sensations on the right side. She had
a progressive loss of strength of the right arm and leg. She also complained
of seizures of the right side of the face, and the last weeks prior to admission of loss of vision in the right visual field and difficulties in swallowing.
Her medical history revealed an accommodation paresis since the age of 15 years.
On examination she had numerous pigmented naevi on the right arm. Her vision
was diminished and there was a horizontal nystagmus. The right cornea reflex
was absent and there was a right facial paresis. A right spastic hemiparesis
and hypaesthesia were found. There was ankle clonus and a positive Babinski
sign on the right. She had slight difficulties in finding words and her speech
was slow and monotone. During her admission she suffered progressive headaches
and vomiting. Roentgenograms of the skull showed signs of elevated intracranial
pressure and an abnormal configuration (*Turmschädel*).
At operation a greyish-red tumour of the left temporo-parietal region was
partly removed.
She died approximately 10 months later, four months after a second operation.

Autopsy: Not performed.

Microscopic study: Glioblastoma multiforme.

Diagnosis: Left temporo-parietal glioblastoma multiforme.

Case 3 (son)

History: This 31-year-old male was admitted to hospital after a three-week
period of severe right-sided headaches. He had complained of minor headaches
for several years. He had suffered from impotence for 8 months. At the age of
16 years he had suffered a head injury resulting in a Horner syndrome.
On examination he had a tongue paresis and possibly a Babinski sign on the
right. There was a slight hypermetria of the left leg. Ventriculography showed
an abnormality of the left lateral ventricle.
The patient died 9 days after admission with signs of brain stem compression.

Autopsy: showed a tumour in the right temporal lobe.
Autopsy of the body revealed no pathology.

Microscopic study: Cystic glioblastoma.

Diagnosis: Right temporal cystic glioblastoma.

Family:

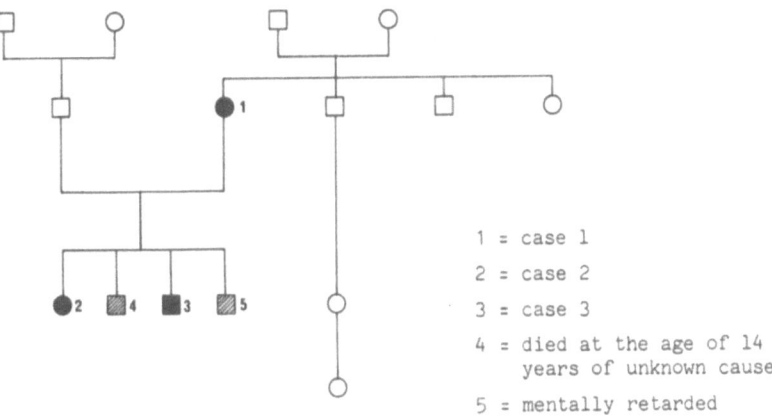

1 = case 1
2 = case 2
3 = case 3
4 = died at the age of 14
    years of unknown cause
5 = mentally retarded

The mother had four normal parturitions, one child dying in the first year
of life. One of her 3 male children died at the age of 14 years of unknown
cause (4). Another was mentally retarded and disappeared when serving as

a soldier in Russia (5). The father in this family was an alcoholic who died
at the age of 42 years.

COMMENT

Microscopic study of the tumour in case 1 was not discussed in the article.
Diagnosis of glioma was apparently based upon autopsy findings.
The pigmented naevi found by examination in case 2 may indicate some relation-
ship to neurofibromatosis.

VII.C.1.3. <u>Mackay 1952 - Leiden, The Netherlands</u> (153)

An uncle and nephew. Dutch.

The uncle died at the age of 57 years of a glioblastoma situated in the right fronto-parietal and corpus callosum regions.
The nephew died at the age of 7 years of a left frontal gigantocellular astrocytoma.
No further information is given in regard to these cases.

VII.C.1.4. <u>Koch 1954 - München, Germany</u> (127)

An uncle and niece. German.

The uncle (1) died of a cystic glioblastoma of the left temporal lobe at the age of 50 years.
His niece (2) died at the age of 28 years of a spongioblastoma with neurino-matous elements of the left precentral region. She had a left temporal naevus pigmentosus vinosus.
Both brain tumours in these cases were histologically verified.
The father of the niece died of a lung tumour.

<u>Family</u>:

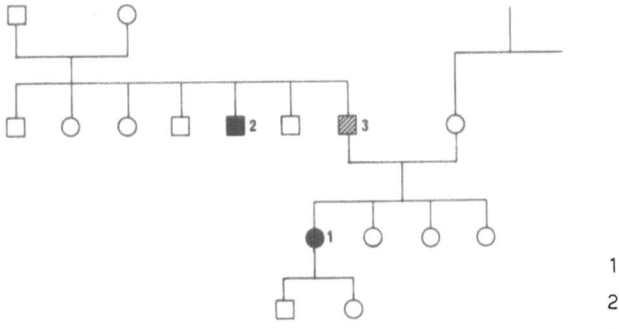

1 = case 1
2 = case 2
3 = lung tumour

VII.C.1.5. <u>Munslow and Hill 1955 - Texas, U.S.A.</u> (182)

Two brothers and a nephew. American.

<u>Case 1</u> (brother)

   <u>History</u>: This white male was admitted to hospital at the age of 52 years.
*Approximately 2 months previously he had had slurring of speech and for the
last 2 weeks he had had right facial numbness. Twitching attacks followed by
transient aphasia had occurred.*
On examination *the patient was right-handed, with right facial hypesthesia and
paresis, slurring of speech and absent abdominal and cremasteric reflexes.*
At operation an infiltrating tumour was found in Broca's area. *A small piece
of tissue just anterior to Broca's area was removed for diagnosis, and a
large ... decompression was performed.*
Death occurred soon after operation.
   <u>Microscopic study</u>: *The surgical specimen contained no neoplastic cells.*
Although lacking histological verification the tumour was identified as a
glioma by the operating surgeon.
   <u>Diagnosis</u>: Glioma in Broca's area (left frontal).

<u>Case 2</u> (brother)

   <u>History</u>: This white male was admitted to hospital at the age of 64 years.
*Eight weeks previously he had suffered a sudden coma of 6 hours' duration with
residual, rapidly receding, hemiparesis. After a 4-week interval of relatively
good health there was onset of progressive aphasia, confusion, vomiting and
headache.*
On examination he *had a right hemiparesis, sensory aphasia, astereognosis of
the right hand and blurred disc margins. Roentgenograms of the skull were
normal. Electroencephalograms discovered a left temporoparietal focus. Initial
pressure on lumbar puncture was 296 mm.; the fluid contained 61 mg. per cent
total protein.*
The patient refused a craniotomy and died a few weeks later.
   <u>Autopsy</u>: revealed a large infiltrating left frontal tumour.
   <u>Microscopic study</u>: The histological diagnosis was grade III astrocytoma.
   <u>Diagnosis</u>: Left frontal astrocytoma grade III.

<u>Case 3</u> (paternally related nephew of cases 1 and 2)

   <u>History</u>: This male entered the hospital at the age of 46 years. *He presented
a 3-month history of personality change, headaches and left-sided paresthesias.*
On examination *the patient was right-handed, with definite evidence of increased*

intracranial pressure, left astereognosis and dysesthesias. Spinal fluid pressure and protein were elevated. Ventriculography suggested a right intraventricular tumor.

At craniotomy a right paraventricular tumor was encountered and grossly removed.

The patient died 2 months after admission.

Microscopic study: *The tumor was a malignant glioma varying from a protoplasmic astrocytoma to a glioblastoma multiforme in character.*

Diagnosis: Right paraventricular glioblastoma multiforme.

Family: The two brothers had four siblings and a paternally related half sibling. The family of case 3 was large with the majority of family members being under the age at which most gliomas occur.

COMMENT

The histological nature of the tumour in case 1 was not verified. It was identified as a glioma by the operating surgeon.

The authors also report a personal communication from Klemme, who had identified gliomas in two members of a family. No further details are given regarding these cases.

VII.C.1.6. Voûte 1958 – The Netherlands
              (personal communication in Van der Wiel 1959) (286)

A mother, daughter and son. Dutch.

The mother died of a glioma at the age of 56 years. Her daughter died at the
age of 36 years of an astrocytoma, and her son died at the age of 34 years of
a gliomatosis cerebri.
The tumours of the daughter and son were histologically verified; this is
doubtful in the case of the mother.
No further information is available regarding these cases.

COMMENT

This case is described by Van der Wiel (1959) as a personal communication.
Personal inquiry by this author revealed no further information.

VII.C.1.7. <u>Kjellin et al. 1960 - Stockholm, Sweden</u> (123)

A father, daughter and son. Swedish.

Case 1 (father)
    <u>History</u>: This 31-year-old man was admitted to hospital because of mental changes existing since one year. *During the last 2 months weakness in the right arm and leg, headache, uncinate fits of smell and taste, and gradual impairment of vision developed.*
He died 22 days after admission.
    <u>Autopsy</u>: *revealed a grayish, gelatinous tumor situated mainly within the depths of the left cerebral hemisphere, but extending from the left to the right thalamus and reaching the lateral ventricles on both sides.*
    <u>Microscopic study</u>: showed a malignant glioma of the astrocytoma group.
    <u>Diagnosis</u>: Astrocytoma grade II-III of the thalamus region.

Case 2 (daughter)
    <u>History</u>: This woman was hospitalized at the age of 23 years. She *reported headache, vomiting, dizziness, paraesthesia in the right side of the face and, occasionally, dimness of vision of 3 months' duration.*
On examination she showed a *slight left-sided facial weakness of central type and bilateral papilledema.*
At operation a *centrally situated tumor was partially removed.* The tumour *originated in the corpus callosum and spread into the cerebral hemispheres, especially on the right side.*
The patient died 6 weeks after operation.
    <u>Autopsy</u>: *revealed that only a small part of the tumor remained.*
    <u>Microscopic study</u>: Histological diagnosis was malignant glioma of the astrocytoma group.
    <u>Diagnosis</u>: Astrocytoma grade II-III of the corpus callosum.

Case 3 (son)
    <u>History</u>: This 19-year-old man was admitted to hospital having had mental changes and headaches for the last 3 months.
On examination a homonymous hemianopia on the right side and bilateral papilloedema were found, and the patient was mentally deteriorated.
At operation a cystic tumour was removed from the left occipital lobe.
The patient died two and a half years after operation.
    <u>Autopsy</u>: Not performed.
    <u>Microscopic study</u>: Malignant glioma of the astrocytoma group.

Diagnosis: Left occipital astrocytoma grade II-III.

Family: There were two other healthy siblings of cases 2 and 3.

COMMENT

The histological features were similar in all three cases, showing a moderate degree of malignancy.

VII.C.1.8. <u>Kjellin et al. 1960 - Stockholm, Sweden</u> (123)

A mother and daughter. Swedish.

<u>Case 1</u> (mother)

<u>History</u>: This woman was hospitalized at the age of 54 years. She *reported*
headache and vomiting about one week prior to admission. The symptoms
increased rapidly, she became stuporous, and ... unconscious ....
She died on the day of admission.

<u>Autopsy</u>: *A brown-grayish, poorly-defined cystic tumor was found in the*
right frontal lobe.

<u>Microscopic study</u>: showed a malignant glioma of the astrocytoma group.

<u>Diagnosis</u>: Right frontal astrocytoma grade IV.

<u>Case 2</u> (daughter)

<u>History</u>: This 30-year-old woman was hospitalized because of *headache,*
disturbance of speech, and weakness and decreased sensibility in the right
half of the body of three weeks' duration.
On examination she demonstrated *aphasia, bilateral papilledema, and right-*
sided hemiparesis and hemihypaesthesia.
At operation *a grayish-red, rather soft, poorly-defined, partly cystic and*
necrotic tumor was removed ....
The patient died 7 months after operation.

<u>Autopsy</u>: Not performed.

<u>Microscopic study</u>: Malignant glioma of the astrocytoma group.

<u>Diagnosis</u>: Left fronto-parietal astrocytoma grade IV.

<u>Family</u>: There was one other healthy sibling of case 2.

<u>COMMENT</u>
The histologic pictures were similar and indicated a high degree of
malignancy.

VII.C.1.9. <u>Kjellin et al. 1960 - Stockholm, Sweden</u> (123)

A mother and son. Swedish.

<u>Case 1</u> (mother)

<u>History</u>: This 72-year-old woman was hospitalized because of complaints of headache and difficulties in finding words which had existed for one and a half years.

On examination *she was mentally deteriorated, and had a right-sided palsy of the facial nerve of central type.*

At operation *a dark reddish-gray tumor was partially removed from the anterior part of the left temporal lobe.*

The patient died 3 months after operation.

<u>Autopsy</u>: *demonstrated a soft, partly necrotic, poorly-defined tumor with signs of older and recent hemorrhages in the left temporal lobe of the brain.*

<u>Microscopic study</u>: *showed an extremely cellular, pleomorphic tumor with many mitoses, which were frequently atypical. There was endothelial proliferation in the numerous blood vessels. Tumor cells were arranged in palisade fashion close to irregular strips of necrotic tissue.* A diagnosis of malignant glioma of the astrocytoma series was made.

<u>Diagnosis</u>: Left temporal astrocytoma grade IV.

<u>Case 2</u> (son)

<u>History</u>: This boy was first admitted to hospital at the age of 6 years. He had *started to vomit, and became clumsy in using arms and legs, had poor balance, speech difficulties, and increasing stupor 3 months before ... admission ....*

On examination *he was stuporous and had bilateral papilledema, slight dysarthria, impairment of gait, a tendency to fall to the left, decreased hearing and caloric excitability on the right side, and was clumsy in both arms and legs.*

A cerebellar cyst was punctured. This procedure was repeated 2 years later. At the age of 15 years a third operation was performed. *The cerebellum contained a large cyst filled with brown-green, thick fluid. In the wall of the cyst a solid mushroom-like growth was found. The tumor was apparently removed completely.* At the age of 19 years he underwent a fourth and last operation. *A dense, solid, well-defined yellow-brown tumor originating in the roof of the fourth ventricle was removed.*

The postoperative course was uneventful until he drowned at the age of 24 years.

Autopsy: Not performed.

Microscopic study: *showed a fairly cellular tumor made up of astrocyte-like cells. It contained many blood vessels and edematous microcysts but no necrotic regions.*

Diagnosis: Cerebellar astrocytoma grade I-II.

Family: The son was the oldest of 4 children.

COMMENT

The histologic appearance of both tumours was entirely different, as stated by the authors.

VII.C.1.10. <u>King and Eisinger 1966 - Elmira, U.S.A.</u> (122)

A father and daughter. American.

<u>Case 1</u> (father)

<u>History</u>: This 50-year-old white male was hospitalized *with the complaint of headache of roughly six months duration, and double vision of about a month's duration.* A few days before admission *he noticed fluid dripping out of the left side of his mouth.* Previous history revealed typhoid fever, a head injury and an appendectomy.

On examination *there was a left hemiparesis with weakness of the central type, of the left side of the face. ... his general mental state was certainly slow and groggy ....* A ventriculogram showed a large right frontal lobe tumour At operation a right frontal tumour with a large subcortical cyst was found extending backward into the temporal and parietal lobes.

The patient did poorly following operation and died on the third postoperative day.

<u>Autopsy</u>: Was unsuccessful as result of error.

<u>Microscopic study</u>: The material obtained at operation disclosed a glioma multiforme.

<u>Diagnosis</u>: Right fronto-temporo-parietal glioma multiforme.

<u>Case 2</u> (daughter)

<u>History</u>: This 34-year-old white female was hospitalized with a history of progressive headaches existing since four months. *She had vomited several times during the past month.* Her neck had become stiff and there was a general slowing of pace in her activities, together with inability to concentrate. *On the day before admission, she had suddenly fainted while sitting in a chair, struck her face and received a 'black eye'. She had not been rousable since. On examination one could get her to respond to simple questions by pinching .... There was papilledema of at least four diopters .... the right arm and leg did not seem to work quite as well as that on the left and the plantar responses were bilaterally extensor.* Her speech was *thick and slurred ....* Bilateral carotid arteriograms *indicated a mass near the midline, high in the left posterior frontal lobe.*

At operation *a large cystic subcortical tumor was removed ....*

The postoperative course was good and the patient made a satisfactory improvement.

<u>Microscopic study</u>: Typical of a glioma multiforme.

Diagnosis: Left posterior frontal glioma multiforme.

Family: The father's *maternal grandmother had died of cancer, as had his father, but the sites of the neoplasms were unknown*. The maternal grandmother of the daughter died of *'cancer of the bowel'*.

VII.C.1.11. Bromowicz et al. 1971 - Lodz, Poland (34)

A mother and son. Polish.

Case 1 (mother)

History: This 30-year-old woman was admitted to hospital because of
progressive weakness of the legs occurring since one year.
On examination a spastic paresis of the legs and anaesthesia below the
level Th_4 was discovered.
The Queckenstedt test was pathological and myelography showed an obstruction
at the level of Th_8.
At operation a tumour located in the meninges below the arachnoid extending
from Th_4 to Th_6 was removed.
Postoperatively the neurological condition of the patient improved remarkably.

Microscopic study: revealed an ependymoma.

Diagnosis: Spinal ependymoma at Th_4 to Th_6.

Case 2 (son)

History: This 8-year-old boy was admitted to hospital with a history of
headaches and vomiting occurring since one year, and disturbances of equilib-
rium since two weeks.
On examination a first grade nystagmus and disorders of balance were found.
Ventriculography revealed a symmetrical internal hydrocephalus and a tumour
in the vermis of the cerebellum.
At operation a tumour of the cerebellum that compressed the fourth ventricle
was removed.
The postoperative course was uneventful.

Microscopic study: Astrocytoma.

Diagnosis: Cerebellar astrocytoma (of the vermis).

VII.C.1.12. <u>Kaufman and Brisman 1972 - New York, U.S.A.</u> (116)

Two first cousins. American.

Case 1
   <u>History</u>: This 4-year-old boy was admitted to hospital *with a 1½ year*
history of headaches, vomiting, ataxia, and signs of pressure and left cere-
bellar dysfunction.
At operation *a cystic cerebellar* tumour *of the vermis and left cerebellar*
hemisphere was subtotally removed.
Postoperatively the patient continued to suffer a fixed cerebellar deficit,
which was exacerbated by presumed muscular dystrophy.
   <u>Microscopic study</u>: showed an astrocytoma.
   <u>Diagnosis</u>: Cerebellar astrocytoma of the vermis and left cerebellar hemisphere. Muscular dystrophy?

Case 2 (first cousin of case 1)
   <u>History</u>: This 14-year-old boy was admitted to hospital because of headaches,
vomiting, and ataxia.
Air, positive contrast, and arteriographic studies indicated a lower brain
stem mass.
At operation a biopsy of a pontine mass was taken.
He improved with radiotherapy but died 18 months later.
   <u>Microscopic study</u>: Malignant astrocytoma.
   <u>Diagnosis</u>: Malignant astrocytoma of the brain stem.

   <u>Family</u>: No further information is given in the article.

VII.C.1.13. <u>Scharrer and Brunngraber 1973 - Köln-Merheim, Germany</u> (230)

A father and son. German.

<u>Case 1</u> (father)

  <u>History</u>: This bricklayer was admitted to hospital at the age of 46 years with a few weeks history of severe, progressive headaches, tinnitus and vertigo.

On examination the patient showed psychomotor retardation. Bilateral papilloedema, a homonymous hemianopia and a slight hemisyndrome on the right were found. The EEG showed focal disturbances in the left temporal region. Left carotid angiography revealed displacement of the medial cerebral artery to the right without obvious vessel pathology.

At craniotomy a round, well demarcated tumour the size of an apple was totally removed from the left occipito-temporal region.

The patient died 7 weeks after operation.

  <u>Autopsy</u>: demonstrated a left temporo-occipital tumour.

  <u>Microscopic study</u>: showed a polymorphous oligodendroglioma with malignant histological features, classified as grade III.

  <u>Diagnosis</u>: Left temporo-occipital oligodendroglioma.

<u>Case 2</u> (son)

  <u>History</u>: This 30-year-old fireman complained of severe headaches, vomiting and short periods of loss of consciousness occurring since a few weeks.

On examination slight bilateral papilloedema was found, more on the left than on the right. No other neurological abnormalities were present. A brain scan demonstrated a diffuse left temporal lesion. Carotid angiography revealed a left temporal tumour without vessel pathology.

At craniotomy a cystic, reddish, nodular tumour was partially removed.

The postoperative course was uneventful and the patient was treated with irradiation. Two years later there were no signs of tumour recurrence.

  <u>Microscopic study</u>: showed a polymorphous oligodendroglioma with malignant development to a glioblastoma, which was classified as grade III.

  <u>Diagnosis</u>: Left temporal oligodendroglioma.

  <u>Family</u>: No information concerning the family members is available.

315

VII.C.1.14. Isamat et al. 1974 - Barcelona, Spain (109)

A father and daughter. Spanish.

Case 1 (father)

History: This male underwent operation of a post-central brain tumour at the age of 56 years. His blood-group was A, Rhesus positive.

Microscopic study: The histological diagnosis was astrocytoma grade IV.

Diagnosis: Post-central astrocytoma grade IV.

Case 2 (daughter)

History: This female underwent a stereotaxic biopsy of a brain tumour located in the third ventricle at the age of 20 years. She had blood-group A, Rhesus positive.

Microscopic study: The histological diagnosis of the biopsy was astrocytoma grade III.

Diagnosis: Astrocytoma grade III in the third ventricle.

Family: No gliomas were found in more distant relatives. Further information is not available.

VII.C.1.15. <u>Isamat et al. 1974 - Barcelona, Spain</u> (109)

A mother and son. Spanish.

<u>Case 1</u> (mother)

<u>History</u>: At the age of 61 years this female underwent operation of a frontal brain tumour. She had blood-group B, Rhesus positive.

<u>Microscopic study</u>: showed an astrocytoma grade IV.

<u>Diagnosis</u>: Frontal astrocytoma grade IV.

<u>Case 2</u> (son)

<u>History</u>: This male was operated upon because of a temporal brain tumour at the age of 39 years. His blood-group was A, Rhesus positive.

<u>Microscopic study</u>: The histological diagnosis was astrocytoma grade II.

<u>Diagnosis</u>: Temporal astrocytoma grade II.

<u>Family</u>: No gliomas were found in the more distant relatives. Further information is not available.

VII.C.1.16. Isamat et al. 1974 - Barcelona, Spain (109)

A mother and son. Spanish.

Case 1 (mother)

   History: This female had a glioma of the right frontal lobe unsuccessfully removed at the age of 38 years.

   Diagnosis: Right frontal glioma.

Case 2 (son)

   History: This male was operated upon because of a parathalamic tumour at the age of 58 years. His blood-group was A, Rhesus positive.

   Microscopic study: The histological diagnosis was ependymoblastoma.

   Diagnosis: Parathalamic ependymoblastoma.

   Family: No gliomas were found in the more distant relatives. Further information is not available.

COMMENT

No further specification of the histological character of the tumour in case 1 is given in the article.

VII.C.1.17. Isamat et al. 1974 - Barcelona, Spain (109)

An aunt and nephew. Spanish.

Case 1 (aunt)

History: This female was operated upon at the age of 50 years because of a frontal brain tumour. Her blood-group was AB, Rhesus positive.

Microscopic study: showed an astrocytoma grade IV.

Diagnosis: Frontal astrocytoma grade IV.

Case 2 (nephew)

History: This male underwent operation of a temporal brain tumour at the age of 29 years. His blood-group was A, Rhesus positive.

Microscopic study: showed an astrocytoma grade I.

Diagnosis: Temporal astrocytoma grade I.

Family: No gliomas were found in other relatives. Further information is not available.

VII.C.1.18. Lynch et al. 1978 - Omaha Neb., U.S.A. (151)

Six cases of primary brain tumours in three generations.

Case 1 (brother, third generation)
This male had a brain tumour at the age of 18 years. The histological diagnosis
was glioblastoma multiforme. He died at the age of 20 years.

Case 2 (sister, third generation)
This female died of a histologically verified glioblastoma multiforme at the
age of 3 years.

Case 3 (paternal cousin, third generation)
This male had a primary malignant brain tumour at the age of 4 years. He died
one year later.

Case 4 (paternal uncle, second generation)
This male died of a brain tumour at the age of 6 years. A histological
diagnosis of glioma was made.

Cases 5 and 6 (distant relatives)
A male of the first generation and a female of the third generation also died
of histologically verified glioblastoma multiforme, respectively at the age
of 51 and 10 years.

COMMENT
The authors report a family with remarkable cancer aggregation of sarcoma,
breast cancer and brain tumours, leukaemia and adrenal cortical carcinoma.
This hereditary tumour complex, designated as the SBLA cancer syndrome is due
to an autosomal dominant factor. Twenty-nine tumours occurred in twenty-six
individuals. No stigmata of phacomatous disorder were present in any of the
cases. The authors suggest *that the cancer-prone genotype interacts with one
or more exogenous factors in causing this familial tumor association*.
It is noteworthy that most of the tumours in these cases occurred at an
early age.

VII.C.1.19. <u>Turowski 1978 - Lublin, Poland</u> (268)

A father and son. Polish.

<u>Case 1</u> (father)

    <u>History</u>: This 60-year-old male was hospitalized with a three-month-history
of headaches, speech disturbances and weakness of the right extremities.
Neurological examination showed papilloedema, sensory and motor aphasia and
right hemiparesis with a positive Babinski sign. The patient's blood-group
was A, Rhesus positive. Carotid angiography revealed a tumour in the left
temporal region.

Operation was performed.

The day after operation a complete paralysis of the left eye was discovered.
The patient was again operated upon and an haematoma in the area of previous
operation removed.

The further postoperative period was uneventful and the patient was discharged
home in satisfactory condition. He remained aphasic, had a partial right hemiparesis and complete paralysis of left eye movements.

    <u>Microscopic study</u>: revealed a glioblastoma multiforme.

    <u>Diagnosis</u>: Left temporal glioblastoma multiforme.

<u>Case 2</u> (son)

    <u>History</u>: This 37-year-old male was admitted to hospital with a seven-month-
history of headaches and weakness of the left extremities.

On examination a slight hemiparesis of the left side was discovered. The
patient's blood-group was A, Rhesus positive. An EEG showed focal changes in
the right temporal region. Carotid angiography revealed a tumour mass in the
right parietal lobe.

Operation was performed.

At first the postoperative condition of the patient was good, but after eight
days he acutely suffered respiratory and circulatory difficulties, and died.

    <u>Autopsy</u>: demonstrated bleeding and oedema of the brain at the site of
operation, and lung oedema.

    <u>Microscopic study</u>: revealed a glioblastoma multiforme.

    <u>Diagnosis</u>: Right parietal glioblastoma multiforme.

<u>COMMENT</u>

This article also reports two sisters with optic nerve glioma, but these
tumours have not been included in this register.

VII.C.1.20. Van der Drift 1980 - The Hague, The Netherlands
           (personal communication)

A mother and daughter. Dutch.

The mother had an occipitally localized astrocytoma grade IV and the daughter
a cerebellar astrocytoma. Both tumours were histologically verified.
No further details concerning these cases are available.

VII.C.1.21. Van der Wiel 1980 - Gouda, The Netherlands
           (personal communication)

A father and daughter. Dutch.

Case 1 (father)
    History: This 60-year-old male was admitted to hospital because of a left-
sided hemiparesis and a disturbed mental condition.
At operation a right frontal tumour was found.
He died three weeks after operation.
    Autopsy: Not performed.
    Microscopic study: Glioblastoma multiforme.
    Diagnosis: Right frontal glioblastoma multiforme.

Case 2 (daughter)
    History: This female was operated upon because of a left fronto-temporal
brain tumour at the age of 41 years.
Postoperatively she received radiotherapy.
She died seven months after operation at the age of 42 years.
    Autopsy: Not performed.
    Microscopic study: Astrocytoma grade IV.
    Diagnosis: Left fronto-temporal astrocytoma grade IV.

    Family: The father had two unaffected siblings, the daughter was an only
child. No further details regarding the family are available.

VII.C.1.22. Van der Wiel 1980 - Gouda, The Netherlands
              (personal communication)

Two cousins. Dutch.

Case 1

   History: This 36-year-old unmarried female nurse was admitted to hospital
after having had severe headaches for several months.
At operation a right fronto-temporal tumour was partially removed.
Postoperatively she received radiotherapy.
She died 11 weeks after the operation of suicide by sleeping pills.
   Autopsy: No information concerning autopsy is available.
   Microscopic study: Astrocytoma grade IV.
   Diagnosis: Right fronto-temporal astrocytoma grade IV.

Case 2 (first cousin)

   History: This female was operated upon because of a left occipito-temporal
brain tumour.
She died four months postoperatively of a lung embolus.
   Autopsy: No information concerning autopsy is available.
   Microscopic study: Astrocytoma grade II.
   Diagnosis: Left occipito-temporal astrocytoma grade II.

   Family:

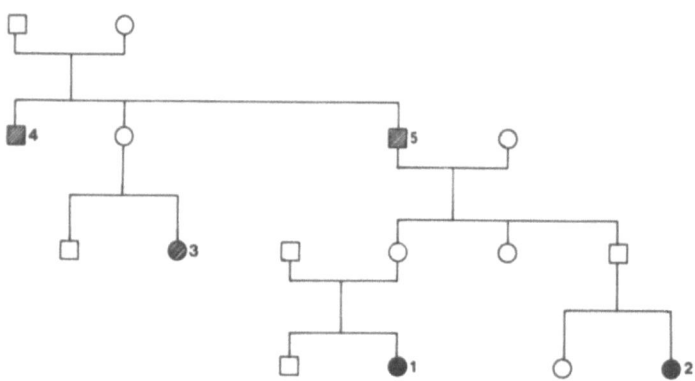

1 = case 1   3 = died of a brain tumour
2 = case 2   4 + 5 = died of carcinoma of the stomach

A third distant relative (3), a daughter of the sister of the grandfather of case 1, was said to have died at the age of 40 years of an inoperable brain tumour in America. This woman was said to have been ill for three years and at autopsy the tumour is said to have been located 'in the middle of the brains' (according to a letter from family in America).

Two other relatives (grandfather (4) and his brother (5)) died of carcinoma of the stomach.

VII.C.1.23. <u>Schianchi and Kraus-Ruppert 1980 - Berne, Switzerland</u> (326)

A father and son. Swiss.

Case 1 (father)

<u>History</u>: This 36-year-old white male was admitted to hospital because of increasing *left-sided spasticity of the limbs and headaches.*
On examination the patient was drowsy and disoriented. He had a left-sided peripheral facial paresis. *Adduction or abduction of the right eye was not possible. Both left extremities showed spasticity with enhancement of the tendon reflexes. Babinski positive on the left. A pneumencephalogram ... showed a communicating internal hydrocephalus. A tumor was located on the floor of the fourth ventricle within the pons cerebri.*
Following the pneumencephalogram respiratory disorders required intubation and the patient died two days later.

<u>Autopsy</u>: *... the brain was markedly enlarged .... hippocampal and cerebellar herniation were noted .... The pons cerebri was extremely distended .... Cross sections through the brainstem revealed a grayish-white tissue, moderately firm, which infiltrated mainly the basilar portion of the pons. ... an intratumoral hemorrhage had penetrated into the fourth ventricle.*

<u>Microscopic study</u>: revealed a low-grade astrocytoma.

<u>Diagnosis</u>: Astrocytoma grade I of the rhombencephalon.

Case 2

<u>History</u>: This 17-year-old male was admitted to hospital after a few weeks of increasing headache *concomitant with nausea, difficulties of gait, disturbances of articulation, and sensory loss in the right cheek.*
On examination he *showed signs of slow cognition and apathy. He had paresis of lateral eye movement on both sides, a right-side oculomotor paresis, a peripheral facial paresis of the left side, and a nystagmus. There was dysarthria, a left-side hemiparesis, an atactic gait, exaggerated reflexes, and positive pyramidal signs bilaterally. The pneumencephalogram ... showed an arc-shaped upward dislocation of the aqueduct. The ventricular system was not visible.*
A vertebral arteriogram showed a space occupying process within the brain stem. The patient had increasing respiratory failure requiring intubation, and he died 16 days after admission.

<u>Autopsy</u>: *... the brain was markedly enlarged .... hippocampal and cerebellar herniation were noted .... The pons cerebri was extremely distended ...* and on cross section revealed a grayish-white moderately firm tissue. The

tumour extended from the mesencephalon to the upper half of the medulla
oblongata.

Microscopic study: showed a low-grade astrocytoma.

Diagnosis: Astrocytoma grade I of the rhombencephalon.

Family: The wife of case 1 (mother of case 2) had multiple sclerosis. A
nephew of case 1 (cousin of case 2) had Cockayne syndrome. Two other nephews
of case 1 (cousins of case 2) died at young age of unspecified cause.

1 = case 1
2 = case 2
3 = multiple sclerosis
4 = Cockayne syndrome
5 = died at 18 months
    of age
6 = died at 8 days

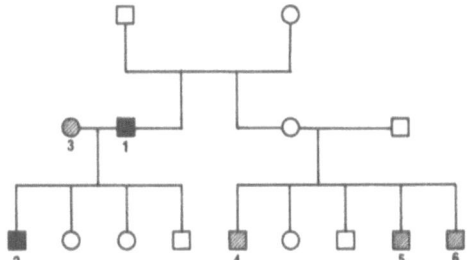

COMMENT

On the basis of their findings in these cases the authors state that *the
possibility of a latent genetic defect of astroglial cell precursors should
... be considered*. The occurrence of multiple sclerosis and of Cockayne
syndrome in this family is of interest. Cockayne syndrome is a rare disorder
of autosomal recessive inheritance beginning in late infancy, and characterized
by dwarfism, premature aging, mental deficiency, microcephaly, intracranial
calcifications, neurological deficits, retinal pigmentation, sensorineural
deafness and photosensitivity.

VII.C.1.24. <u>Koch and Waldbaur 1981 - Nürnberg, Germany</u> (132)

A father and son. German.

<u>Case 1</u> (father)

<u>History</u>: This bricklayer was admitted to hospital at the age of 37 years.
He had complained of progressive headaches and disturbances of vision for
three months.

On examination there was a protrusio bulbi and papilloedema on both sides. The
left pupil did not respond to light. Deep tendon reflexes were brisker on the
left. His gait was slightly disturbed. Roentgenograms of the skull showed
signs of elevated intracranial pressure (enlargement of the sella). The EEG
demonstrated focal disturbances of the right hemisphere and carotid angiography
revealed a tumour mass in the left fronto-basal region.

At operation a deeply situated and diffuse growing tumour of the left frontal
lobe was partly removed.

Postoperatively the patient received radiotherapy. Fourteen months afer operation the condition of the patient deteriorated and he was readmitted to
hospital on suspicion of tumour recurrence.

He died four weeks later at the age of 39 years.

<u>Autopsy</u>: Not performed.

<u>Microscopic study</u>: Spongioblastoma with differentiation to a small cell
astrocytoma.

<u>Diagnosis</u>: Left fronto-basal spongioblastoma with differentiation to a
small cell astrocytoma.

<u>Case 2</u> (son)

<u>History</u>: This merchant was admitted to hospital at the age of 30 years. He
had suffered from left-sided Jacksonian attacks and a loss of strength of the
left hand for two months.

On examination there was a facial and hypoglossal paresis on the left and a
distal paresis of the left arm. Computerized tomography showed a mass in the
right parietal operculum. Right carotid angiography indicated a tumour in the
region of the medial cerebral artery.

At operation a soft, approximately 4 x 4 cm cystical tumour in the temporo-
parietal region was totally removed.

Postoperatively the patient received radiotherapy. He made a good recovery
and 30 months after operation the patient was in a good condition and at work.

<u>Microscopic study</u>: Astrocytoma with signs of malignant degeneration in
small, localized areas.

Diagnosis: Astrocytoma with signs of malignant degeneration in the right temporo-parietal region.

Family: The son was an only child. The father had two healthy siblings.

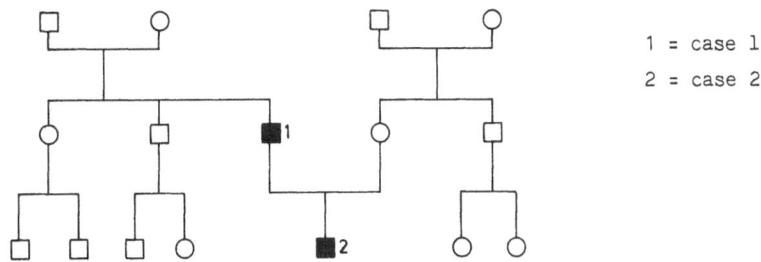

1 = case 1
2 = case 2

COMMENT

In case 2 (the son) a karyogram was made, which showed no abnormalities (46, XY). No signs of phacomatosis or neurofibromatosis were present in either patient.

VII.C.1.25. Thuwe et al. 1981 - Göteborg, Sweden
            (personal communication)

Seven cases in one family, Swedish.
A brother, a sister, a niece and a grand-niece, and three distant relatives.

Case 1 (brother)
    History: This patient was admitted to hospital at the age of 38 years
because of headaches, vomiting and diplopia.
Neurological examination revealed bilateral papilloedema, and hemiparesis of
the right side. The patient was slightly euphoric. He had suffered these
symptoms for two months.
In the hospital he was given radiotherapy and recovered within three weeks.
Two years later he was readmitted to hospital with the same symptoms.
He died three weeks later at the age of 41 years.
    Autopsy: showed a reddish-gray voluminous tumour in the left frontal lobe,
and tumour infiltrations over a large portion of the brain.
    Microscopic study: Not performed.
    Diagnosis: Left frontal tumour cerebri.

Case 2 (sister)
    History: This female died at the age of 25 years apparently of eclampsia
occurring in relation to a first parturition. She had not previously demonstrated symptoms of neurological disease.
    Autopsy: revealed a mandarin size tumour in the right temporal lobe. On
section the surface was white and the tumour was poorly demarcated from the
brain tissue. The dissector found the appearance of the tumour macroscopically
indicative of a glioma.
    Microscopic study: Not performed.
    Diagnosis: Right temporal tumour cerebri.

Case 3 (niece)
    History: This patient was admitted to hospital at the age of 57 years.
Earlier in life she had suffered from migraine until the menopause. At approximately 45 years of age she began complaining of attacks of dizziness and black-
outs which lasted for some minutes. At 55 years she suffered a grand mal
attack and during the following two years had difficulties in work, mostly
because of memory loss and bradyphrenia. She also developed an incontinentia
urinae.
At the age of 57 years she was operated upon and a resection of the right

frontal lobe performed. The tumour had grown through the corpus callosum into the left hemisphere and could not be completely removed.

Postoperatively she received radiotherapy.

She retained symptoms of bradyphrenia and incontinentia but was alive 4 years later.

Microscopic study: Astrocytoma grade I.

Diagnosis: Astrocytoma grade I of the corpus callosum and both frontal lobes.

Case 4 (grand-niece)

History: Since the age of 20 this female had been admitted to psychiatric departments four times because of depressive states. No neurological symptoms occurred until the age of 36, when she had a grand mal attack. After some time she began to suffer from headaches and her visual acuity diminished.

At the age of 37 years whe was operated upon and a cystic tumour of the left frontal lobe removed.

Postoperatively she made a relatively speedy recovery, but two months after operation was readmitted because of a left-sided hemiparesis. A recurrence of tumour on the left side was found with growth into the right hemisphere. There was also a small tumour in the right thalamus.

She died 6 months after operation, at the age of 38 years.

Autopsy: Not performed.

Microscopic study: Astrocytoma grade IV.

Diagnosis: Left frontal astrocytoma grade IV.

Case 5 (distant relative, see pedigree)

History: This male was admitted to hospital at the age of 35 years with complaints of severe headache and nausea, followed in later weeks by vomiting. At operation a tumour of the left frontal lobe was removed.

For two months after operation his condition was rather good but then deteriorated rapidly and he died 4 months postoperatively at the age of 35 years.

Autopsy: Performed.

Microscopic study: Gemistocytic glioblastoma.

Diagnosis: Left frontal glioblastoma.

Case 6 (distant relative, see pedigree)

History: This male began having epileptic seizures at the age of 42 years. Prior to this he had been healthy, although he had experienced some headaches from time to time. At the age of 45 years an angiogram suggested a small expanding process in the left frontal lobe. For various reasons he was not operated upon. In the following years his epileptic seizures continued. At the age of 49 years he again suffered from headaches. He then had symptoms of aphasia and showed a right-sided facial paresis. A new angiogram revealed progression, and the tumour was judged to be inoperable. His symptoms decreased after radiotherapy.

One and a half years later his condition deteriorated, and he died shortly thereafter at the age of 51 years.

Autopsy: Not performed.

Microscopic study: Not performed.

Diagnosis: Left frontal tumour cerebri.

Case 7 (distant relative, see pedigree)

History: From the approximate age of 35 to 40 years this male had suffered periods of insomnia and depression. He also demonstrated a rather high alcohol consumption. At the age of 42 years he increasingly developed headaches and showed changes in his personality. Some months later he had a grand mal attack and was admitted to hospital.

Angiography showed signs of a left-sided temporal expanding process. He then also developed symptoms of aphasia. A second angiogram showed considerable regression and operation was not considered indicated. During the following years the patient was twice admitted to hospital because of episodes of disorientation, dizziness, vomiting and motor weakness. The diagnosis remained unclear.

At the age of 54 years he died at home and was found five days later.

Autopsy: The cause of death was said to be cardial infarction. It is not known whether examination of the central nervous system was performed.

Microscopic study: Not performed.

Diagnosis: Left temporal tumour cerebri?

Family: The brother and sister (cases 1 and 2) had 9 other siblings; two of them died at an early age. The niece (case 3) had one unaffected sibling. The grand-niece (case 4) had 9 unaffected siblings; one brother died from suicide at the age of 24 years. Case 5 had one healthy half-brother. Case 6 had 8 other siblings; one of them died at the age of 22 years from tuberculosis.

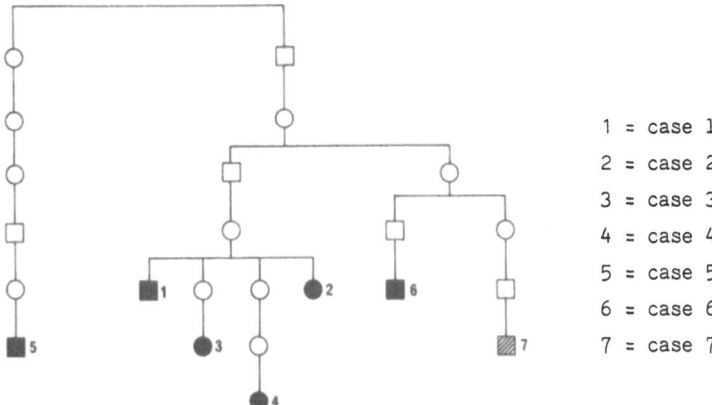

1 = case 1
2 = case 2
3 = case 3
4 = case 4
5 = case 5
6 = case 6
7 = case 7

COMMENT

This family was first described in a preliminary report in 1979 (262). The additional data have been obtained from the authors by personal communication.

VII.C.2.   OTHER GENERATIONS AND DISTANT RELATIVES WITH DISCORDANT TUMOUR

VII.C.2.1. Rados 1946 - Newark, N.J., U.S.A. (324)

Two cousins. American.

Case 1

History: This 5-year-old girl was admitted to hospital with the complaint of vomiting since one month.

On examination *the Babinski sign was present bilaterally. Increased intracranial pressure was suspected, and a suboccipital decompression, with postoperative roentgenologic treatment, was performed.* There was no improvement: the patient did not speak, her right arm and leg were spastic, there was knee clonus on the right and the Babinski sign was present bilaterally. On suspicion of a subdural haematoma a burr hole was made. ... *a tense brain was exposed, without any evidence of subdural hematoma* and a brain cannula was inserted. Ventriculography showed *a symmetric dilatation of the ventricular system up to the aqueduct, which was not visualized, a state presumably indicative of an expanding lesion of the brain stem.*

The condition postoperatively became progressively worse and the patient died one month later.

Autopsy: showed a large brain with flattened gyri. A cystic, whitish, club-shaped tumour was found in the pons and brain stem. The ventricles were greatly distended. No other developmental defects were noted.

Microscopic study: ... *presented the characteristic features of a fibrous astrocytoma in which cyst formation had occurred.*

Diagnosis: Astrocytoma of the pons.

Case 2

History: This boy had his left eye enucleated at the age of 8 months. *The right eye was treated with roentgen radiation and then enucleated three months later.*

Microscopic study: ... *revealed the picture of retinal glioma with formation of true and pseudorosettes, i.e., a neuroepithelioma.*

Diagnosis: Bilateral retinal neuroepithelioma.

Family: The mothers of the two cases were sisters. *The family histories were entirely negative for glioma and for all other forms of malignant growth. Each child was the first and only child of the mother.*

COMMENT

In this family there is an interesting coincidence of cerebral glioma with bilateral retinal neuroepithelioma. Retinal neuroepithelioma and retinoblastoma are considered equivalent in the modern nomenclature. Retinoblastomas may occur on a hereditary basis. The mode of inheritance is assumed to be autosomal dominant with diminished penetrance (330).

VII.C.2.2. Koch 1949 - Münster, Germany (126)

Two brothers and a nephew. German.

Two brothers died of histologically unverified brain tumours at the respective ages of 17 and 65 years. Their nephew - a son of their brother - was operated upon at the age of 35 years because of an astrocytoma of the left temporal lobe. No further details concerning these cases are available.

VII.C.2.3. Blickenstorfer 1951 - Zürich, Switzerland (30)

A brother and sister, grandmother and aunt. Swiss.

Case 1 (proband, brother)

History: The patient worked as a director in industry. He never had been seriously ill until the age of 68 years when he developed a hemiparesis on the left side. The previous months some changes in his character had been noticed: some disorientation and confusion, and an intellectual decline. At the age of 68 he was admitted to hospital.

At operation a large, partly cystic, glioma of the right occipital lobe was found and totally removed by an occipital lobectomy.

Postoperatively the patient received radiotherapy.

His condition gradually declined and he died about 10 months after operation. The cause of death appeared to be recurrence of the tumour.

Autopsy: Was not performed.

Microscopic study: The histological diagnosis of the tumour was undifferentiated glioblastoma multiforme.

Diagnosis: Right occipital glioblastoma multiforme.

Case 2 (sister)

History: This patient was the eldest sister of the proband. She showed the same mental symptoms as her brother in the course of her illness.

She had a frontal meningioma. No further data are given in the article.

Diagnosis: Frontal meningioma.

Case 3 (maternal grandmother)

History: This female began complaining of severe headaches between the ages of 60 and 70 years. She became melancholic, suffered memory disturbances and confusion, and made several suicide attempts.

She was said to have died of a brain tumour at the age of 71 years.

No further information was available.

Case 4 (maternal aunt)

History: This female complained acutely of severe headache at the age of 64 years. She also demonstrated confusion of speech.

She died a year later, following craniotomy for a brain tumour.

No other data are available concerning this case.

Family: The proband had two younger sisters. Fifty-nine members of his family were investigated. Aside from mental disorders no other important diseases were found among the relatives.

VII.C.2.4. <u>Koch 1954 - Münster, Germany</u> (127)

An uncle and niece. German.

The proband (niece) died of an anatomically diagnosed cystic glioma of the
left parieto-occipital lobe at the age of 18 years.
Her uncle had a clinically suspected brain tumour.

    <u>Family</u>: The mother of proband (3) died of cancer of the liver at the age
of 63 years.

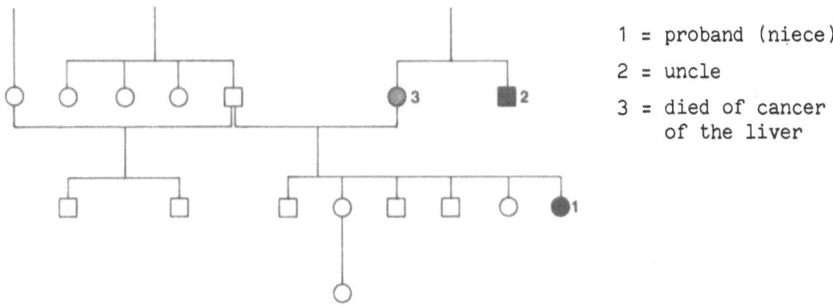

1 = proband (niece)
2 = uncle
3 = died of cancer
    of the liver

<u>COMMENT</u>
No further information concerning the cases is mentioned in the article. The
cases were mentioned in an extensive study of 350 female patients having
brain tumours.

VII.C.2.5. <u>Meyer 1956 - Münster, Germany</u> (172)

An uncle and nephew. German.

<u>Case 1</u> (uncle)

<u>History</u>: This 57-year-old male was admitted to hospital because of vertigo attacks, headaches and vomiting of a few weeks duration.

On examination the patient was bradyphrenic and somnolent. There was slight papilloedema on both sides. A left hemiparesis with lowered tendon reflexes was found. Romberg's sign was positive and there was an ataxia of gait. Cerebrospinal fluid showed elevated protein content. Arteriography revealed a very large tumour in the anterior part of the right hemisphere.

The patient's condition progressively deteriorated and he died some 3 weeks after admission.

<u>Autopsy</u>: showed a tumour in the right frontal and anterior parietal lobe with growth into the corpus callosum.

<u>Microscopic study</u>: Glioblastoma.

<u>Diagnosis</u>: Left fronto-parietal glioblastoma.

<u>Case 2</u> (nephew)

<u>History</u>: This 31-year-old male was admitted to hospital having had progressive headaches and disturbances of memory and concentration for several months. On examination there was slight papilloedema on both sides. Deep tendon reflexes of the legs were brisker on the right. Romberg's sign was positive and diadochokinesis of the left hand was slightly disturbed. His mental condition was apathetic. An encephalogram indicated a tumour mass in the region of the basal ganglia. Cerebrospinal fluid showed a pleocytosis and an elevated protein content.

The condition of the patient gradually deteriorated and he died a few weeks later.

<u>Autopsy</u>: Not performed.

<u>Diagnosis</u>: Brain tumour in the left basal ganglia.

Family:

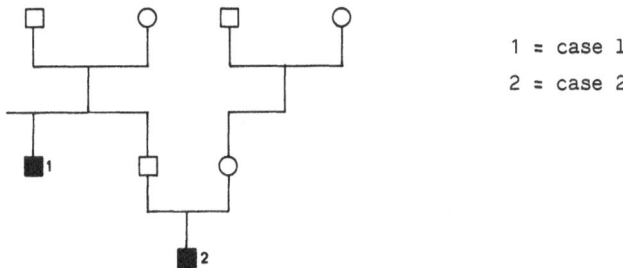

1 = case 1
2 = case 2

COMMENT

Unfortunately no histological diagnosis of the tumour in case 2 was made.
The cases are described in an extensive study of 459 male patients with brain
tumours. Investigation of their relatives revealed 7 families having familial
occurrence of brain tumours.

VII.C.2.6. Meyer 1956 - Münster, Germany (172)

A son, a mother, an aunt and an uncle. German.

Case 1 (son)

History: This 24-year-old textile manufacturer was admitted to hospital because of attacks of unconsciousness, progressive headaches and vomiting occurring since a few weeks.

On examination there was slight papilloedema on both sides. A hemihypaesthesia on the right side was found. Deep tendon reflexes were brisker on the right and there was a positive Babinski sign. Ataxia and dysdiadochokinesis were found on the right. A naevus was discovered in the left nasolabial fold. Cerebrospinal fluid showed an elevated protein content and a slightly elevated cell count. Left-sided arteriography revealed a parasagittal tumour.

At operation a large, grayish, subcortical cystical tumour in the left temporo-parietal region was partially removed.

The patient died two months postoperatively.

Autopsy: Not performed.

Microscopic study: Neuroblastoma, partly consisting of spongioblastic cells, partly of neuroblasts with differentiation to ganglionic cells. A histological diagnosis of immature ganglio-neuroblastoma was made.

Diagnosis: Left temporo-parietal, subcortical, ganglioneuroblastoma.

Case 2 (mother)

History: The mother (of case 1) died at the age of 36 years of a brain tumour.

Case 3 (aunt, sister of case 2)

History: This female died at the age of 26 years of a brain tumour.

Case 4 (uncle, brother of case 2)

History: This male died at the age of 48 years of a brain tumour.

Family:

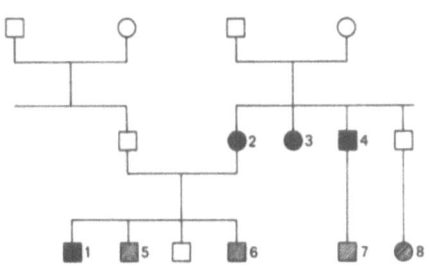

1 = case 1

2 = case 2

3 = case 3

4 = case 4

5 = this brother died at
    the age of 13 years of
    a sarcoma of the kidney

6 = this brother died at
    the age of 8 weeks of
    'Krämpfen'

7 = this cousin died at the
    age of 25 years in a
    depressive state

8 = this cousin suffered
    from seizures

COMMENT

No further information concerning the medical histories of cases 2, 3, and 4
was available.

This report is described in an extensive study on 459 male patients with brain
tumours. Family investigation of these patients revealed 7 families with
familial brain tumour occurrence.

VII.C.2.7. <u>Meyer 1956 - Münster, Germany</u> (172)

A father and son. German.

<u>Case 1</u> (son)

<u>History</u>: This boatman was admitted to hospital at the age of 35 years. At
the age of 33 years he had a motorcycle accident resulting in loss of consciousness for half an hour. A few weeks later he had an 'Attack' of unconsciousness.
This sort attack recurred four times in the following year. A few weeks before
admission he had also complained of disturbances of vision and headaches in the
right face and frontal region.

On examination papilloedema on both sides and a right central facial paresis
were found. Cerebrospinal fluid pressure was slightly elevated. An encephalogram indicated a tumour mass in the left hemisphere, probably of the temporal
lobe. As he was free of complaints the patient was discharged home at his own
request.

He was readmitted three years later because of headaches, tinnitus and recurrence of symptoms. His mental condition had also deteriorated.

Roentgenograms of the skull showed signs of elevated intracranial pressure and
arteriography indicated a tumour in the left frontal lobe.

At operation a very large tumour of the left frontal lobe extending to the
skull base was subtotally removed.

Postoperatively the patient received radiotherapy.

Five months later the patient was again operated upon because of tumour
recurrence, and again received radiotherapy.

His postoperative course was good and he was discharged home a few months later.

<u>Microscopic study</u>: Oligodendroglioma with the characteristic honey-comb
structure.

<u>Diagnosis</u>: Left frontal oligodendroglioma.

<u>Case 2</u> (father)

<u>History</u>: The father died at the age of 56 years of a brain tumour.

Family:

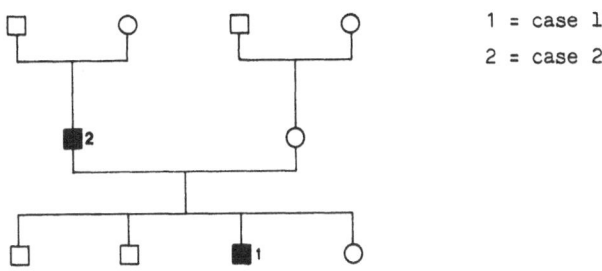

1 = case 1
2 = case 2

COMMENT

No further information concerning the medical history of the father (case 2)
is available.

This family is described in an extensive study of 459 male patients with brain
tumours. Investigation of their relatives revealed 7 families with familial
brain tumour occurrence.

342

VII.C.2.8. <u>Meyer 1956 - Münster, Germany</u> (172)

Two first-cousins. German.

<u>Case 1</u>
   <u>History</u>: This storekeeper was hospitalized at the age of 47 years. He had
complained of headaches and disturbances of vision for a few months. Also a
mental deterioration had been noticed.
On examination there was slight papilloedema of the right fundus and a doubtful
Babinski sign on the right. His gait showed a slight deviation to the left. His
mental condition was retarded and he had difficulties in finding words. Encephalography indicated a tumour in the left hemisphere, which was confirmed by
angiography and localized in the posterior basal frontal lobe.
At operation a deep tumour containing many blood vessels was partially removed
from the left frontal lobe.
The patient died a few hours after operation.
   <u>Autopsy</u>: Not performed.
   <u>Microscopic study</u>: Not performed.
   <u>Diagnosis</u>: Left fronto-basal glioblastoma.

<u>Case 2</u>
   <u>History</u>: This cousin was treated for a brain tumour in another hospital. No
further information on this case is available.

   <u>Family</u>: An aunt (3; sister of the mother of case 1) suffered from melancholia
at older age.

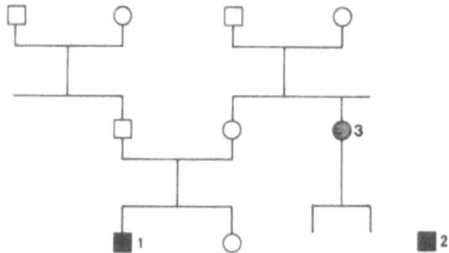

1 = case 1

2 = case 2

3 = aunt with
    melancholia

COMMENT

The diagnosis of the tumour in case 1 was based on the macroscopic findings at operation and was not histologically verified. No medical history of case 2 was available.

This report is described in an extensive study on 459 male patients with brain tumours.

VII.C.2.9. Weersma 1957 - The Netherlands
            (personal communication in Van der Wiel 1959) (286)

A mother and daughter. Dutch or Indonesian.

The daughter died at the age of 45 years of a glioblastoma fusiforme. Her
mother had died at the age of 55 years after a brain operation in Batavia.
She had a malignant brain tumour located in a cerebral hemisphere.
No further information is available concerning these cases.

COMMENT

This case is described by Van der Wiel (286) as a personal communication.

VII.C.2.10. Kemper 1964 - Münster, Germany (117)

An aunt and nephew. German.

Case 1 (aunt)

History: This 47-year-old female was hospitalized because of acute headaches
and dizziness, followed by a loss of strength of the left extremities and pain
in the left leg.

On examination the reaction of the pupils to light was weak. Deep tendon
reflexes were brisker on the left and there was a left positive Babinski sign.
A spastic left hemiparesis was found. Funduscopy showed minimal signs of
papilloedema on the right. Angiography revealed a tumour in the middle of the
right temporal lobe.

In the following weeks the patient suffered from parotitis and pneumonia and
she died two weeks after admission.

Autopsy: showed a tumour in the right temporal lobe.

Microscopic study: Histological diagnosis was glioblastoma multiforme.

Diagnosis: Right temporal glioblastoma multiforme.

Case 2 (nephew)

History: This 19-year-old male was hospitalized because of headaches and
visual disturbances existing since a few months. His medical history revealed
a head injury at the age of 5 years.

On examination papilloedema on both sides was found and there was some disorientation in time. An EEG showed focal disturbances over the left occipito-
temporal region and angiography demonstrated a left temporo-parieto-occipital
tumour.

At operation this tumour was totally removed.

Microscopic study: showed a fibromatous meningioma.

Diagnosis: Left temporo-parieto-occipital fibromatous meningioma.

Family: The father of case 2 was missed during the war, the mother was
alive and healthy. Two sisters were healthy. The mother of case 1 (3) died at
the age of 80 years of apoplexy. No other patients with tumour could be found
in this family.

346

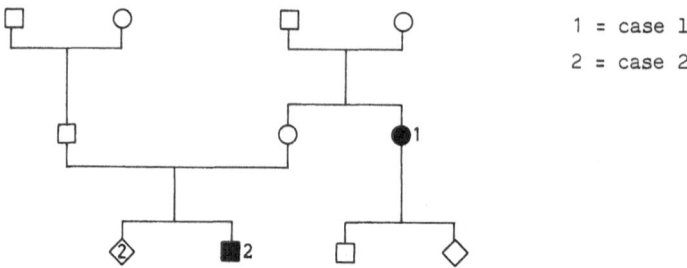

1 = case 1
2 = case 2

COMMENT

This familial occurrence of brain tumours was mentioned in an extensive study
of 254 male and 199 female patients with brain tumours, including 6 pairs of
twins. Six occurrences of familial brain tumours were noted within this study.

VII.C.2.11. Kemper 1964 - Münster, Germany (117)

An uncle and nephew. German.

Case 1 (uncle)

History: This 29-year-old male was hospitalized having had progressive loss of strength of the right arm and leg for 3 months, and disturbances of speech since two weeks.

Roentgenograms of the skull showed no abnormalities, but ventriculography revealed a cystic process in the left parietal region.

At operation a cystic tumour in the left parieto-occipital region was extirpated.

The patient died 4 months postoperatively.

Autopsy: Not performed.

Microscopic study: Cystic glioma.

Diagnosis: Left parieto-occipital cystic glioma.

Case 2 (nephew)

History: This 17-year-old male was hospitalized because of loss of strength, pain and numb feelings of the left leg. A year before he had been diagnosed as having Scheuermann's disease. His further medical history revealed his having had a pyloric stenosis as a baby.

On examination a restriction of the spinal column movements, a slight atrophy of the left leg muscles with paresis, and hypaesthesia below the level of L_3 were found. Deep tendon reflexes were brisk on both sides, more on the left than on the right, and the Babinski sign was bilaterally positive. Lasègue's sign was positive on the left at 40 degrees. Lumbar puncture showed a normal pressure and positive Queckenstedt sign. The CSF was yellow with an elevated protein content. Myelography demonstrated an obstruction at the Th_{11} level.

At operation an extramedullary tumour originating from a dorsal nerve root on the left and compressing the myelum was completely removed.

Postoperatively the patient made a good recovery.

Microscopic study: Neurinoma.

Diagnosis: Neurinoma of the spinal cord (Thoracic X-XII).

Family: A cousin of the mother of case 2 and a cousin of his father had multiple sclerosis. The mother of case 2 suffered from depressions. A brother of case 2 was treated for temporary dysphoric states. There was consanguinity between the grandparents (cousins).

348

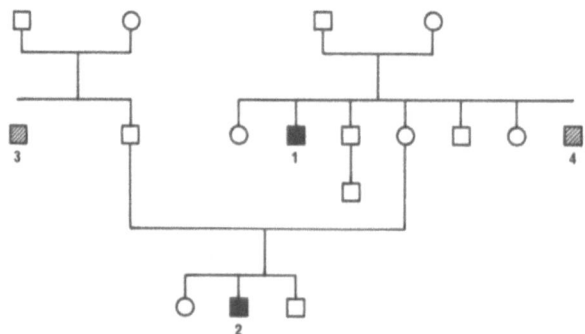

1 = case 1;   2 = case 2;   3 + 4 = multiple sclerosis

COMMENT

No signs of neurofibromatosis were found in the family.

These cases were mentioned in an extensive study of 254 male and 199 female patients having brain tumours; 6 families with familial occurrence of brain tumours were found.

VII.C.2.12.   Walker et al. 1971 - Baltimore, U.S.A. (276)

At the twenty-third Annual Meeting of the American Academy of Neurology the authors presented a large kindred demonstrating malignancies, the most common of which were brain tumours.

The proband and 1 of his 3 siblings died of malignant glioma, while a third died of osteogenic sarcoma.

The proband's paternal uncle and paternal granduncle both died of brain tumor, and many of their respective siblings died of malignancy (carcinoma of the stomach, bowel, breast, and adrenal glands and sarcoma).

Data were collected concerning five generations. *Three generations had two cases of brain tumors in each, with the next most common malignancy being leukemia. In the third generation, a brother and sister of one family married a sister and brother of another family, thus creating two further lines of disease propagation. Both lines have developed malignancy, including brain tumor, in succeeding generations.*

Studies of *chromosome configuration, serum contents, immune responses, and immune electrophoresis ... have been carried out* but the results were not reported.

COMMENT

This family must be considered as a manifestation of the SBLA family cancer syndrome.

VII.C.2.13. Van der Wiel 1980 - Gouda, The Netherlands
            (personal communication)

A grandfather and granddaughter. Dutch.

The grandfather died at the age of 47 years of a glioblastoma multiforme; his
granddaughter died at the age of 5 years of a medulloblastoma.
The son of the grandfather had a large spina bifida occulta. A cousin of the
granddaughter died shortly after birth of anencephaly (see also II.C.2.2).

TABLES

352

TABLE 1 – MONOZYGOTIC TWINS WITH CONCORDANT TUMOUR (VII.A.1)

	case	gender	relationship	number of unaffected siblings	race or nationality	age at symptom occurrence	age at death	location of the tumour
VII.A.1.1. Joughin 1928	1	f	s	?	Jew.	32 y	33 y	R temporal
	2	f	s	?	Jew.	27 y	35 y	L subcortical
VII.A.1.2. Kjellin 1960	1	m	br	4	Swed.	33 y	38 y	R temporal
	2	m	br	4	Swed.	49 y	50 y	R temporal
VII.A.1.3. Fairburn 1971	1	m	br	0	Engl.	3 y	4 y	Brain stem and L cerebellar hemisphere
	2	m	br	0	Engl.	7 y	7 y	L fronto-parietal
VII.A.1.4. Clarenbach 1979	1	m	br	1 br 2 s	Germ.	22 y	–	4th ventricle
	2	m	br	1 br 2 s	Germ.	22 y	–	4th ventricle

TABLE 2 – MONOZYGOTIC TWINS WITH DISCORDANT TUMOUR (VII.A.2)

	case	gender	relationship	number of unaffected siblings	race or nationality	age at symptom occurrence	age at death	location of the tumour
VII.A.2.1. Hoppe 1952	1	m	br	?	Germ.	35 y	–	L sphenoidal
	2	m	br	?	Germ.	53 y	53 y	L fronto-central
VII.A.2.2. Koch 1957	1	m	br	1 br 4 s	Germ.	47 y	48 y	R temporal
	2	m	br	1 br 4 s	Germ.	35 y	47 y	R basomedial

diagnosis	biopsy	autopsy	associated physical or mental conditions	family	comment
Glioma	+	+	–	–	No histological description of the glioma
Glioma	+	–	–		
Astrocytoma I	+	–	–	–	–
Astrocytoma I-II	+	+	–		
Mixed glioma	+	+	–	–	Both mixed glioma with oligodendroglial and astrocytic elements
Mixed glioma	+	+	–		
Subependymoma	+	–	–	–	Same twins as described by Voigt & Marquardt in 1979
Subependymoma	+	–	–		

diagnosis	biopsy	autopsy	associated physical or mental conditions	family	comment
Meningioma	+	–	Pointed head form	Several twins in family of mother	Case 1 first reported by Pedersen & Geyer in 1938. Case 2 healthy at that time
Glioblastoma	+	–	Pointed head form		
Glioblastoma multiforme	+	–	Septum pellucidum cyst	1 sister liver-cirrhosis; 1 sister lung-tuberculosis	Case 2: clinical diagnosis
Septum pellucidum cyst	–	–	–		

TABLE 3 - SIBLINGS WITH CONCORDANT TUMOUR (VII.B.1)

	case	gender	relationship	number of unaffected siblings	race or nationality	age at symptom occurrence	age at death	location of the tumour
VII.B.1.1. Besold 1896	1	f	s	0 ?	Germ.	16 y	17 - 18 y	3rd ventricle
	2	f	s	0 ?	Germ.	11 y	14 y	3rd ventricle
VII.B.1.2. Böhmig 1918	1	m	br	0	Germ.	23 y	24 y	L fronto-parietal
	2	f	s	0	Germ.	37 y	38 y	R frontal
VII.B.1.3. Hoffmann 1919	1	m	br	3 s	Germ.	30 y	33 y	L gyrus hippo-campi
	2	m	br	3 s	Germ.	48 y	48 y	R gyrus hippo-campi
VII.B.1.4. Bender 1932 Hallervorden 1936	1	m	br	6 s 1 br	Germ.	56 y	60 y	central; lateral and 3rd ventricles
	2	m	br	6 s 1 br	Germ.	41 y	46 y	diffuse, with accumulation in R temporal lobe
	3	m	br	6 s 1 br	Germ.	47 y	47 y	?
VII.B.1.5. Glauberman 1936	1	m	br	?	?	56 y	?	L temporal
	2	m	br	?	?	51 y	?	L temporal

diagnosis	biopsy	autopsy	associated physical or mental conditions	family	comment
Sarcomatous tumour of ependymal origin	-	+	Thyroid gland cysts, pancreatic haemorrhages, double L ureter, open foramen ovale	Grandmother died of a brain suppuration	Histological diagnosis anaplastic ependymoma
Sarcomatous tumour of ependymal origin	-	+	Pneumonia as a child		
Glioma	-	+	Convulsions at the age of 3 months	Father died of paralysis	Microscopic study of case 1 was not mentioned in the article
Glioma	-	+	Agoraphobia, anaemia		
Glioma	-	+	-	Father epilepsia tarda, died of CVA, a sister feeble-minded and suffering from hysterical (?) convulsions, 2 offspring in both cases died very young	-
Glioma	-	+	Slight rheumatic complaints		
Spongioblastoma	-	+	Alcoholic, impotent, depression, lipoma, pes caves, naevi	2 sisters oligophrenic, 1 br and 1 s naevi, 1 s pes caves. 54 relatives investigated: 4 oligophrenic, 1 epilepsy, 2 pes caves, 5 naevi	Autopsy and histological diagnosis of case 2 described by Hallervorden in 1936. Case 3 clinical diagnosis. Relationship with neurofibromatosis complex.
Glioblastomatosis	-	+	Alcoholic, depression, psychosis, naevus, pes caves, skin tumours		
Brain tumour	-	-	Naevi, pes caves		
Spongioblastoma multiforme	?	?	?	?	Cited by Manuelidis 1972
Spongioblastoma multiforme	?	?	?		

TABLE 3 - continued

	case	gender	relationship	number of unaffected siblings	race or nationality	age at symptom occurrence	age at death	location of the tumour
VII.B.1.6. Pass <u>1938</u>	1	f	half s	5 s 3 br	Germ.	?	49 y	frontal
	2	f	half s	0	Germ.	?	46 y	temporal
VII.B.1.7. Geyer <u>1939</u>	1	m	br	?	Germ.	?	43 y	frontal
	2	f	s	?	Germ.	?	44 y	frontal
VII.B.1.8. Halpern <u>1943</u>	1	m	br	?	?	42 y	?	L peduncle
	2	m	br	?	?	43 y	?	L temporal
VII.B.1.9. Riese <u>1944</u>	1	m	br	?	Amer.	50 y	50 y	R fronto-parietal
	2	f	s	?	Amer.	39 y	39 y	R temporal
VII.B.1.10. Lange-Cosack <u>1949</u>	1	f	s	?	?	?	?	?
	2	f	s	?	?	?	?	?
VII.B.1.11. Zülch <u>1951</u>	1	m	br	?	?	?	54 y	parieto-occipital region
	2	m	br	?	?	?	61 y	parieto-occipital region
VII.B.1.12. Almeida Lima <u>1954</u>	1	m	br	?	?	?	?	?
	2	m	br	?	?	?	?	?
VII.B.1.13. Koch <u>1954</u>	1	f	s	4 s	Germ.	47 y	?	R lateral ventricle
	2	m	br	4 s	Germ.	53 y	?	R fronto-temporal
VII.B.1.14. Appelman <u>1956</u>	1	m	br	?	Dutch	?	?	?
	2	m	br	?	Dutch	?	?	?

diagnosis	biopsy	autopsy	associated physical or mental conditions	family	comment
Glioma	?	?	?	Mother died of an oesophagus carcinoma, 2 sisters died as young children	No further specification of histological diagnosis.
Glioma	?	?	?		Study on 30 families of patients with brain tumours
Glioblastoma multiforme	?	+	?	?	Diagnosis of case 2 made macroscopically at autopsy
Glioblastoma multiforme	?	+	?		
Astroblastoma	?	?	?	?	Cited by Peyser and Beller 1951 and Manuelidis 1972
Astroblastoma	?	?	?		
Glioblastoma multiforme	-	+		-	
Glioblastoma multiforme	+	+	Bronchiogenic lung carcinoma, leiomyomata uteri		
Glioma	?	?	?	?	Cited by Van der Wiel 1959
Glioma	?	?	?		
Glioblastoma	?	?	?	?	Cited by Koch 1954
Glioblastoma	?	?	?		
Astrocytoma	?	?	?	?	Personal communication in Koch 1954
Astrocytoma	?	?	?		
Ependymoma	?	?	-	-	Study of 350 female patients with CNS tumour
Cystic glioma	?	?	-		
Glioblastoma	?	?	?	-	Personal communication in Van der Wiel 1959
Glioblastoma	?	?	?		

TABLE 3 - continued

case	gender	relationship	number of unaffected siblings	race or nationality	age at symptom occurrence	age at death	location of the tumour
VII.B.1.15. Noetzel 1959							
1	m	br	-	Germ.	43 y	43 y	L parieto-occipital
2	f	s	-	Germ.	28 y	32 y	R frontal
VII.B.1.16. Noetzel 1959							
1	m	br	7	Germ.	49 y	49 y	posterior corpus callosum
2	m	br	7	Germ.	59 y	60 y	L parieto-occipital
VII.B.1.17. Grosz 1960							
1	m	br	3	Isr.	50 y	51 y	L temporal
2	f	s	3	Isr.?	32 y	32 y	L temporal
VII.B.1.18. Symonds 1960							
1	m	br	?	Engl.	35 y	35 y	corpus callosum and L frontal
2	f	s	?	Engl.	34 y	-	L frontal
VII.B.1.19. Koch 1960							
1	f	s	6 br 4 s	Germ.	54 y	54 y	R fronto-parietal
2	f	s	6 br 4 s	Germ.	51 y	51 y	R temporal
3	f	s	6 br 4 s	Germ.	50 y	50 y	L temporal
VII.B.1.20. Parkinson 1962							
1	m	br	?	Can.	33 y	-	L frontal
2	m	br	?	Can.	30 y	-	Subfrontal, 3rd and lateral ventricles
VII.B.1.21. Metzel 1963							
1	m	br	?	Germ.	approx. 9 y	approx. 9 y	R hemisphere
2	m	br	?	Germ.	9 y	9 y	R ventricle

diagnosis	biopsy	autopsy	associated physical or mental conditions	family	comment
Glioblastoma multiforme	-	+	"Lappung" kidneys, nodular goiter, head injury 43 y	-	
Glioblastoma multiforme	-	+	Depressive		
Glioblastoma	-	+	40 y: enucleation of R eye after shell splinter injury	Mother died of tuberculosis	-
Glioblastoma fusiforme	+	-	Head injury 59 y		
Glioblastoma multiforme	+	-	Musical prodigy, withdrawn	Family of musicians	No details about histological structure of case 2;
Glioma	+	-	Talented musician		died in Vienna 22 y before her brother
Glioblastoma	-	+	"Schizophrenic psychosis"	-	-
Oligodendro-glioma	+	-	"Schizophrenic psychosis"		
Brain tumour	-	-	-	Mother diabetic at older age, 2 brothers died 2 y of age of unknown cause	PA in case 1 not histologically verified, glioblastoma multiforme suspected
Glioblastoma multiforme	+	-	-		
Glioblastoma multiforme	+	-	Feeble-minded, rheumatic complaints		
Oligodendro-glioma	+	-	-	?	PA of case 2: some areas of the tumour indistinguishable from highly malignant glioma of the astro-cytic type
Oligodendro-glioma	+	-	-		
Ependymoma	-	+	-	Mother suffered from seizures	Diagnosis of case 2 based on cytological examination of CSF. Age of case 1 approx. same as case 2
Ependymoma	-	-	-		

TABLE 3 - continued

	case	gender	relationship	number of unaffected siblings	race or nationality	age at symptom occurrence	age at death	location of the tumour
VII.B.1.22. Metzel 1964	1	f	s	?	Germ.	?	28 y	4th ventricle
	2	m	br	?	Germ.	?	?	?
VII.B.1.23. Armstrong 1969	1	m	br	6	Can.	64 y	64 y	R temporal
	2	m	br	6	Can.	50 y	50 y	L temporal
	3	f	s	6	Can.	57 y	57 y	R temporal
VII.B.1.24. Baughman 1969	1	f	s	2 s	Amer.	12 y	14 y	white matter of both hemispheres
	2	m	br	2 s	Amer.	25 y	26 y	caudate nucleus and L temporal lobe
	3	m	br	2 s	Amer.	12 y	12 y	L fronto-parietal subcortical
	4	f	s	2 s	Amer.	21 y	-	L frontal
VII.B.1.25. Blaauw 1971	1	m	br	1 br	Dutch	15 y	21 y	cervical cord
	2	m	br	1 br	Dutch	18 y	18 y	cervical cord
VII.B.1.26. Kaufman 1972	1	m	br	2 br 1 s	Amer.	38 y	38 y	L thalamus to brain stem
	2	m	br	2 br 1 s	Amer.	50 y	50 y	R cerebellar hemisphere
VII.B.1.27. Isamat 1974	1	f	s	?	Span.	55 y	?	anterior 3rd ventricle
	2	f	s	?	Span.	57 y	?	post-frontal

diagnosis	biopsy	autopsy	associated physical or mental conditions	family	comment
Ependymoma	-	-	-	Son of case 1 was operated at 19 y because of arachnoidal cyst of the cisterna magna	Study of 393 patients with verified gliomatous brain tumours showed 3 familial occurrences in siblings
Glioblastoma	+	-	-		
Astrocytoma II-III	+	-	-	-	-
Astrocytoma II-III	+	-	-		
Astrocytoma II-III	+	-	-		
Glioblastoma multiforme	+	+	1 café-au-lait spot, 1 pigmented naevus, polyposis of colon	76 family members of five generations investigated. No additional case of polyposis or occurrence of neurofibromatosis. 3 y old female maternal 2nd cousin had a posterior-fossa ependymoma	Manifestation of glioma-polyposis syndrome. Relationship with neurofibromatosis
Glioblastoma multiforme	-	+	Abundant pigmented naevi, polyposis of colon		
Glioblastoma multiforme	+	-	4 café-au-lait spots		
Glioblastoma multiforme	+	-	2 polyps of the colon		
Subependymoma	-	+	Syringomyelic cavity; haemophilia	Other haemophiliacs	Coincidence of familial CNS tumours with familial haemophilia
Subependymoma	+	+	Haemophilia		
Glioblastoma multiforme	-	+	-	Mother diabetic, 1 br diabetic, 1 s migraine	The article also mentions two 1st cousins with astrocytoma (VII.C.1.12)
Glioblastoma multiforme	+	+	-		
Astrocytoma	+	-	Blood-group A	-	
Astrocytoma III	+	-	Blood-group A		

TABLE 3 - continued

case	gender	relationship	number of unaffected siblings	race or nationality	age at symptom occurrence	age at death	location of the tumour
VII.B.1.28. Isamat 1974							
1	m	br	?	Span.	49 y	?	bifrontal corpus callosum
2	m	br	?	Span.	48 y	?	temporal
VII.B.1.29. Schoenberg 1975							
1	m	br	1 br	Amer.	12 y	13 y	aqueduct of Sylvius
2	f	s	1 br	Amer.	6 y	-	R temporo-parietal
3	f	s	1 br	Amer.	12 y	12 y	L frontal
VII.B.1.30. Li 1977							
1	m	br	2 br	White Amer.	6 y	6 y	4th ventricle
2	m	br	2 br	White Amer.	11 y	12 y	frontal
VII.B.1.31. Pelgrom von Motz 1977							
1	f	s	3 br 3 s	Dutch	69 y	69 y	insular region
2	f	s	3 br 3 s	Dutch	52 y	53 y	L parieto-occipital
3	f	s	3 br 3 s	Dutch	73 y	73 y	R frontal and L parietal
VII.B.1.32. de Tribolet 1979							
1	m	br	?	Swiss	50 y	50 y	L temporal
2	m	br	?	Swiss	69 y	69 y	R temporal
VII.B.1.33. Sulla 1979							
1	m	br	6	Czech	61 y	61 y	R temporal
2	m	br	6	Czech	59 y	59 y	R frontal
VII.B.1.34. Schouwink 1980							
1	m	br	?	Dutch	59 y	59 y	R frontal
2	m	br	?	Dutch	51 y	51 y	L frontal

diagnosis	biopsy	autopsy	associated physical or mental conditions	family	comment
Astrocytoma IV	+	-	Blood-group A	A nephew aque-ductal stenosis, presumably due to gliosis	
Astrocytoma IV	+	-	Blood-group A		
Brain tumour	-	-	-	Brother medias-tinal cystic hydroma. Grandfather prostatic cancer. Grandmother kidney disease	-
Astrocytoma II and III	+	-	-		
Astrocytoma III	+	-	Presacral lipoma at 6 y		
Glioma	-	-	Meningocoele, acute leukemia	Brother myelo-genous leukemia, haemangioma, multiple nevo-xanthoendothe-liomas; brother cardiac mal-formations, squamous papill-oma; father polio	Von Recklinghausen's neurofibromatosis or other inherited cancer syndrome?
Glioblastoma multiforme	+	-	Café-au-lait spot, pigmented naevi, lymphocytic lymphoma		
Astrocytoma III	-	+	-	Many malignan-cies in the family (lung, breast, stomach, uterus)	No connection between two tumours in case 3. Both were microscopic-ally identical
Astrocytoma III	+	-	-		
Astrocytoma III	-	+	-		
Glioblastoma	+	+	-	?	-
Glioblastoma	+	+	-		
Astrocytoma II	+	-	Blood-group AB, Rh +	-	-
Astrocytoma III	+	-	Blood-group AB, Rh +		
Astrocytoma	-	+	Luetic infection and tabes dorsalis	3rd brother died at younger age supposedly of brain tumour	Personal communication
Astrocytoma	-	+	-		

364

TABLE 3 - continued

	case	gender	relationship	number of unaffected siblings	race or nationality	age at symptom occurrence	age at death	location of the tumour
VII.B.1.35. Spit 1980	1	f	s	?	Dutch	64 y	64 y	R temporal
	2	m	br	?	Dutch	61 y	61 y	R frontal
VII.B.1.36. Todd 1981	1	f	s	0	Amer.	17 y	19 y	L frontal
	2	m	br	0	Amer.	10 y	12 y	R temporo-parieto-occipital
	3	m	br	0	Amer.	18 y	23 y	L frontal

diagnosis	biopsy	autopsy	associated physical or mental conditions	family	comment
Astrocytoma III-IV	+	-	-	?	Personal communication
Astrocytoma III	+	-	-		
Glioblastoma multiforme	+	-	-	Maternal grandfather carcinoma of the stomach	Manifestation of Turcot syndrome (glioma-polyposis syndrome)
Astrocytoma III	+	+	Hodgkin's disease; polyposis coli		
Glioblastoma multiforme	+	+	Polyposis coli; adenocarcinoma coli		

TABLE 4 - SIBLINGS WITH DISCORDANT TUMOUR (VII.B.2)

	case	gender	relationship	number of unaffected siblings	race or nationality	age at symptom occurrence	age at death	location of the tumour
VII.B.2.1. Oehler 1936	1	m	br	8	Germ.	26 y	29 y	L fronto-temporal
	2	m	br	8	Germ.	32 y	38 y	hypophysis
VII.B.2.2. Hallervorden 1936	1	m	br	2 s	Germ.	44 y	47 y	diffuse
	2	f	s	2 s	Germ.	-	42 y	-
VII.B.2.3. Peyser 1951	1	m	br	4	Isr.	14 y	15 y	L frontal horn
	2	m	br	4	Isr.	14 m	20 m	R cerebral hemi-sphere
VII.B.2.4. Koch 1954	1	m	br	1 br	Germ.	?	45 y	R temporal
	2	f	s	1 br	Germ.	?	57 y	L frontal
VII.B.2.5. Henschen 1955	1	m	br	?	?	55 y	?	temporal
	2	f	s	?	?	42 y	?	
VII.B.2.6. Turcot 1959	1	f	s	-	Can.	21 y	21 y	L frontal lobe
	2	m	br	-	Can.	17 y	17 y	medulla spinalis
VII.B.2.7. Hauge 1960	1	f	s	8 br	Dan.	-	55 y	R temporal
	2	m	br	8 br	Dan.	-	45 y	?
	3	m	br	8 br	Dan.	-	46 y	?
	4	f	s	8 br	Dan.	-	49 y	?

diagnosis	biopsy	autopsy	associated physical or mental conditions	family	comment
Glioblastoma multiforme	+	+	Multiple pigmented naevi, papilloma of the tongue	Mother died of uterus cancer	Case 2: clinical diagnosis
Hypophysis tumour					
Glioblastoma-tosis	-	+	Fibroma on the back, head injury	Mother died of intestinal cancer	Case 2: clinical diagnosis
Brain tumour	-	-	-		
Glioblastoma multiforme	+	-	-	-	
Choroid plexus papilloma	-	+	Pertussis at 4 m and bilateral otitis at 8 m		
Glioma	?	?	?	A brother died of a liver carcinoma	Case 2: no histological diagnosis
Brain tumour	-	-	?		
Glioblastoma	?	?	?	?	Cited by Kemper 1964
Brain tumour	-	-	?		
Glioblastoma	-	+	Polyposis colon, chromophobe adenoma hypophysis	-	Glioma-polyposis syndrome
Medulloblastoma	-	+	Polyposis colon with adenocarcinoma		
Astrocytoma	?	?	-	Father: suicide. 1 br died in infancy from unknown cause; 1 br died from malaria and possible cerebral abscess	Case 3 histologically verified?
Brain tumour	?	?	-		
Gliomatosis (?)	?	?	-		
Brain tumour	?	?	-		

TABLE 4 - continued

case	gender	relationship	number of unaffected siblings	race or nationality	age at symptom occurrence	age at death	location of the tumour
VII.B.2.8. Kjellin 1960							
1	m	br	7	Swed.	11 y	12 y	R occipital
2	f	s	7	Swed.	25 y	25 y	L basal ganglia
VII.B.2.9. Metzel 1963							
1	m	br	?	Germ.	42 y	42 y	L temporal
2	m	br	?	Germ.	-	55 y	L temporal
VII.B.2.10. Kemper 1964							
1	f	s	3 s 3 br	Germ.	64 y	64 y	L occipital
2	f	s	3 s 3 br	Germ.	?		?
VII.B.2.11. Colafranceschi 1970							
1	m	br	3 s 3 br	Ital.	50 y	51 y	L temporal
2	m	br	3 s 3 br	Ital.	57 y	57 y	R frontal
VII.B.2.12. Chen 1970							
1	f	s	3 s 7 br	Guam.	?	13 y	-
2	f	s	3 s 7 br	Guam.	?	7 y	-
3	m	br	3 s 7 br	Guam.	?	5 y	L hemisphere
4	m	br	3 s 7 br	Guam.	?	5 y	paraventricular and R hemisphere
VII.B.2.13. De Tribolet 1979							
1	m	br	?	Swiss	21 y	-	R frontal
2	f	s	?	Swiss	15 y	15 y	R thalamus

diagnosis	biopsy	autopsy	associated physical or mental conditions	family	comment
Astrocytoma	+	-	-	?	Histological diagnosis of case 2 is lacking, a glioma is assumed
Brain tumour	-	-	-		
Astrocytoma	+	+	-	?	A gliomatous tumour in case 2 is assumed by the author. No histological verification
Brain tumour	?	-	-		
Glioblastoma multiforme	-	+	-	Brother died at 38 y of carcinoma of stomach; sister tumour of face	Extensive study of 254 male and 199 female patients with brain tumours. No medical history of case 2
Brain tumour	?	?	-		
Glioblastoma multiforme	+	-	Blood-group 0, Rh -	Brother of M, brother of F, nephew of F: carcinoma of stomach; brother of F: leukaemia	A glioma is assumed in case 2 by the authors
Brain tumour	-	-	Blood-group 0, Rh -		
Medulloblastoma	?	+	Black naevi on the back, hypoplasia of corpus callosum	Two sibs with leukaemia, some sibs with black naevi and café-au-lait spots. Two grandfathers hepatoma; great-uncle laryngeal cancer; 2 relatives ALS	Relationship with phacomatoses complex and/or SBLA cancer syndrome
Medulloblastoma	?	+	Café-au-lait spots, haemangiomata of leg and spleen		
Glioblastoma	?	+	Café-au-lait spots on the back		
Haemangioma	?	+	-		
Glioblastoma multiforme	+	-	-	?	A diagnosis of glioblastoma multiforme in case 2 is assumed by the authors
Brain tumour	-	-	-		

TABLE 4 - continued

	case	gender	relationship	number of unaffected siblings	race or nationality	age at symptom occurrence	age at death	location of the tumour
VII.B.2.14. Blattner 1979	1	m	br	2 s	Amer.	33 y	–	R temporal
	2	m	br	2 s	Amer.	2 y	2 y	4th ventricle

diagnosis	biopsy	autopsy	associated physical or mental conditions	family	comment
Astrocytoma I-II	+	-	-	Sister: seizure; distant rel.: cerebellar tumour (metastatic?); many relatives with cancer: breast, sarcomas, leukaemia	Manifestation of SBLA cancer syndrome (same as II.B.2.3)
Medulloblastoma	-	+	-		

TABLE 5 - OTHER GENERATIONS AND DISTANT RELATIVES WITH CONCORDANT TUMOUR (VII.C.1)

	case	gender	relationship	number of unaffected siblings	race or nationality	age at symptom occurrence	age at death	location of the tumour
VII.C.1.1. Ostertag 1948	1	f	m	?	Germ.	?	23 y	parieto-occipital
	2	f	d	?	Germ.	?	dead at birth	parieto-occipital
VII.C.1.2. Koch 1949	1	f	m	2 br 1 s	Germ.	51 y	51 y	L parieto-occipital
	2	f	d	2 br	Germ.	23 y	23 y	L temporo-parietal
	3	m	son	2 br	Germ.	31 y	31 y	R temporal
VII.C.1.3. Mackay 1952	1	m	uncle	?	Dutch	?	57 y	R fronto-parietal and corpus callosum
	2	m	neph	?	Dutch	?	7 y	L frontal
VII.C.1.4. Koch 1954	1	m	uncle	4 br 2 s	Germ.	?	50 y	L temporal
	2	f	niece	2 s	Germ.	?	28 y	L praecentral
VII.C.1.5. Munslow 1955	1	m	br	4, 1 half	Amer. white	52 y	52 y	L frontal (Broca's area)
	2	m	br	4, 1 half	Amer. white	64 y	64 y	L frontal
	3	m	neph	many	Amer. white	46 y	46 y	R paraventricular

diagnosis	biopsy	autopsy	associated physical or mental conditions	family	comment
Glioblas-tomatosis	?	?	?	?	Personal communication in Koch 1949. Case 2 premature child, dead at birth
Glioblas-tomatosis	?	?	?		
Glioma	−	+	−	Father alcoholic; 1 child died in first year; 1 son mentally retarded; 1 son died at 14 y of unknown cause	PA of case 1 histologically verified?
Glioblastoma multiforme	+	−	Pigmented naevi L arm, pointed head form		
Cystic glio-blastoma	−	+	Contusio cerebri with traumatic Horner at 16 y		
Glioblastoma	?	?	?	?	
Astrocytoma	?	?	?		
Cystic glio-blastoma	?	+	Epilepsy	Father of case 2 died of lung tumour	Study on 350 female patients with brain tumour
Spongioblas-toma	?	+	Naevus pigmentosus vinosus L temporal		
Glioma	+	−	−		PA of case 1 not histologically verified. Anatomical diagnosis at operation. Cites personal communication from Klemme: glioma in 2 members of a family
Astrocytoma III	−	+	−		
Glioblastoma multiforme	+	−	−		

TABLE 5 - continued

	case	gender	relationship	number of unaffected siblings	race or nationality	age at symptom occurrence	age at death	location of the tumour
VII.C.1.6. Voûte 1958	1	f	m	?	Dutch	?	56 y	?
	2	f	d	?	Dutch	?	36 y	?
	3	m	son	?	Dutch	?	34 y	?
VII.C.1.7. Kjellin 1960	1	m	f	?	Swed.	31 y	31 y	L and R thalamus
	2	f	d	2	Swed.	23 y	23 y	corpus callosum
	3	m	son	2	Swed.	19 y	21 y	L occipital
VII.C.1.8. Kjellin 1960	1	f	m	?	Swed.	54 y	54 y	R frontal
	2	f	d	1	Swed.	30 y	30 y	L fronto-parietal
VII.C.1.9. Kjellin 1960	1	f	m	?	Swed.	70 y	72 y	L temporal
	2	m	son	3	Swed.	6 y	24 y	cerebellar
VII.C.1.10. King 1966	1	m	f	?	Amer.	50 y	50 y	R fronto-temporo-parietal
	2	f	d	?	Amer.	34 y	?	L frontal
VII.C.1.11. Bromowicz 1971	1	f	m	?	Pol.	29 y	-	Spinal Th_{4-6}
	2	m	son	?	Pol.	7 y	-	vermis cerebellum
VII.C.1.12. Kaufman 1972	1	m	cous	?	Amer.	3 y	-	vermis and L cerebellar hemisphere
	2	m	cous	?	Amer.	14 y	15 y	lower brain stem

diagnosis	biopsy	autopsy	associated physical or mental conditions	family	comment
Glioma	?	?	?	?	Tumour of case 1 histologically verified? Personal communication in Van der Wiel 1959
Astrocytoma	?	+	?		
Gliomatosis	?	+	?		
Astrocytoma II-III	-	+	-	-	
Astrocytoma II-III	+	+	-		
Astrocytoma II-III	+	-	-		
Astrocytoma IV	-	+	-	-	
Astrocytoma IV	+	-	-		
Astrocytoma IV	+	+	-	-	Different histological appearance of tumours. Case 2 drowned at 24 y
Cerebellar astrocytoma	+	-	-		
Glioma multiforme	+	+	Typhoid fever, head injury, appendectomy	Maternal grandmother and father case 1: cancer. Maternal grandmother case 2: cancer of the bowel	
Glioma multiforme	+	-	-		
Ependymoma	+	-	-	?	
Astrocytoma	+	-	-		
Cystic astrocytoma	+	-	Muscular dystrophy (?)	?	
Malignant astrocytoma	+	-	-		

TABLE 5 - continued

	case	gender	relationship	number of unaffected siblings	race or nationality	age at symptom occurrence	age at death	location of the tumour
VII.C.1.13. Scharrer 1973	1	m	f	?	Germ.	46 y	46 y	L temporo-occipital
	2	m	son	?	Germ.	30 y	-	L temporal
VII.C.1.14. Isamat 1974	1	m	f	?	Span.	56 y	?	post-central
	2	f	d	?	Span.	20 y	?	3rd ventricle
VII.C.1.15. Isamat 1974	1	f	m	?	Span.	61 y	?	frontal
	2	m	son	?	Span.	39 y	?	temporal
VII.C.1.16. Isamat 1974	1	f	m	?	Span.	38 y	?	R frontal
	2	m	son	?	Span.	58 y	?	parathalamic
VII.C.1.17. Isamat 1974	1	f	aunt	?	Span.	50 y	?	frontal
	2	m	neph	?	Span.	29 y	?	temporal
VII.C.1.18. Lynch 1978	1	m	br	2 br	Amer.	18 y	20 y	?
	2	f	s	2 br	Amer.	3 y	3 y	?
	3	m	cous	1 br 1 s	Amer.	4 y	5 y	?
	4	m	uncle	4 br 2 s	Amer.	6 y	6 y	?
	5	m	dist. rel.	?	Amer.	?	51 y	?
	6	f	dist. rel.	?	Amer.	?	10 y	?
VII.C.1.19. Turowski 1978	1	m	f	?	Pol.	60 y	?	L temporal
	2	m	son	?	Pol.	37 y	37 y	R parietal

diagnosis	biopsy	autopsy	associated physical or mental conditions	family	comment
Oligodendro-glioma	+	+	-	-	
Oligodendro-glioma	+	-	-		
Astrocytoma IV	+	-	Blood-group A, Rh +	?	
Astrocytoma III	+	-	Blood-group A, Rh +		
Astrocytoma IV	+	-	Blood-group B, Rh +	?	
Astrocytoma II	+	-	Blood-group A, Rh +		
Glioma	+	-	-	-	No further PA specification of tumour of case 1 available
Ependymo-blastoma	+	-	Blood-group A, Rh +		
Astrocytoma IV	+	-	Blood-group AB, Rh +	-	
Astrocytoma I	+	-	Blood-group A, Rh +		
Glioblastoma multiforme	?	?	-	Family with SBLA cancer syndrome, 29 tumours in 26 individuals. No signs of phacomatosis	Manifestation of SBLA cancer syndrome, a hereditary tumour complex
Glioblastoma multiforme	?	?	-		
Primary malignant brain tumour	?	?	-		
Glioma	?	?	-		
Glioblastoma multiforme	?	?	-		
Glioblastoma multiforme	?	?	-		
Glioblastoma multiforme	+	-	Blood-group A, Rh +	?	Another family with two sisters with optic nerve glioma also reported in this article
Glioblastoma multiforme	+	+	Blood-group A, Rh +		

378

TABLE 5 - continued

	case	gender	relationship	number of unaffected siblings	race or nationality	age at symptom occurrence	age at death	location of the tumour
VII.C.1.20. Van der Drift 1980	1	f	m	?	Dutch	?	?	occipital
	2	f	d	?	Dutch	?	?	cerebellar
VII.C.1.21. Van der Wiel 1980	1	m	f	2	Dutch	60 y	60 y	R frontal
	2	f	d	0	Dutch	41 y	42 y	L fronto-temporal
VII.C.1.22. Van der Wiel 1980	1	f	cous	1 br	Dutch	36 y	36 y	R fronto-temporal
	2	f	cous	1 s	Dutch	?	?	L occipital-temporal
VII.C.1.23. Schianchi 1980	1	m	f	1 s	Swiss	36 y	36 y	rhombencephalon
	2	m	s	2 s 1 br	Swiss	17 y	17 y	rhombencephalon
VII.C.1.24. Koch 1981	1	m	f	1 br 1 s	Germ.	37 y	39 y	L fronto-basal
	2	m	son	0	Germ.	30 y	-	R temporo-parietal

diagnosis	biopsy	autopsy	associated physical or mental conditions	family	comment
Astrocytoma IV	?	?	?	?	Personal communication
Astrocytoma	?	?	?		
Glioblastoma multiforme	+	-	-	-	Personal communication
Astrocytoma IV	+	-	-		
Astrocytoma IV	+	?	Committed suicide	Distant relative brain tumour; grandfather and his brother died of carcinoma of the stomach	Personal communication
Astrocytoma II	+	?	Lung embolus		
Astrocytoma I	-	+	-	Mother case 2: mult. sclerosis. Nephew case 1: Cockayne syndrome. 2 nephews of case 1 died at an early age	
Astrocytoma I	-	+	-		
Spongioblastoma	+	-	Appendectomy	-	Case 2: normal karyogram
Astrocytoma	+	-	Appendectomy		

TABLE 5 - continued on the following page

TABLE 5 - continued

	case	gender	relationship	number of unaffected siblings	race or nationality	age at symptom occurrence	age at death	location of the tumour
VII.C.1.25. Thuwe 1981	1	m	br	9	Swed.	38 y	41 y	L frontal
	2	f	s	9	Swed.	-	25 y	R temporal
	3	f	niece	1	Swed.	45 y	-	corpus callosum, R + L frontal
	4	f	grand-niece	9	Swed.	36 y	38 y	L frontal
	5	m	dist. rel.	1	Swed.	35 y	35 y	L frontal
	6	m	dist. rel.	8	Swed.	42 y	51 y	L frontal
	7	m	dist. rel.	?	Swed.	42 y	54 y	L temporal

diagnosis	biopsy	autopsy	associated physical or mental conditions	family	comment
Glioma (?)	-	+		Two siblings died at early age	No microscopic study, glioma suggested at autopsy
Glioma (?)	-	+	Eclampsia	Two siblings died at early age	No microscopic study, glioma suggested at autopsy
Astrocytoma I	+	-	Migraine	-	-
Astrocytoma IV	+	-	Depressive states	One brother died from suicide at 24 y	-
Glioblastoma	+	+	-	-	-
Brain tumour	-	-	-	One sibling died of TBC at 22 y	Clinical diagnosis
Brain tumour	-	-	Alcoholic, depressions	-	Tumour clinically suspected

TABLE 6 - OTHER GENERATIONS AND DISTANT RELATIVES WITH DISCORDANT TUMOUR (VII.C.2)

	case	gender	relationship	number of unaffected siblings	race or nationality	age at symptom occurrence	age at death	location of the tumour
VII.C.2.1. Rados 1946	1	f	cous	–	Amer.	5 y	5 y	brain stem
	2	m	cous	–	Amer.	8 m	–	both retinas
VII.C.2.2. Koch 1949	1	m	br	?	Germ.	?	17 y	?
	2	m	br	?	Germ.	?	65 y	?
	3	m	neph	?	Germ.	35 y	?	L temporal
VII.C.2.3. Blickenstorfer 1951	1	m	br	1 s	Germ.	68 y	69 y	R occipital
	2	f	s	1 s	Germ.	?	?	frontal
	3	f	grand-m	?	Germ.	60 y	71 y	?
	4	f	aunt	?	Germ.	64 y	65 y	?
VII.C.2.4. Koch 1954	1	f	niece	3 br 2 s	Germ.	?	18 y	L parieto-occipital
	2	m	uncle	?	Germ.	?	?	?
VII.C.2.5. Meyer 1956	1	m	uncle	?	Germ.	57 y	57 y	L fronto-parietal
	2	m	neph	0	Germ.	31 y	31 y	L basal ganglia
VII.C.2.6. Meyer 1956	1	m	son	3 br	Germ.	24 y	24 y	L temporo-parietal, subcortical
	2	f	m	1 br	Germ.	?	36 y	?
	3	f	aunt	1 br	Germ.	?	26 y	?
	4	m	uncle	1 br	Germ.	?	48 y	?

diagnosis	biopsy	autopsy	associated physical or mental conditions	family	comment
Astrocytoma	-	+	-	-	-
Neuroepithelioma	+	-	-		
Brain tumour	?	?	?	?	No histological diagnoses of cases 1 and 2
Brain tumour	?	?	?		
Astrocytoma	+	?	?		
Glioblastoma	+	-	-	59 relatives investigated. Apart from mental disorders no other relevant diseases	No histological diagnoses of cases 3 and 4
Meningioma	+	-	-		
Brain tumour	?	?	-		
Brain tumour	?	?	-		
Cystic glioma	?	?	-	Mother of case 1 died of cancer of the liver at 63 y	Case 2: brain tumour clinically suspected. Extensive study of 350 female patients with brain tumour
Brain tumour	?	?			
Glioblastoma	-	+	-	-	Case 2: no histological diagnosis. Extensive study of 459 male patients with brain tumour, 7 families with brain tumour occurrence were found
Brain tumour	?	?	Rachitis		
Ganglioneuro-blastoma	+	-	Chronic otitis media, naevus L nasolabial fold	Brother died at 13 y of sarcoma of kidney; brother died at 8 w of "krampfen"; cousin died at 25 y in depressive state; cousin: epilepsy	No histological diagnoses of cases 2 - 4. Same study as VII.C.2.5.
Brain tumour	?	?	?		
Brain tumour	?	?	?		
Brain tumour	?	?	?		

384

TABLE 6 - continued

case	gender	relationship	number of unaffected siblings	race or nationality	age at symptom occurrence	age at death	location of the tumour
VII.C.2.7. Meyer 1956								
1	m	son	6	Germ.	33 y	-	L frontal
2	m	f	?	Germ.	?	56 y	?
VII.C.2.8. Meyer 1956								
1	m	cous	7	Germ.	47 y	47 y	L fronto-basal
2	m	cous	?	Germ.	?	?	?
VII.C.2.9. Weersma 1957								
1	f	d	?	Dutch Indones.?	?	45 y	?
2	f	m	?	Dutch Indones.?	?	55 y	hemisphere
VII.C.2.10. Kemper 1964								
1	f	aunt	?	Germ.	47 y	47 y	R temporal
2	m	neph	2 s	Germ.	19 y	-	L temporo-parieto-occipital
VII.C.2.11. Kemper 1964								
1	m	uncle	2 br 3 s	Germ.	29 y	30 y	L parieto-occipital
2	m	neph	1 br 1 s	Germ.	15 y	-	thoracic
VII.C.2.12. Walker 1971	A family with two cases of brain tumours in each of three generations, in one generation two siblings with malignant glioma.							

diagnosis	biopsy	autopsy	associated physical or mental conditions	family	comment
Oligodendro-glioma	+	-	Motor accident with head injury at 33 y	-	No histological diagnosis of case 2. Same study as VII.C.2.5.
Brain tumour	?	?	?		
Glioblastoma (?)	+	-	-	Aunt melancholia at older age	Diagnosis case 1 based on macroscopic findings at operation. No histological diagnosis of case 2. Same study as VII.C.2.5.
Brain tumour	?	?	?		
Glioblastoma fusiforme	+	-	?	?	Cited by Van der Wiel 1959 as a personal communication
Brain tumour	+	?	?		
Glioblastoma multiforme	-	+	-	Mother of case 1 died at 80 y of apoplexy	Study of 453 patients with brain tumour; 6 cases of familial brain tumour occurrence were found
Fibromatous meningioma	+	-	Head injury at 5 y		
Cystic glioma	+	-	-	Consanguinity grandparents. Cousin mother and cousin father case 2: mult.scler.; mother case 2 depressive; brother case 2 mental disturbances	Same study as VII.C.2.10.
Neurinoma	+	-	Pyloric stenosis, Scheuermann's disease		
				Many malignancies in other relatives: leukaemia, carcinoma of stomach, bowel, breast, adrenal gland and sarcoma	SBLA family cancer syndrome

TABLE 6 - continued

	case	gender	relationship	number of unaffected siblings	race or nationality	age at symptom occurrence	age at death	location of the tumour
VII.C.2.13. Van der Wiel 1980	1	m	grand-f	?	Dutch	47 y	47 y	?
	2	f	grand-d	0	Dutch	?	5 y	?

diagnosis	biopsy	autopsy	associated physical or mental conditions	family	comment
Glioblastoma multiforme	+	-	-	Son of case 1: spina bifida occulta; cousin case 2 died after birth with anencephaly	Personal communication
Medulloblastoma	+	-	-		

GENERAL ASPECTS OF GLIOMA

Gliomas are primary intracranial tumours derived from parenchymatous elements of the central nervous system, primary intracranial neoplasms comprising approximately 8 to 15% of the malignant tumours in man (20, 201, 234, 279) and 28 to 57% of these being gliomas (20, 234). The discrepancy in percentages of occurrence found in large series can be largely explained by the use of varying classifications of brain tumours and differing epidemiological approaches and data collection by the different investigators.

An overall age-adjusted incidence rate for gliomas diagnosed before death (Rochester, Minnesota) was shown to be 4.0 per 100,000 population among males and 4.1 among females; of all autopsies on subjects aged 55 years and older approximately 1% confirmed or discovered the presence of gliomas (7). In most studies the incidence of glioma was found to be somewhat higher in males than in females, and higher in caucasians than in negroes (97, 305, 312).

The classification of gliomas is complicated and many attempts at description and classification of these tumours have been made.

In 1926 Bailey and Cushing (13) introduced a classification system based upon the morphology of the neoplastic cell, comparing it to that of differentiated normal glial cells of the central nervous system. Their classification remains the basis of most modern classification systems of glioma. The most important modifications in classification have been made by Kernohan et al. (118, 119), Zülch (299) and Rubinstein (225). Kernohan et al. (118), considering the degree of malignancy, incorporated biological aspects of the cerebral neoplasms in their classification. The suggested classification was based on degrees of anaplasia of the adult cell types in the central nervous system: astrocytes, ependymal cells, oligodendroglial cells and nerve cells. A grading system of 1 to 4 proved satisfactory for the astrocytomas, but was less suitable for other groups. A problem of the grading system is the basis of diagnosis upon the most malignant portion of the neoplasm, variance in biopsy sampling possibly leading to an undergrading in diagnosis. Zülch (299) included such aspects as site of origin and age at manifestation in his classification and divided neuroepithelial brain tumours into four main groups: medulloblastoma, glioma, paraglioma and gangliocytoma. A widely used modification of the classification of Bailey and Cushing has been proposed by Rubinstein (225). The four classifications are reviewed in table I.

Table I. CLASSIFICATIONS OF GLIOMA

Rubinstein 1972	Zülch 1956	Kernohan 1952	Bailey 1926
I. Tumours of neuro-glial cells:	I. Neuroepithelial tumours		
A. 1. Astrocytomas (fibrillary, proto-plasmic gemistocytic, pilocytic, giant cell, gliomatosis)	A. Glioma 1. Spongioblastoma 2. Astrocytoma (fibrillary, proto-plasmic, giant cell, malignant, astroblastoma)	A. Astrocytoma grade 1 – 4	Astrocytoma
2. Spongioblastoma polare			Spongioblastoma polare
3. Astroblastoma			Astroblastoma
4. Malignant astro-cytoma	3. Glioblastoma (fusiforme, multi-forme, globuliforme) grade 3 grade 4		Glioblastoma multiforme
5. Glioblastoma multiforme			
B. Oligodendrogliomas	4. Oligodendroglioma	B. Oligodendroglioma grade 1 – 4	Oligodendroglioma
C. Ependymomas (subependymomas, malignant ependymo-blastoma)	B. Paraglioma 1. Ependymoma 2. Plexus papilloma 3. Pinealoma 4. Neurinoma	C. Ependymoma grade 1 – 4	Ependymoma Neuroepithelioma
II. Tumours of neuronal cells:			
A. Medulloblastomas	C. Medulloblastoma 1. Retinoblastoma 2. Medulloblastoma	D. Medulloblastoma	Medulloblastoma
B. Neuroblastoma	3. Pineoblastoma 4. Sympathicoblastoma	E. Neuroastrocytoma grade 1 – 4	Neuroblastoma
C. Ganglioneuroma and ganglioglioma	D. Gangliocytoma		Ganglioneuroma

Table II.   NEW HISTOLOGICAL CLASSIFICATION OF TUMOURS OF THE CENTRAL
NERVOUS SYSTEM (WHO)   (Zülch KJ, 1980 (302))

	Grade
I. Tumours of neuroepithelial tissue	
A. Astrocytic tumours	
1. Astrocytoma	II
a. fibrillary	
b. protoplasmic	
c. gemistocytic	
2. Pilocytic astrocytoma	I
3. Subependymal giant cell astrocytoma (ventricular tumour of tuberous sclerosis)	I
4. Astroblastoma	II-IV?
5. Anaplastic (malignant) astrocytoma	III
B. Oligodendroglial tumours	
1. Oligodendroglioma	II
2. Mixed oligoastrocytoma	II
3. Anaplastic (malignant) oligodendroglioma	III
C. Ependymal and choroid plexus tumours	
1. Ependymoma	I
Variants:	
a. Myxopapillary ependymoma	I, II
b. Papillary ependymoma	I
c. Subependymoma	I
2. Anaplastic (malignant) ependymoma	III, IV
3. Choroid plexus papilloma	I
4. Anaplastic (malignant) choroid plexus papilloma	III, IV
D. Pineal cell tumours	
1. Pineocytoma (pinealocytoma) isomorphous	I-III
2. Pineoblastoma (pinealoblastoma)	IV
E. Neuronal tumours	
1. Gangliocytoma	I
2. Ganglioglioma	I, II
3. Ganglioneuroblastoma	III
4. Anaplastic (malignant) gangliocytoma and ganglioglioma	III, IV
5. Neuroblastoma	IV
F. Poorly differentiated and embryonal tumours	
1. Glioblastoma)	
Variants:)	
a. Glioblastoma with sarcomatous component) (mixed glioblastoma and sarcoma))	IV
b. Giant cell glioblastoma)	
2. Medulloblastoma	IV
Variants:	
a. Desmoplastic	III, IV
b. Medullomyoblastoma	III, IV
3. Medulloepithelioma	IV
4. Primitive polar spongioblastoma	IV
5. Gliomatosis cerebri	?

In 1959 in an attempt at achieving a uniform international classification the International Cancer Society (269) proposed a histological nomenclature for human tumours, including neoplasms of the nervous system, but this has not been generally accepted. This classification was illustrated in 1965 (270) and reviewed in 1969 (271).

Recently the World Health Organization (WHO) requested the development of a new classification of brain tumours to standardize nomenclature and attempt international agreement on this subject. Both classification and prognosis aspects through a system of grading have been incorporated in this work (302). The histological classification for the glioma group is shown in table II. Grade I is 'benign', grade II 'semi-benign', grade III 'less malignant', and grade IV 'highly malignant'. This classification system appears appropriate for use by members of the neurosciences. Classification of tumours in the section on familial aspects of glioma in this text has been based upon this system.

The four most frequently occurring glioma types, astrocytoma, glioblastoma, oligodendroglioma and ependymoma, require more description in detail.
Astrocytomas are neoplasms originating from the astrocyte, the principal supporting cell of the central nervous system. They account for 6 to 17% of all intracranial tumours, and for 20 to 30% of tumours in the glioma group (2, 70, 225, 227, 300). In an examination of 54,946 autopsies astrocytomas formed 28.4% of CNS neoplasms (280). The varying percentages found in the literature reflect differences in classification systems.

Astrocytomas occur at any age but are most frequently found between the ages of 30 and 50 years (70, 225, 280, 299). Cerebellar and pontine astrocytomas are mainly found in childhood and adolescence. Most studies of astrocytomas indicate a slightly greater incidence in males than in females (28, 225, 280, 299). Astrocytomas may occur anywhere in the brain, but are predominantly found in the frontal, temporal and parietal lobes (238, 280, 298). Less frequent locations are the cerebellar, thalamic, midbrain, pontine and spinal cord regions (298). Multiple occurrence of astrocytoma is rare but has been reported (51, 252, 260). Astrocytomas can also occur in combination with other brain tumours such as meningioma, pituitary adenoma and sarcoma (51, 164, 184, 228). Other disease entities such as neurofibromatosis, tuberous sclerosis (the subependymal giant cell type), and syringomyelia (spinal cord astrocytoma) have been found in association with astrocytoma occurrence (see familial aspects). The development of astrocytomas in demyelinating disease is rare, but has been reported (6). The symptomatology of astrocytomas varies to a considerable degree according to

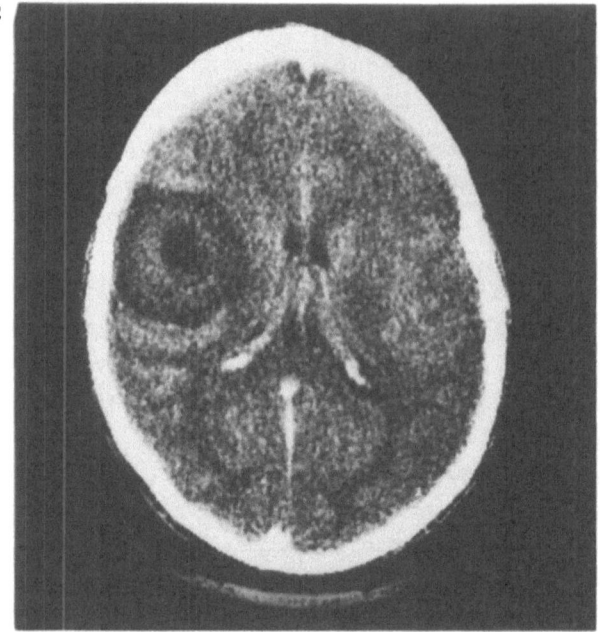

Fig. 1. CT-scan of a right parietal low grade astrocytoma (enhanced)

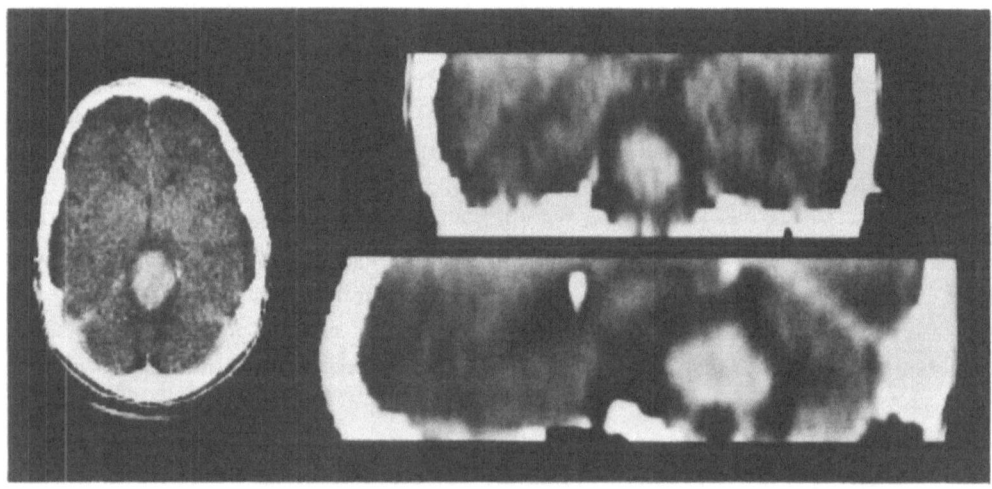

Fig. 2. CT-scan with coronal and sagittal reformatting of a spongioblastoma
        of the brain stem (enhanced)

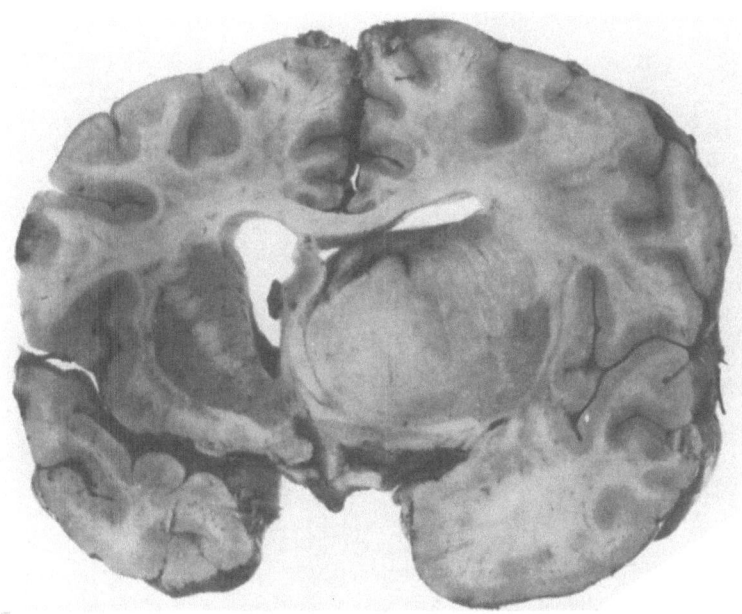

Fig. 3. Cross-section of an astrocytoma located in the region of the right
basal ganglia

their localization. Epileptic seizure has been the presenting symptom in 40 to 75%
of the cases in different series (70), and may be the only symptom for many years.
Other clinical features may be personality changes, disorders of speech, cranial
nerve disorders, hemiparesis of the limbs and signs of raised intracranial pressure.

The gross appearance of astrocytomas depends upon their degree of differentiation. They generally occur superficially in the hemispheres from which they infiltrate into the central white matter. Pronounced demarcation from the normal brain
tissue occurs infrequently. The neoplasm is rather firm with a pinkish-gray or
yellowish-white colour and may contain cysts (70, 225, 227).

Microscopically astrocytomas demonstrate a modest cellularity with homogeneous
distribution, their blood vessels forming an inconspicuous capillary network.
Mitotic figures and vascular endothelial proliferation are absent in the low grade
types, but common in the malignant varieties. Calcification rarely occurs and
necrosis may be found in the malignant types (70, 225, 227, 299). On the basis of
cytological features astrocytomas may be subdivided into: 1. a fibrillary, most
frequently occurring type characterized by very small cells and many fibrils;
2. a protoplasmic type composed of small stellate non-fibrillated astrocytes with
delicate processes forming a cobweb matrix; 3. a gemistocytic type; 4. a pilocytic
type; 5. an anaplastic type (70, 225, 227, 302).
The gemistocytic type demonstrates large, often multinucleated cells sometimes
forming pseudorosettes similar to those seen in astroblastomas, tumours originally

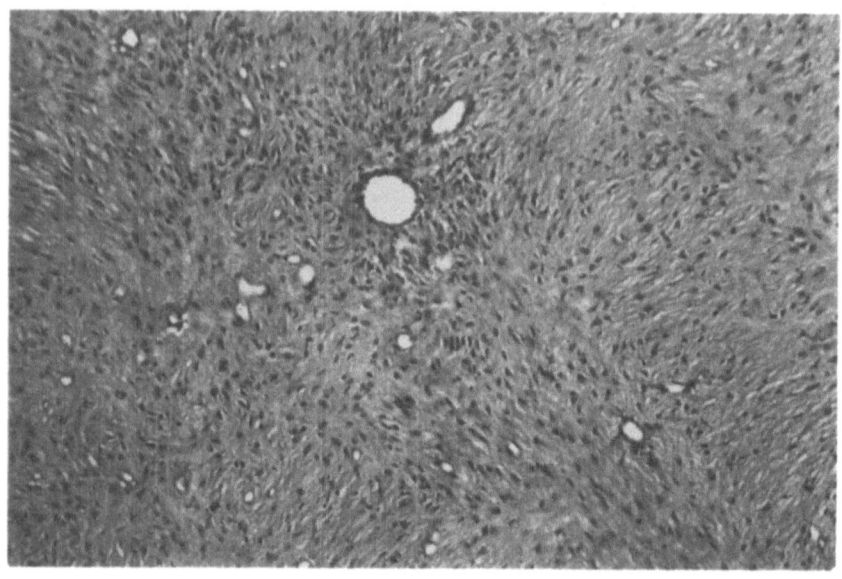

Fig. 4. Microscopic appearance of a low grade fibrillary cerebellar astrocytoma
HE, 75x

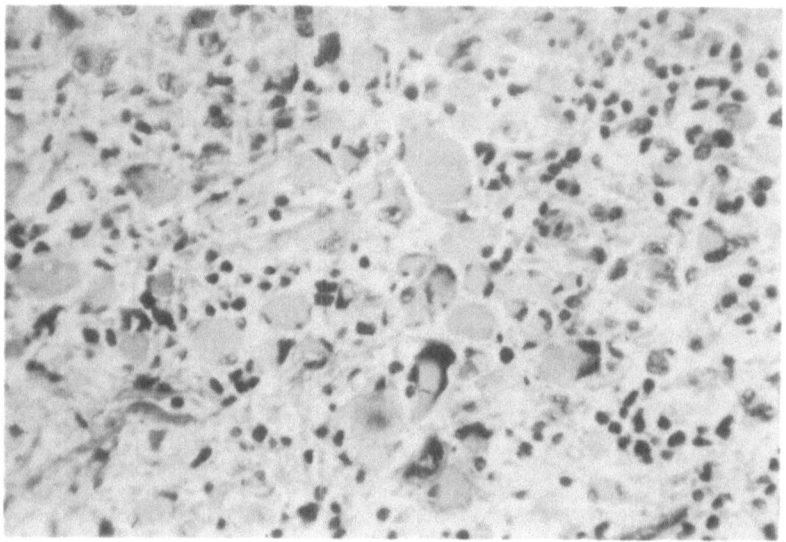

Fig. 5. Microscopic appearance of a gemistocytic astrocytoma grade II
HE, 150x

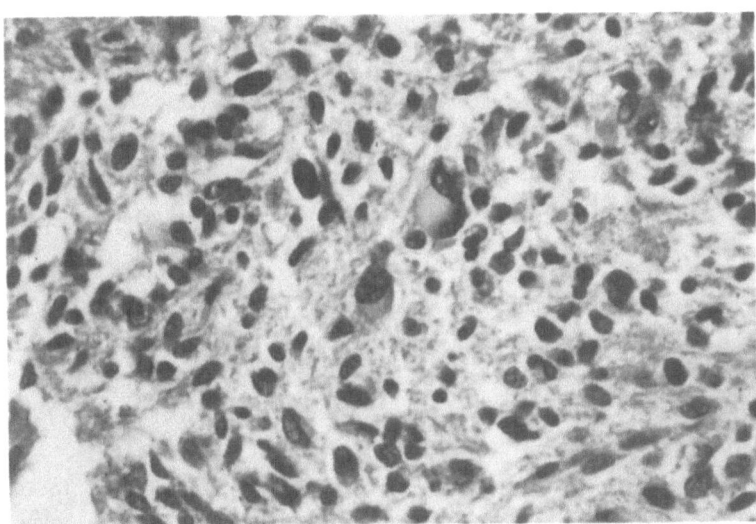

Fig. 6. Microscopic appearance of an anaplastic astrocytoma
HE, 300 x

described by Bailey and Cushing and included in the classification of Kernohan
among the second grade astrocytomas. Gemistocytic astrocytomas are predominantly
found in the cerebral hemispheres in adults (70, 225, 227).
The pilocytic type, described under the term spongioblastoma polare by Bailey and
Cushing, and Zülch, is characterized by elongated often bipolar fusiform cells,
Rosenthal fibres and granular bodies (302). It is most frequently seen occurring
in children and adolescents in the third ventricle, the brain stem and cerebellum.
Anaplastic astrocytoma - corresponding in the classification of Kernohan to grade
3 astrocytoma - show moderate cellular pleomorphism, a variable degree of vascular endothelial proliferation, a variable number of mitotic figures, abnormal
stroma reaction, and dedifferentiation and necrosis with or without pseudopalisading of nuclei (107, 225, 227, 302).
The problem of malignancy in astrocytomas is as yet unresolved. Some authors stress
the malignant degeneration of astrocytomas, and some degree of anaplastic change
has been demonstrated in autopsy cases (227, 231). Others maintain the primary
malignant character of astrocytomas, regarding malignant degeneration of primarily
benign gliomas as an exception (70).
While focal invasion of the leptomeninges by astrocytoma frequently occurs, metastatic spread through the cerebrospinal fluid pathways is rare (225, 293, 299).
Extraneural astrocytoma metastases may occur, primarily to the lungs and pleurae
(196).

The prognosis for patients with astrocytoma varies according to the tumour type, grade and location. Surgical treatment of astrocytomas is dependent upon the location of the tumour. Literature reports concerning the value of radiation therapy have been inconsistent but most seem to indicate radiation therapy to be an important determinant in postoperative survival. Survival benefit as the result of cytostatic agent treatment of astrocytoma has not been definitely demonstrated (205, 220, 285, 311).

Glioblastomas, designated as astrocytomas grade 3 and 4 in the classification of Kernohan and Sayre (119), are highly malignant neoplasms of the central nervous system originating from astrocytic cells. As stated earlier they may arise from malignant change in low-grade astrocytomas (225, 231) or may occur as primary malignant neoplasms (70, 111, 301).

Glioblastomas account for approximately 50% of the gliomas and represent 15 to 20% of all intracranial tumours (111, 152, 235). The tumours may occur at any age but are rare in children and adolescents, the majority manifesting between the ages of 40 and 60 years (73, 111, 152, 225, 227, 274). Men are more often affected than women, the incidence in males as compared to females being 1 1/2 or 2 to 1 (73, 235, 274, 301).

All parts of the brain and spinal cord may be affected but glioblastomas predominantly occur in the cerebral hemispheres. Most authors report a preferential site

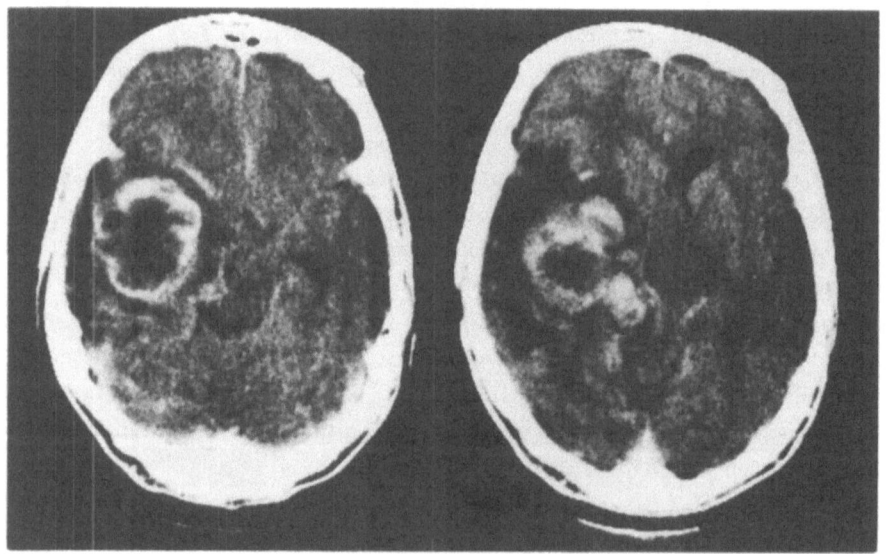

Fig. 7. CT-scan of a right temporal glioblastoma (enhanced)

in the frontal and temporal lobes (73, 225, 227, 274), but some report an equal distribution among the four different lobes (235). There is no preference for the left or right hemisphere. The basal ganglia and the commissural pathways are also sites of frequent occurrence, but location in the cerebellum or spinal cord is rare (85, 111, 247). Multiple localization of glioblastoma occurs in about 14% of the cases (17, 178, 260). Association of glioblastoma with meningiomas and sarcomas has been reported (68, 164, 225, 256).

Other reported associated diseases are neurofibromatosis, tuberous sclerosis and demyelinating diseases (6, see also familial aspects).

The glioblastoma is a rapidly growing tumour and therefore the clinical history of most patients is short (73). In a study on 550 cases of glioblastoma Vogt reported in two thirds of the patients the interval between onset of symptoms and diagnosis as being three months at the most. Headaches and vomiting, cerebral seizures and mental changes are the most frequent early signs and symptoms, followed by papilloedema, aphasia and stroke-like onset (73, 274). Mental disorders occur most often in association with tumours in the temporal and frontal lobe and the corpus callosum.

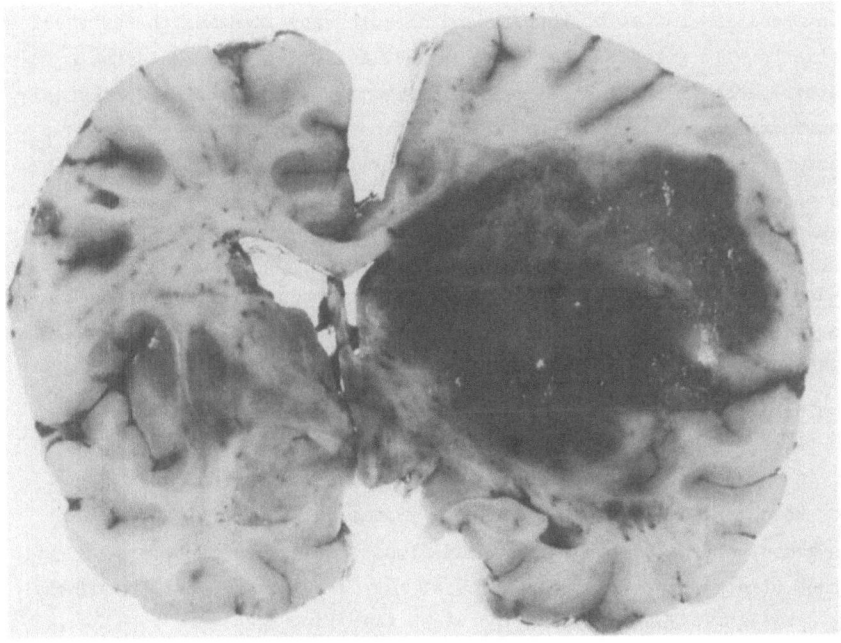

Fig. 8. Cross-section of a glioblastoma of the right hemisphere

On gross examination the most characteristic feature is the great variation seen on cross section of the neoplasm from which its name 'multiforme' is derived: areas of necrosis, fatty degeneration, haemorrhages, cysts, and a variety in colouring (grayish-pink, creamy yellow, reddish). While seeming to be round and well circumscribed these neoplasms are in fact poorly demarcated from the normal brain tissue (111, 152, 225).

Microscopically the most striking feature is the variety of cell forms and the differences between parts of the tumour. Cytologically only a few cells remain distinguishable as astrocytes. Histological features are a marked hypercellularity, extreme nuclear pleomorphism, a variable number of mitotic figures, pseudopalisading around areas of necrosis, and marked endothelial hyperplasia of the capillaries (107, 111, 225, 227). Histological variants are: giant cell glioblastomas with a predominance of bizarre, highly multinucleated giant cells, and glioblastomas with sarcomatous components (or mixed glioblastoma and sarcoma), the stroma of which appears to consist of 'malignant transformed' elements (111, 225, 302).

Glioblastomas have a poor prognosis regardless of the therapy given and no definite examples of cure are reported in the literature (73, 111, 152, 225). The only benefit of present treatment is to influence the quality and duration of survival, most patients dying within two years after the onset of the disease (152, 229). Adequate postoperative radiation therapy and chemotherapy increase the survival time for patients with glioblastoma (98, 99, 205, 242, 244, 311). Metastatic spread to other parts of the central nervous system by way of the cerebrospinal fluid is not uncommon and occurs in 5 to 20% of the cases (111, 152, 225, 235, 293). Distant extracranial metastases especially to the lungs or pleura, lymph nodes, bone and liver have been reported (196, 248, 249). Most of these patients had previous craniotomy or a shunt operation (134, 196).

Oligodendrogliomas are the third most commonly occurring gliomas, after astrocytomas and glioblastomas, accounting for 3 to 8% of all gliomas (54, 159, 194, 225, 227, 236). The tumours originate from oligodendrocytes and were first described by Bailey and Cushing in 1926 (13). This was followed by the classical description of 13 cases of oligodendrogliomas by Bailey and Bucy three years later (12). In subsequent series of oligodendrogliomas figures on sex and age distribution have varied. Most authors report a somewhat greater frequency in men than in women, estimates ranging from an almost equal distribution to a ratio of two to one. Oligodendrogliomas can occur at any age, but are most frequently encountered between the ages of 30 and 50 years (43, 105, 158, 194, 236). Chin et al. (43) in a series of 54 patients also reported a small peak of incidence between the ages of 6 and 12 years.

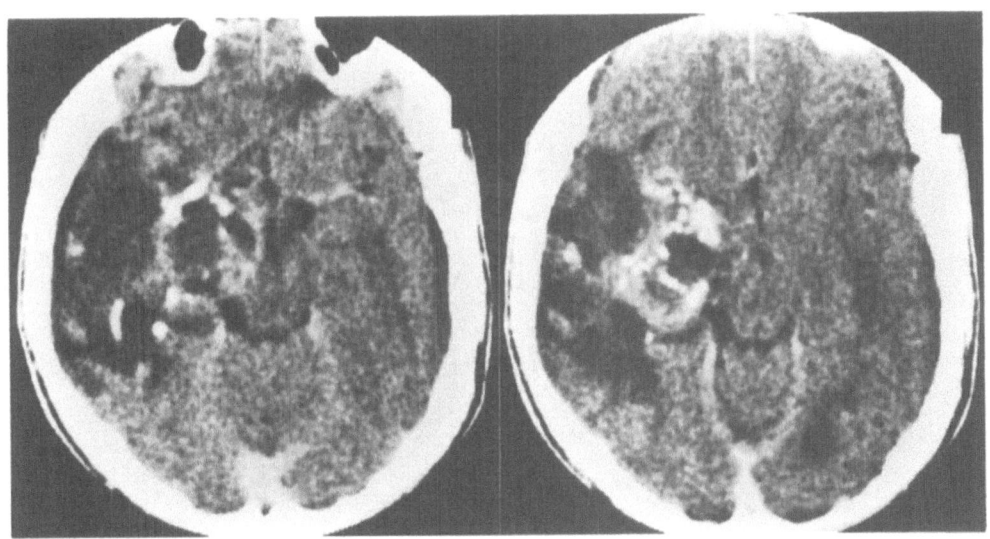

Fig. 9. CT-scan of a right temporal oligodendroglioma (enhanced)

Oligodendrogliomas demonstrate slow growth and are therefore often diagnosed after a long time period. Epileptic seizures are the most common clinical manifestations, appearing in 50 to 87% of the cases (43, 194). The patients often show a long clinical history with treatment for supposed primary epilepsy before the tumour is discovered, a pattern which will probably change as a result of the introduction of the CAT-scan which facilitates early diagnosis. Other common findings, especially in an advanced stage, are signs of raised intracranial pressure such as headache, vomiting, visual disturbance and papilloedema (159). These symptoms are related to the location of the tumour which is typically situated in the frontal or fronto-temporal area of either cerebral hemisphere. Approximately 50% of the cases in different series have been found occurring in these areas (64, 105, 158, 194, 236). Oligodendroglioma may be primarily located in the lateral and third ventricles, or they may secondarily invade the ventricle system. Signs of raised intracranial pressure are frequent in intraventricular examples. Cerebellar and spinal cord oligodendrogliomas may also occur, but are very rare (136, 210). Association of oligodendroglioma and meningioma has been reported (51, 57).

Grossly these tumours are usually well circumscribed, multilobar neoplasms situated in the white matter. They have a pinkish-gray colour and often a soft consistency. They may vary greatly in size and may grow to considerable proportions. Cystic formation is found in one out of five cases (64, 158) and foci of

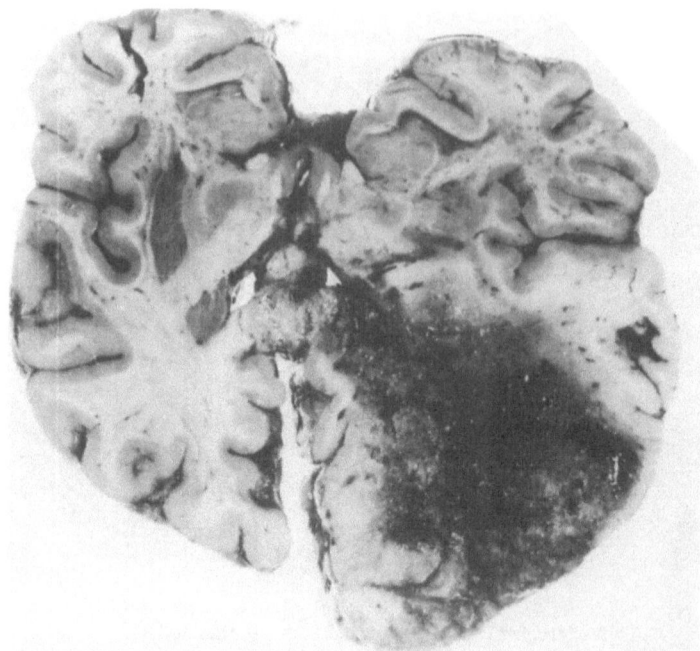

Fig. 10. Cross-section of a right temporal oligodendroglioma

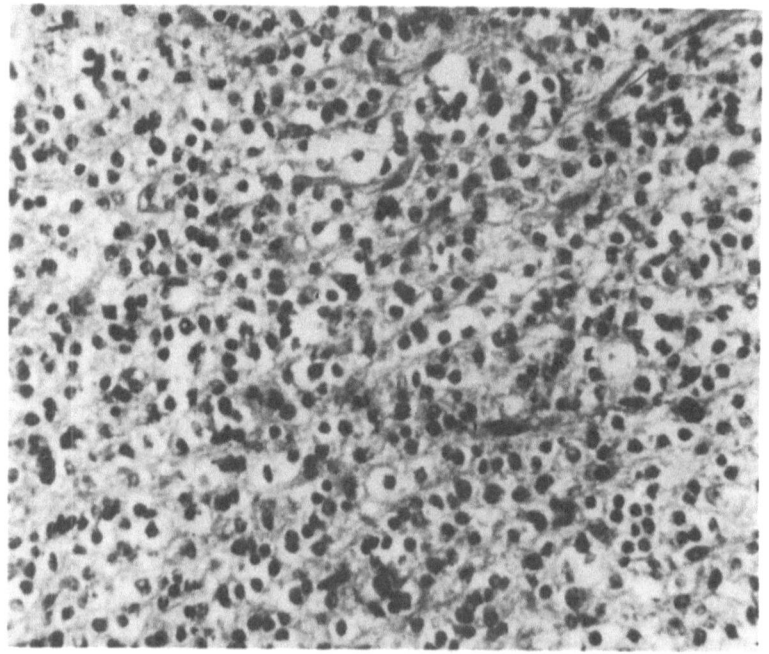

Fig. 11. Microscopic appearance of an oligodendroglioma
HE, 200x

calcification and haemorrhage are often present (159, 225, 227).

In most cases histological diagnosis is not difficult as the tumour has a characteristic microscopic appearance showing a monotonous, highly cellular pattern of
uniform cells grouped in compact masses. The tumour cells are of various size with
round, darkly staining nuclei surrounded by a clear halo, a very typical feature.
Mitotic figures can vary but calcifications are often present (159, 225). The anaplastic (malignant) variant is characterized by cellular pleomorphism, necrotic
zones with pseudopalisading and proliferation of vessels (14, 302).

Transitional forms to astrocytoma (mixed oligoastrocytoma) may give problems in
diagnosis (225, 302). Attempts at grading the malignancy of oligodendrogliomas
have not been successful as a valid correlation between the microscopic appearance
of the tumour and its clinical evolution has not been established (14, 119, 159,
225). Metastatic spread of oligodendroglioma through the cerebrospinal fluid pathways has been reported (23, 213).

Treatment with radical surgery, where possible, and postoperative radiation
therapy is recommended (43, 159).

Ependymomas are neuroepithelial tumours originating from ependymal cells and
subependymal glia cells. In the literature up to 1924, when they were first separated as a group by Bailey (11), they are frequently described under the name
neuroepithelioma. Zülch (299) registered these neoplasms within the group of para-
gliomas, but most other authors have classified them among the gliomas.

In different series they account for 2 to 6% of all intracranial glioma (9, 16,
225, 227). They constitute about 10% of the brain tumours occurring in children
under the age of 16 years (9, 58). This type of tumour appears to be more common
in Japan and India, accounting for 12.7% of gliomas in these countries (55, 115).
Ependymoma arise from the ependyma lining the cerebral ventricular system and the
central canal of the spinal cord, occurring at any level of the central nervous
system from the frontal region to the cauda equina. Supratentorial examples, however, are less frequent than infratentorial ones with a respective ratio of
approximately 30 to 40% as compared to 60 to 70% (72, 227), infratentorial tumours
occurring most frequently in the fourth ventricle (16, 72, 227). Next in frequency
are the spinal ependymomas, most often found in the lumbosacral segments or cauda
equina, constituting 5 to 30% of the cases in different series (63, 72, 225).
Association of spinal ependymomas with neurofibromatosis and syringomyelia has
been reported (see familial aspects).

Ependymoma may occur at any age. Zülch (299) maintained that cerebral ependymomas
most frequently occur in youth, those of other sites appearing later, particularly
during the third and fourth decades. This has been contradicted by other authors

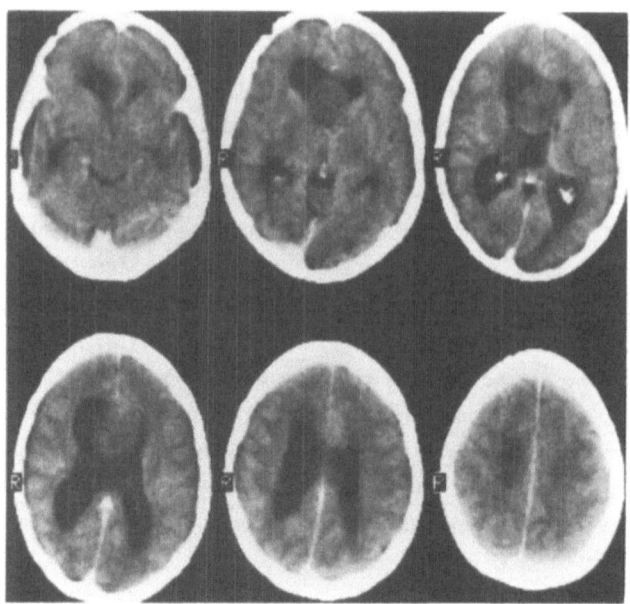

Fig. 12. CT-scan of an ependymoma in the left lateral ventricle (enhanced)

who found no age difference between patients with supra- or infratentorial tumours or even a somewhat higher mean age in the supratentorial group (9, 16, 72, 219). Most series indicate supratentorial ependymomas to be equally distributed throughout all age groups, whereas the infratentorial tumours show a predominance in the first decade (9, 16, 72, 219). Spinal cord ependymomas show a peak of incidence between the ages of 20 and 50 years (63, 72, 247). Sexual differences in incidence have not been clearly established. Some series show a slight predominance of occurrence in males but in others there is an equal distribution or even a female predominance (9, 16, 58, 72, 299).

Ependymomas are generally slow growing tumours, the clinical symptoms being related to the location of the neoplasm. The most common symptoms of the cerebrally located tumours are headache, nausea, vomiting, ataxia, diplopia, seizure, vertigo and paresis. The most common physical findings are papilloedema, ataxia, cranial nerve palsies, paresis, nystagmus and dysmetria (9, 16, 58, 72).

Grossly, ependymomas are well-circumscribed lobular tumours with a grayish-red colour. They may achieve large size as in the lateral ventricles, but in the fourth ventricle they may produce severe symptoms even when relatively small. Cystic degeneration of these neoplasms is not uncommon and foci of calcification may be found (9, 72, 225, 227).

Microscopically the ependymomas are composed of closely grouped polygonal cells. The nuclei have a regular oval or rounded shape and are surrounded by a distinct

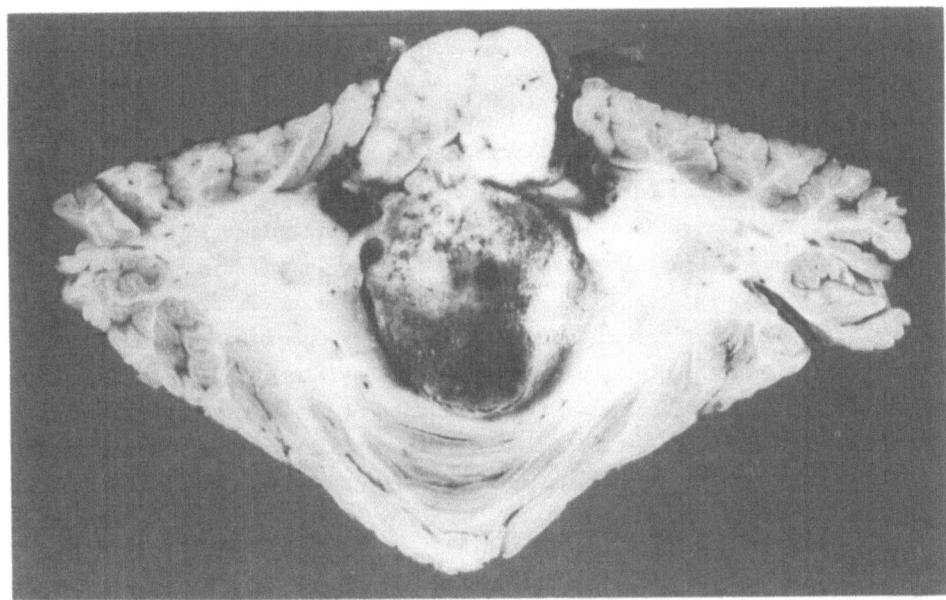

Fig. 13. Cross-section of an ependymoma in the fourth ventricle

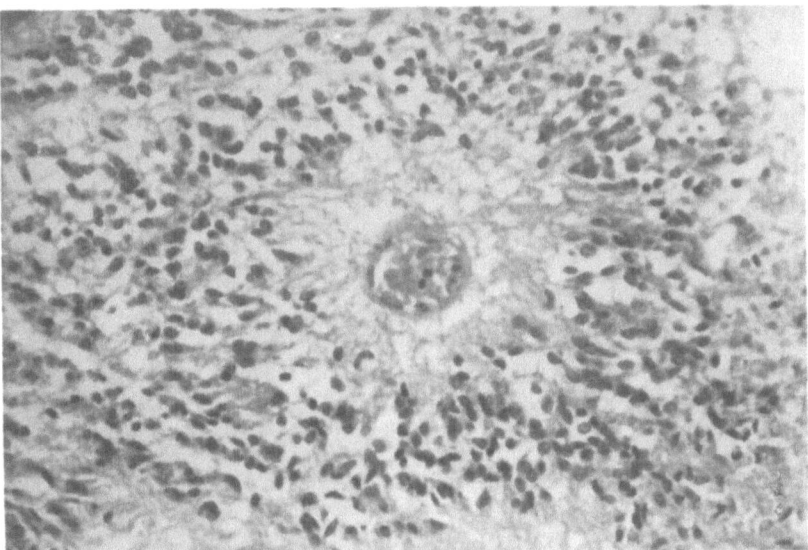

Fig. 14. Microscopic appearance of an ependymoma with a perivascular
pseudorosette
HE, 150x

nuclear membrane. Highly characteristic features of ependymoma are the presence
of ependymal rosettes, groupings of ependymal cells around circular cavities which
must be differentiated from Bailey's pseudorosettes found in medulloblastomas, and
perivascular pseudorosettes. Perivascular pseudorosettes, perivascular arrangements of ependymal cells into coronal structures, can also be found in astroblastomas (9, 41, 72, 225, 227, 299, 302). Blepharoblasts can be demonstrated in the
cytoplasm of ependymoma cells in most cases by special staining methods.
Microscopically, varieties of ependymoma may be distinguished into a cellular type,
fibrillary type, myxopapillary type, papillary type, subependymoma and an anaplastic
(malignant) ependymoma (41, 72, 225, 302). Subependymoma are regarded as a variant
of ependymoma strongly resembling the fibrillary type. The majority is found in the
fourth ventricle in middle-aged or elderly patients (225). The myxopapillary type
of ependymoma is found exclusively in the region of the cauda equina and filum
terminale (41, 72, 225, 302). The malignant ependymomas, also called ependymoblas-
tomas, are characterized by the presence of many mitoses, micronecrosis and proliferation of vascular endothelium (41, 225). They tend to occur above the tentorium.

Metastases of ependymoma occur rarely, generally by spread along the cerebrospinal fluid pathways, although extraneural metastases have been incidentally
reported (16, 72, 82, 198, 225, 226, 249). Treatment of ependymoma consists of
radical operative removal followed by radiation therapy, especially in those cases
where removal has been incomplete (9, 16, 58, 72).

Pathogenesis

Many theories concerning the pathogenesis of gliomas have been postulated but
in fact little is known about the origin of these neoplasms.
One hypothesis, mainly suggested by early reports, is based on the theory that
gliomas arise from abnormalities of embryonal origin. This dysontogenetic theory,
first suggested by Ostertag (192), supposed gliomas to be the result of developmental disturbances of the central nervous system. The association of the phacomatoses and other malformations (i.e. syringomyelia) with glioma, and the existence
of congenital examples would favour this explanation. Except for the case of certain midline tumours of infancy and early childhood (blastomas), this theory of the
origin of glioma has not been generally accepted. The theory is discussed in the
chapter on familial aspects as germinal genetic factors may play a role in this
hypothesis.
A second, somewhat more supported hypothesis, suggests that the majority of gliomas
arise from neoplastic transformation of adult glial elements (225, 330). According
to this theory the tumours originate during life in pre-existent normal glial

tissue. The malignant cell transformation (somatic genetic alteration) is assumed
caused by certain not as yet specified endogenous or exogenous influences.
A third explanation might be a combination of both hypotheses, hereditary factors
and concomitant endogenous or exogenous influences determining the development of
these tumours (see also chapter I). The different incidences of brain tumours
found in various animal species, also after induction with carcinogens, may support
this theory (330). Janisch et al., for example, demonstrated that genetically
determined metabolic patterns influence the susceptibility of the brain to tumour
induction in various species (317).

A number of influences have been found to play a possible role in tumour development. In experimental animal studies there is conclusive evidence that brain
tumours can be induced by chemical carcinogens. Nitrosamines have induced gliomas
in the rat (60, 61, 124, 125, 282, 291), and gliomas in mice have been induced by
intracerebral implantation of aromatic polycyclic hydrocarbons (214, 296). The
subject of chemically induced experimental brain tumours has been extensively reviewed by Janisch and coworkers (110, 317). Especially tumours resembling human
oligodendrogliomas, glioblastomas and ependymomas have been found in experimental
animal studies (110, 282). The relevance of these experimental studies to the
human situation is not yet clear (168, 311).
A high incidence of CNS tumours and glioblastomas has been reported among workers
in the rubber industry (157, 319).
Brooks (35), who studied the geographic distribution of 612 brain tumour patients
in the state of Kentucky found a geographic cluster in the eastern area of this
state. The incidence of gliomas within this area was 4.4 times higher than
expected; 66.1% of the cases were located along major tributaries of the Kentucky
and Licking rivers. The possibility of water contamination with chemical carcinogens was suggested by the author. A follow-up study, however, did not conform
these findings (328).
Reports of lead poisoning associated with human astrocytomas have been made (237),
but an autopsy control study of nine patients with brain tumour (glioblastomas,
astrocytomas, meningiomas, pituitary adenoma, neuroblastoma) demonstrated no difference in mean cerebral lead concentration (294).
The etiological role of barbiturates in the development of brain tumours has been
postulated (309, 310, 313). Gold et al. (313) stated that *as many as 8% of brain
tumours in children may be attributable to use of barbiturates either by the child
or prenatally by the mother*. The histological types of brain tumours in the children in their study were astrocytoma (five cases), ependymoma (two cases),

medulloblastoma (two cases), glioma (one case), and oligodendroglioma (one case)
(314). Others, however, were not able to confirm this association (306).
The copper content of astrocytomas and glioblastomas was investigated by Kaiser
and Gullotta (318). They found the peritumoural tissue of glioblastomas to contain
more copper than the tumour tissue itself, while in astrocytomas more copper was
detected in the central parts of the tumour.
In a case-control study of risk factors in the development of brain tumours in
children by Gold et al. (315) children with brain tumours were found to have had
more exposure to insecticides than had normal children. No significant difference
between groups with regard to maternal smoking during pregnancy was found. Factors
such as smoking and alcohol consumption were also investigated by Choi et al. (47),
and showed no association with brain tumour occurrence.
The association of other chemical compounds with human brain tumour occurrence has
not as yet been demonstrated.

The role of oncogenic viruses and other infectious agents in the development of
human tumours is a matter of great interest in modern research. In experimental
animal studies intracranial tumours have been induced by viruses such as the Rous
sarcoma virus induced gliomas in hamsters, rabbits and dogs (206, 207, 208, 209),
the Simian virus 40 (SV40) induced tumours of the ependyma in hamsters (62, 287),
and gliomas developing in owl monkeys inoculated with a human polyoma virus (JC-
virus) (320). The literature on virus-induced brain tumours up to 1975 has been
extensively reviewed by Janisch and Schreiber (110).
Smith et al. (250) reviewed the possible relationship between oncogenic viruses
and brain tumours in humans, listing a number of possible reasons for such an
association: 1. certain types of brain tumours have common tumour-specific antigens,
suggesting a common etiology; 2. brain tissue maintains *a privileged sanctuary from
the host's immunological defences*; 3. brain tumour tissue surgically removed can be
cultured in vitro; 4. *several viruses produce brain tumours in experimental animals*;
5. *at least one 'C' type virus is known to be neurotropic*.
SV40 related DNA sequences were found in one (a glioblastoma multiforme) of a
series of seven human brain tumours removed at craniotomy (167). Farwell et al.
(67) studied the effect of SV40 contaminated polio vaccine on the incidence and
type of CNS neoplasms in children. They demonstrated a strong association between
antenatal exposure and the development of medulloblastoma, and there was suggestive
evidence that SV40 was associated with the occurrence of gliomas.
Heinonen et al. (95) made a prospective study of 50,987 pregnancies to explore the
possible relationship between immunization against influenza and poliomyelitis

during pregnancy, and subsequent malignancies in the offspring and found a relative risk of 12.7 to 1 for neural malignancies among children of women who had received killed polio vaccine as compared to those who had not.

An association between toxoplasma gondii infections and tumours of the CNS in humans has been demonstrated (239). The correlation was particularly high for astrocytomas. A relationship between cerebral glioma and previous tuberculosis has been suggested (278), but this was contradicted in a large controlled study of 300 cases (154).

In the previously mentioned study on risk factors for brain tumours in children by Gold et al. (315) children with brain tumours were found to have had more exposure to farm animals and ill pets than unaffected children suggesting a possible etiological role of animal viruses.

Intracranial gliomas have also been reported occurring in association with demyelinating disease, particularly multiple sclerosis. The tumours probably develop from neoplastic transformation of glia in areas of demyelination, but a definite causal relationship has not yet been established (6, 227, 325).

Evidence of glioma induction by irradiation in experimental animal studies is rare, only Haymaker et al. (94) succeeding in producing glioblastoma multiforme in monkeys following total body irradiation. Few reports of human glioma occurrence following therapeutic irradiation are available in the literature. Sogg et al. (251) reported a malignant astrocytoma following radiotherapy of a craniopharyngioma; Clifton et al. (47) described a spinal cord glioblastoma following irradiation of Hodgkin's disease; a frontal lobe astrocytoma occurring after radiotherapy for medulloblastoma was reported by Cohen et al. (48). These instances are insufficient as proof of radiation induction of glioma as the simultaneous occurrence of different brain tumours is an accepted phenomenon.

A retrospective study of 11,000 children receiving radiation of the head for tinea capitis demonstrated a relative risk of brain tumour of seven to one among irradiated children as compared to the general population and sibling controls (176). The radiation-induced intracranial neoplasms found here were mostly sarcomas or meningiomas (108, 181, 187, 275, 281).

Choi et al. (45) and Gold et al. (315) investigated the influence of prenatal exposure to X-rays (diagnostic or therapeutic) and found no differences between tumour cases and control groups.

Many case reports and studies concerning the relationship of head injury to the development of glioma are available in the literature. In reviewing the data

and in accord with the findings of most authors there is no evidence that trauma
plays a significant role in the subsequent development of these tumours. Zülch
and Mennel (303, 304) in their analysis of this subject state that *it appears
unlikely that any traumatic factors cause tumour development. However, the hypothesis that the regenerative processes following trauma may act synergically in
carcinogenesis is attractive though still unproven.* In accord with this statement
Morantz and Shain (179) in an experimental study on rats found that trauma may act
as a carcinogen and enhance glioma formation in the presence of exposure to a
potent carcinogen. In rats exposed transplacentally to ethylnitrosourea 62% of 28
animals randomly allocated to open brain trauma developed gliomas in comparison
with 47% of a control group.

Perinatal period. Choi et al. (45) described a case-control study of 22 glioma
patients examining relationships between perinatal factors and central nervous
system neoplasms. The brain tumour patients in this study were under 20 years of
age. No statistically significant differences in parameters such as average
birth weight, premature birth, delivery complications, history of prenatal illness and mothers age were found. In the patient group more abortions had occurred
in pregnancies prior to patient birth as compared to the control group, this
disparity disappearing if abortions in subsequent pregnancies were included in
the calculations.
Gold et al. (315) studied risk factors in a case-control study of 84 children with
brain tumours and found a greater tendency of first births and a higher birth weight
in children with brain tumours as compared to normal children. These findings, however, must be interpreted with caution in regard to the size of the groups and the
indirect collection method of data. Further investigations and validation of these
findings would appear useful.

Blood-groups. Results of studies on the distribution of ABO blood-types in
glioma occurrence have shown some disparity. Yates et al. (290) found a slight
reduction in the proportion expected of group 0 in their group of 473 astrocytoma
patients, and Selverstone and Cooper (241) reported a highly significant decrease
in their 139 astrocytoma patients of serum anti-A-factor, corresponding to the
blood-groups 0 and B. Turowski and Czochra (329) statistically compared the distribution of ABO blood-groups in 271 patients treated for glioblastoma multiforme
with a control group of 500 patients treated for craniocerebral trauma. A statistically significant difference was observed between these groups with a higher
frequency of type A and a lower frequency of type 0 in the tumour patient group.

Most other large studies, however, show no significant differences in distribution
of the different blood-types among glioma patients (45, 75, 165). Choi et al.
noted a somewhat lower proportion of Rh positives within the astrocytoma group,
but this was not statistically significant (45).

Immunobiology. There is evidence in the literature supporting the theory that
immunological mechanisms play a role in the development of gliomas. Research on
the relationship of immunological factors and gliomas suggests that glioma-
associated antigens are present. These tumour-associated antigens have been demonstrated in several studies (90, 133, 138, 221, 243). Study results, however, are
difficult to interpret as both normal brain and glial tumours have shared antigenic components.

In recent years several investigations have attempted to prove that gliomas give
rise to a host immune response in man. Patients with gliomas have been shown to
have circulating tumour-specific cytotoxic lymphocytes (80, 138, 141). Another
indication of immune response is the observation that lymphocytic infiltration is
present in about a third of the cases of fatal glioma (217). Also elevated serum
IgM levels are found in many patients with glioblastomas (155).

Impairment of the general host immunocompetence of patients with malignant gliomas
has been reported. A humoral immunosuppressive factor, an inhibitory factor that
depresses cell-mediated immunity, i.e. lymphocytic activity, has been reported
(36, 38, 169). An impairment of cutaneous delayed-type hypersensitivity and a
reduced number of circulating thymus-derived lymphocytes in glioma patients has
been found (36, 37, 39, 80, 155).

These data suggest that the host produces a cellular and humoral immune response
to glioma-associated antigenic components, but that especially the cell-mediated
immune response appears depressed. In contrast Garson et al. (76), who investigated the humoral immune response to autologous gliomas in 16 patients, demonstrated an inhibition of IgM complement-fixing activity on cultured glioma cell
membranes by autologous IgG. According to the authors this competitive IgG/IgM
interaction may represent one of the means by which these tumours are able to
evade effective immune surveillance in the host.

The significant work dealing with the relationship between the immune system and
intrinsic glial neoplasms has been recently reviewed (8).

HLA-typing of glioma patients has also been studied and showed no significant
evidence of an HLA-linked susceptibility gene as a main etiological factor (26).
However, an association between some specific subgroup and antigens Bw35 and DRw1
has been suggested (177).

Clinical studies on the relationship between glioma and immunological factors are rare and no conclusions can be drawn from them. Patients with primary immunodeficiency syndromes or immunosuppressive therapy have a far greater risk of developing malignancies, especially lymphoreticular and haematological malignancies, but tumours of the central nervous system (astrocytoma, glioma, medulloblastoma, neuroblastoma) are also known to occur (120, 323). Renal-transplant recipients with immunosuppression also have shown a raised frequency of primary malignant tumour occurrence in the brain, but all of these were lymphoreticular malignancies (233, 254). Gold et al. (315) in their epidemiological study on risk factors for brain tumours in children reported fewer children with brain tumours having had tonsillectomies as compared to normal children.

Thus far the treatment of glioma by immunochemotherapeutic approaches has not successfully produced significant beneficial effects (1, 8, 31, 156, 191, 266, 311).

FAMILIAL ASPECTS OF GLIOMA

In the literature a number of established genetic diseases have been associated with the occurrence of nervous system tumours. These are neurofibromatosis (Von Recklinghausen's disease), tuberous sclerosis (Bourneville's disease), retino-cerebral angiomatosis (Von Hippel-Lindau's disease) and the multiple nevoid basal cell carcinoma syndrome (Gorlin's disease). As skin and eye lesions are also present among these disease entities they have been designated under the term phacomatoses (Greek phakos = lentil-shaped spot) (100, 101). Bielschowsky (25), who first associated tuberous sclerosis with neurofibromatosis, described them as dysplasias with a tendency to blastoma formation. Other synonyms are hamartoses, hamartoblastoses, neurocutaneous syndromes and neuroectodermal dysplasias. The phacomatoses are congenital conditions with a dominant mode of inheritance.

Apart from cases of glioma associated with genetic disease, the influence of genetic factors in the development of gliomas is uncertain. Separation of a small group of familial cases from the larger group of gliomas unassociated with genetic disease has been attempted by some authors (87, 126, 127, 128, 170). Topographically these tumours were located in the region of the ventricular germinal centres, i.c. deeply situated within the brain. On the basis of histological resemblance Hallervorden (87) concluded that these cases of familial gliomatosis-glioblastomatosis constitute a special form within the group of dysplasias with blastomatous features (25). Transitional forms between this entity and some of the phacomatoses have been reported (21, 87, 127, 170, 197, 286).

The possible relationship between hereditary factors and development of gliomas has been mainly based on the dysontogenetic theory of the pathogenesis of gliomas. This theory, first described by Ostertag in 1936 (192), was derived from Cohnheim-Ribbert's theory concerning the origin of tumours (49, 215, 304). It postulates that gliomas arise as the result of disturbances in embryonic development. Primitive, multipotent, undifferentiated cells persist and/or dedifferentiate from normal tissue in early embryonic development and can be stimulated to tumour growth in later life by certain factors. Corresponding to this theory Koch (126, 127) thought two factors at least necessary for the formation of a glioma: 1. a local hereditary influence: neuroglial dysplasia in the region of the ventricular germinal centres with a tendency to tumour degeneration; he suggested a mutation in a pleiotropic gene to be responsible for this local disturbance. 2. a second

or several general factors, exogenous or endogenous, that initiate oncogenesis
in these predisposed areas.

Analogous to the criteria for the cancer family syndrome established by Lynch
et al. (321), Koch and Waldbaur (132) recently proposed to designate the familial
brain tumours as a 'brain tumour family syndrome'.

In order to examine the relationship between genetic factors and glioma development the available literature was reviewed. The subject was examined from a
number of points of reference:

I. Twin studies,
II. Familial occurrence in siblings (case reports and serial studies of siblings),
III. Familial occurrence in other generations and distant relatives (case reports
    and relative studies),
IV. Association with hereditary disease and congenital disorders,
V. Cytogenetic studies.

In reviewing the literature some antiquated diagnoses were encountered. As
stated earlier in the chapter on general aspects, no general agreement in classification of gliomas exists or existed. In the description of the case reports we
have cited the diagnosis as stated by the authors. In this discussion we have
adapted, where possible, these diagnoses according to the recently proposed
classification of the World Health Organization, which is described in the previous
section. In some cases the available information permitted diagnosis adaptation, in
others difficulties of interpretation arose. Reports in which the brain tumour was
not verified histologically or at autopsy, were regarded in principle as discordant
occurrences.

Earlier reviews of familial cases of brain tumours have been published by Koch
(127), Van der Wiel (286), Kurland et al. (139), Metzel (170), Kemper (117),
Manuelidis (322), Schoenberg et al. (327), and Mulcahy and Harlan (180).

I. TWIN STUDIES

Case reports

The first report of concordant occurrence of glioma in twins was made by
Joughin in 1928. He described two identical female twins with gliomas that
presented at approximately the same age. Unfortunately the exact histological
nature of the gliomas was not reported in the article (VII.A.1.1). Subsequently
three other reports of monozygotic twins with concordant glioma appeared in

the literature. The relevant data concerning these cases are given in table 1. A fifth case has been cited in a few reports (81, 127) concerning a monozygotic male twin pair with gliomatosis, as being described by McFarland and Meade in 1932 (166). This case, however, could not be verified from the original article. Twins with subependymomas reported by Clarenbach et al. (47), are the same as those reported by Voigt and Marquardt (273). They separately described the angiographic diagnostic features of these cases. Examining the parameters of the reported concordant gliomas one finds:

Gender:

    female 2   male 6

A male predominance is suggested but the populations are too small for statistical reliability.

Histological diagnosis:

unspecified glioma	2
astrocytic tumour	2
oligodendroglial tumour	2
ependymal tumour	2

Location of the tumour:

temporal	3
4th ventricle	2
subcortical	1
fronto-parietal	1
cerebellar and brain stem	1

It is of interest that in the four twin pairs the histological nature of the tumours was identical in both twins. The age at symptom occurrence was the same in three pairs and the location of the tumour coincided in two of the four pairs. Information on associated conditions or family disorders revealed no further data of relevance.

In the discordant group (table 2) Koch et al. (130) described monozygotic twins both having a large septum pellucidum cyst; one of the twins also had a glioblastoma of the right temporal region. According to the authors the association of such abnormalities with a glioblastoma may be an indication of the possible existence of a pleitropic gene responsible for their origin. Another report of discordant tumour was originally described by Pedersen and Geyer in 1938 (199), only one twin then having a meningioma. Fourteen years later Hoppe (104) reported a glioblastoma multiforme occurring in the other member.

The chance occurrence of such tumours in twins seems unlikely. The similarity in age, location and histological diagnosis reported by Clarenbach et al. (46), for example, has led these authors to suggest a prenatal origin of the tumours and to favour the view that this tumour type is of maldevelopmental origin. It may also be relevant that concordant glioma occurrence in dizygotic twins has not as yet been reported. The interpretation of such infrequent occurrences, however, remains tenuous.

Serial studies of twins

Studies on serial selections of twins have also been performed. Within a series of 10,000 patients with tumours of the central nervous system Thums (261) found 83 patients that were one of a twin pair. In 43 of these cases the tumours were histologically verified; in 19 cases the diagnosis was glioma. In 25 pairs of twins who could be examined, 7 of whom were identical, both members of one pair of identical twins had been operated upon for a histologically unverified brain tumour occurring at approximately the same age. In the other cases the twin partners did not demonstrate cerebral neoplasms.

Kuhnen (137) studied 266 twin pairs among an unselected series of 27,504 patients. Ninety-six of these twins had lost their partner at birth or during the neonatal period. Among the remaining 170 pairs a histologically verified glioma was present in one pair only (dizygotic twin); three others (two monozygotic and one dizygotic twin) had a clinical diagnosis of glioma. The second twin in each of these four pairs had no cerebral tumour.

Koch (127) reported an additional 10 twin pairs selected from the same Neurological Clinic in Münster. Six twins (two dizygotic, four unspecified) had a clinical diagnosis of glioma. Of the 10 twin partners one had epilepsy, one had an apoplexy, one had a blood disease and another microcephaly, but no brain tumours were encountered. In this article the author also reviewed the findings on monozygotic twin pairs, one twin in each pair demonstrating a glioma, from the literature.

In her thesis on the occurrence of brain tumours in twins and families Meyer (172) found nine twin pair members in an unselected series of 459 male patients with brain tumours. In three twins (one monozygotic, one dizygotic, one unspecified) a histologically verified glioma was present; in three others (one dizygotic, two unspecified) gliomas were clinically suspected. Among the co-twins no cerebral tumours were found. Some of the twins mentioned in this study were the same as those reported earlier by Koch in 1954 (127).

Harvald and Hauge (89) studied the relatives of 169 patients with histologically verified glioblastoma. Three of the probands were twins (one monozygotic, two dizygotic) and in all three cases the co-twin was healthy. In

a follow-up study of 6,757 relatives of 641 patients with intracranial
tumours by the same authors in 1960 (92), 11 twin pairs (three monozygotic,
eight dizygotic) with histologically verified glioma were found. None of
the co-twins had a cerebral tumour; one of the twin partners died at 76 years
of age from cancer of the mammae. Five other twins (two mono- and three dizygotic) in the study died from a cerebral tumour of unknown type, but none
of their partners had a cerebral neoplasm.

Van der Wiel (286) drew attention to the fact that strikingly few glioma
patients are members of a twin pair. Only one patient with a (dizygotic)
twin, a healthy girl, could be found among 380 patients with gliomas, whereas
4 or 5 would have been expected. This excess of single-births in glioma
patients has also been reported by Kuhnen (137).

In an unselected twin-birth cohort of 145,708 individual twins born in
California, Norris and Jackson (188) found 52 instances of childhood cancer
deaths other than from leukaemia. Twenty-one of these cases had brain tumours,
two spinal cord tumours, five neuroblastomas and one a retinoblastoma. Two of
the co-twins had signs of central nervous system disease - one drowned at the
age of 14 years after an epileptic seizure; one died at six weeks of a cerebral haemorrhage - but none of the partners had cerebral tumours. Monozygotic
twins were not underrepresented among the brain tumour deaths compared to
single-born children.

Miller (175) studied the deaths from childhood leukaemia and solid tumours
among twins and siblings in the United States from 1960 to 1967. He found one
pair of male twins who died of a neuroblastoma at 13 days and 16 months of
age respectively, and a pair of female twins who died at 14 years of age: one
of a glioblastoma multiforme and the other of leukaemia after removal of a
limb for osteosarcoma. No instances of concordant gliomas in twins were encountered.

Koch (127) made a longitudinal study of a series of 450 monozygotic and dizygotic twin pairs. He found three monozygotic twins with unspecified brain
tumours; one of the co-twins had another unspecified brain tumour, the other
two co-twins did not have cerebral tumours.

The information obtained from these studies seems to indicate that genetic
factors are not of major importance in the etiology of gliomas in twins. It
is further noted that zygocity was not always adequately documented within
the studies.

II. FAMILIAL OCCURRENCE IN SIBLINGS

Case reports

1. Concordant cases

The influence of genetic factors in the development of cerebral tumours was first discussed in 1896 by Besold (22) who reported two sisters with brain tumours which were then described as haemangioblastomas or so-called periepitheliomas (VII.B.1.1). According to the histological description in this article these tumours would now best be classified as ependymal tumours in the modern nomenclature. Since this time a number of reports on concordant gliomas in siblings have been published. The relevant and available data from these reports are illustrated in table 3. Thirty-two reports of two affected siblings, three reports (possibly six reports if VII.B.1.4, B.1.19 and B.1.29 are included) of three affected siblings, and one report of four affected siblings are registered.

Two other familial occurrences of brain tumours in siblings have been reported. De la Torre (264) described a brother who died of a papilloma of the choroid plexus at the age of 9 months, and a sister who died of an ependymoma of the lateral ventricle at the age of 5 months. According to the modern classification of brain tumours by the World Health Organization these cases may be classified as concordant ependymal tumours. The histological differentiation between ependymomas and choroid plexus papillomas can be very difficult. Choroid plexus papillomas are discussed in a separate chapter, and as a choice this report has been registered among the familial choroid plexus papillomas (IV.B.1.1). Keuter (121) is cited in a table by Van der Wiel (286) as having reported two brothers with astrocytoma. We could not, however, find these cases in the original article.

On the basis of an age-adjusted incidence rate of 4.0 per 100,000 population per year for gliomas (7), and a mean age at death of 50 years, the chance of occurrence of gliomas in more than one sibling in a family can be calculated (fig. 1).

Risk of occurrence:

two	affected siblings in a sibship of two							:	0.8	in 100,000
two	"	"	" "	"	"	five	:	8		in 100,000
two	"	"	" "	"	"	ten	:	36		in 100,000
three	"	"	" "	"	"	three:	0.0048		in 100,000	
three	"	"	" "	"	"	five	:	0.048		in 100,000
three	"	"	" "	"	"	ten	:	0.577		in 100,000

417

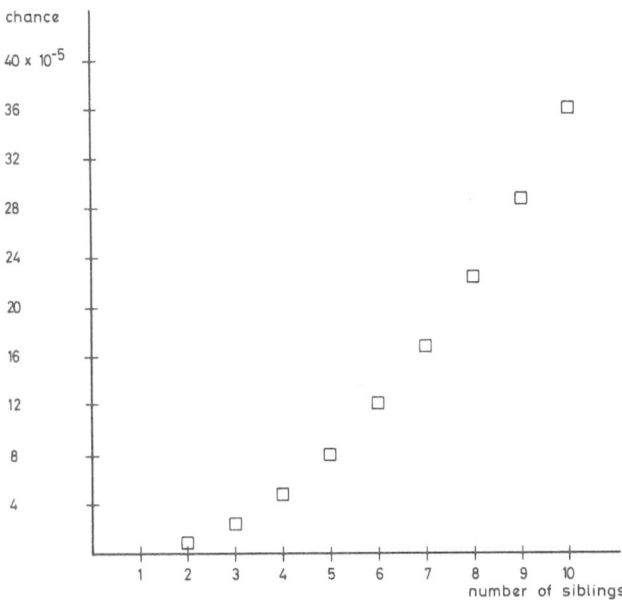

Fig. 1. The chance of glioma occurrence in two siblings of one family

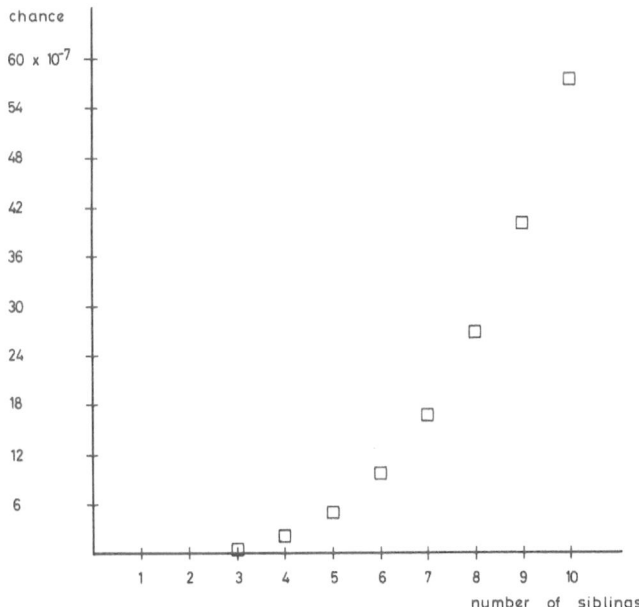

Fig. 2. The chance of glioma occurrence in three siblings of one family

Based on statistical calculations the ratio of occurrence of gliomas in
two as compared to three siblings in a family is approximately 1:100, so
for every report of three siblings with gliomas, 100 reports of two
siblings should be expected. The actual ratio, however, is 3 (possibly 6):
32, which is approximately 9 (or 18) times more than expected.

Examination of the parameters registered in table 3 revealed the following:

Gender:

    female patients: 29 (36.25%)
    male patients : 51 (63.75%)

A predominance of the male sex among the familial cases of glioma is found.
This is in contrast to the sex-ratio found in isolated cases which is
approximately equal or shows a slightly higher incidence in females (see
general aspects). The gender of the affected siblings in each family reported was the same in 24 of the 36 reports.

Histological diagnosis:

    A. Astrocytic tumours: 21 cases
       - Astrocytoma (not graded)   5
       - Astrocytoma II   1
       - Astrocytoma III   13
       - Astroblastoma   2

    B. Oligodendroglial tumours: 3 cases
       - Oligodendroglioma   3

    C. Ependymal tumours (without
       choroid plexus tumours):
       - Ependymoma   4
       - Subependymoma   2
       - Ependymoblastoma   2

    D. Poorly differentiated and
       embryonal tumours
       (without medulloblastoma):   35 cases
       - Glioblastoma   33
       - Glioblastomatosis   1
       - Spongioblastoma   1

    E. Unspecified glioma: 11 cases

On a percent basis for the cases in which the histological nature of the
glioma is specified one found:

poorly differentiated tumours (glioblastomas) 52.3%, astrocytic tumours
31.3%, ependymal tumours 11.9%, and oligodendroglial tumours 4.5%.

In comparison to statistics on isolated cases of glioma the mutual percentages are approximately identical, most cases being glioblastomas and
(high grade) astrocytomas (83.6%), with the exception of the ependymal
tumours, which seem somewhat overrepresented within the familial group.
It is noteworthy that the histological nature of the gliomas in the
affected siblings of each family was identical in 30 (85.7%) of the 36

reports; in 5 reports it was different and in one uncertain. In the reports
on three and four affected siblings the histological nature was identical
in affected siblings in all but one case; this, however, showed a minor
difference: astrocytoma grade III instead of glioblastoma (VII.B.1.36).

Location of the tumour:

A. Astrocytic tumours: 21 cases
   - temporal   8
   - frontal   7
   - parieto-occipital   2
   - parietal   2
   - third ventricle   1
   - peduncle   1

B. Oligodendroglial tumours: 3 cases
   - frontal   3

C. Ependymal tumours: 8 cases
   - lateral ventricle   3
   - third ventricle   2
   - fourth ventricle   1
   - cervical cord   2

D. Poorly differentiated tumours: 35 cases
   - temporal   10
   - frontal   7
   - fronto-parietal   3
   - parieto-occipital   4
   - corpus callosum   3
   - diffuse   3
   - thalamus   1
   - cerebellar   1
   - unknown   3

E. Unspecified glioma: 11 cases
   - temporal   4
   - frontal   2
   - fronto-parietal   1
   - fronto-temporal   1
   - fourth ventricle   1
   - unknown   2

All gliomas: 78 cases
   - temporal   22
   - frontal   19
   - fronto-temporal   1
   - fronto-parietal   4
   - parieto-occipital   6
   - parietal   1
   - corpus callosum   3
   - diffuse   3
   - thalamus   1
   - lateral ventricle   3
   - third ventricle   3
   - fourth ventricle   2
   - cerebellar   1
   - peduncle   1
   - cervical cord   2
   - unknown   5

Familial cases of glioma occurred predominantly in the frontal, temporal, and less frequently the parieto-occipital regions. The parietal and occipital lobes in these cases are rarely involved compared to the statistics on isolated cases of glioma (see general aspects). In most cases the tumours were situated deeply in the brain and not near the surface. There was no difference in frequency of occurrence within the right and left hemispheres. The appearance of multiple gliomas was seen in only one of the familial cases (VII.B.1.31). The location of the tumour in affected siblings within one family was the same in 16 of the 36 reports, different in 16 and unknown in 4 reports.

Age:

	mean age at symptom occurrence	mean age at death
Astrocytic tumours	48.9 y	-
Oligodendroglial tumours	32.3 y	-
Ependymal tumours	19.1 y	-
Poorly differentiated tumours	42.3 y	42.6 y
Unspecified glioma	33.6 y	34.5 y

The mean age of symptom occurrence in the familial cases of glioma was approximately the same as the age at which 'isolated' gliomas frequently occur (see general aspects). Specifically, the mean age of manifestation of the astrocytic group, however, was somewhat higher, and that of the glioblastomas perhaps somewhat lower in comparison to the nonfamilial group. The mean survival time for the unspecified glioma group was very short, which suggests that most of these tumours were of the malignant type. The mean survival time of the glioblastomas did not differ from that expected for isolated occurrences.

Associated physical or mental conditions:

Some of the affected siblings had associated *congenital anomalies*. Autopsy of one of the sisters described by Besold (VII.B.1.1) revealed a double left ureter, thyroid gland cysts and an open foramen ovale. The brother reported by Noetzel (VII.B.1.15) had a persisting foetal 'Lappung' of the kidneys and a nodular goiter. One of the siblings reported by Li et al. had a meningocoele and acute leukaemia, the other a café-au-lait spot, pigmented naevi and a lymphocytic lymphoma (VII.B.1.30). This last report may be regarded as some form of a *cancer family syndrome* or of Von Recklinghausen's *neurofibromatosis*. Bender and Panse, and Haller-vorden described two brothers with diffuse gliblastomatosis mainly affecting the temporal lobes (VII.B.1.4). The affected brothers also had pes caves, naevi and skin tumours, disorders that were also seen in other family members. A third brother died of a clinically suspected brain tumour, but no autopsy was performed. From these and other observations Hallervorden concluded this familial gliomatosis to be a disease entity constituting a special form of dysontogenetic process with blastomatous features (*phacomatosis*).

Two of the four brothers with glioblastoma reported by Baughman et al. also had polyposis of the colon and pigmented naevi; another had café-au-lait spots and the fourth two polyps of the colon (VII.B.1.24). This family and a family with three affected siblings described by Todd et al. (VII.B.1.36) manifest the *glioma-polyposis* or Turcot syndrome, a probably autosomal recessive disorder which is discussed later in this chapter.

In both brothers described by Blaauw and Schenk a coincidence of subependymoma with *haemophilia*, an X-linked recessive disorder, was present (VII.B.1.25). One of the brothers also had a syringomyelic cavity, an association that has been reported earlier by Poser (204).

Associated *tumours* were found in two affected siblings. The female with a glioblastoma described by Riese et al. (VII.B.1.9) also had a bronchiogenic lung carcinoma and leiomyomata uteri. One of the sisters with astrocytomas reported by Schoenberg et al. (VII.B.1.29) had undergone excision of a presacral lipoma.

Data on *blood-groups* were available in six affected siblings: four had blood-group A and two had blood-group AB.

Previous *head injury* was noted in three of the affected siblings.

Other incidence of *disease* reported were: rheumatic complaints (2 cases), luetic infection with tabes dorsalis (1 case), pneumonia (1 case), convulsions as a baby (1 case), frontal sinusitis (1 case), and anaemia (1 case). Associated *mental conditions* were: agoraphobia (1 case), alcoholism (2 cases), depression (3 cases), schizofrenic psychosis (2 cases), and feeble-mindedness (1 case).

Family:

The findings of naevi, pes caves and oligophrenia in a number of family members of the brothers reported in the previously mentioned study by Bender and Panse, and Hallervorden (VII.B.1.4) suggest a relationship with the *neurofibromatosis* complex.

Signs of *phacomatosis* were also seen in family members of the siblings reported by Li et al. (VII.B.1.30). This family also showed occurrence of multiple primary malignancies, especially haematologically, and cardiac malformations, and must be regarded as a form of neurofibromatosis or a *cancer family syndrome*.

Congenital abnormalities were present in the family members reported by Metzel (VII.B.1.22). A son of the female with an ependymoma underwent operation on an arachnoidal cyst of the cisterna magna at the age of 19 years. According to the author this coincidence supports the dysontogenetic theory of the development of gliomas.

Haemophilia was also seen in family members of the two brothers reported by Blaauw and Schenk (VII.B.1.25).

In three reports a third sibling with a histologically unverified *brain tumour* was clinically diagnosed (VII.B.1.4, B.1.19, B.1.29), and in one report a third brother died at an early age, supposedly of a brain tumour (VII.B.1.34).

An aqueduct stenosis, presumably due to gliosis, was found in a nephew of the two brothers reported by Isamat (VII.B.1.28).

Family *deaths of unknown cause occurring at an early age* were reported in three cases: in two reports concerning two other siblings of affected patients (VII.B.1.6 and VII.B.1.19); in the third report concerning two children of each of two siblings having gliomas (VII.B.1.3).

Other *malignancies* (lung, breast, stomach and uterus) were reported among family members by Pelgrom von Motz et al. (VII.B.1.31). Three other instances of malignancies among relatives, a carcinoma of the oesophagus and a carcinoma of the stomach, and prostatic cancer, were registered.

Seizures are mentioned in two relatives of affected siblings.

Other incidental diseases among family members are listed in table 3.

2. Discordant cases

Fourteen reports on siblings with discordant CNS tumour, one sibling having a glioma, are available in the literature (table 4). In one of these 14 publications (92) an uncertain diagnosis of gliomatosis is reported for a sibling of a patient having an astrocytoma. Although concordant occurrence is implied, this case has been registered as discordant because of insufficient validation. Twelve reports concerned two siblings and two reports four siblings. The male-female ratio was 5:3.

Histological diagnosis and number of gliomas found:

glioblastoma	9
astrocytoma	4
unspecified glioma	1

The discordant CNS tumours encountered in the siblings were:

uncertain histological nature	12
medulloblastoma	4
plexus papilloma	1
meningioma	1
haemangioma	1

A generally short survival time after symptom occurrence is noted for patients having brain tumours of uncertain histological nature (table 4), possibly reflecting their malignant character.

Associated conditions and family:

The patient with a glioblastoma described by Oehler (VII.B.2.1) had multiple pigmented naevi and a papilloma of the tongue; one with glioblastomatosis reported by Hallervorden (VII.B.2.2) also had fibroma on the back. These stigmata suggest a possible relationship with *neurofibromatosis*.

Chen et al. (VII.B.2.12), investigating the clinical and genetic patterns of neurological disease on Guam, reported a family having brain tumours associated with stigmata of the *phacomatoses complex*. Other forms of cancer such as leukaemia, hepatoma, and laryngeal cancer also occurred among the relatives, possibly suggesting a relationship with the *SBLA family cancer syndrome*. The brothers reported by Blattner et al. (VII.B.2.14) were certainly members of a family with this SBLA syndrome.

The siblings reported by Turcot et al. (VII.B.2.6) had polyposis of the colon and in one case a hypophysal chromophobe adenoma. This family manifests the *glioma-polyposis syndrome,* to which Turcot gave his name. Other *malignancies* found in relatives of affected siblings were: uterus cancer (1 case), intestinal cancer (1 case), liver cancer (1 case), stomach cancer (4 cases), and leukaemia (1 case). The family reported by Colafranceschi and Mennonna (VII.B.2.11) is noteworthy in this respect, family members having a high frequency of carcinoma of the stomach.

In both concordant and discordant cases no other information was available concerning parameters of interest, as e.g. pregnancy and birth influences.

Serial studies of siblings

Statistical studies on the occurrence of brain tumours in siblings have been performed. While generally not specific for gliomas, these studies have been registered here in regard to the high frequency of glioma occurrence. Miller (174, 175) investigated the deaths from childhood leukaemia and solid

tumours among siblings in the United States in the years 1960 to 1967. He
found brain tumours in eight sibling pairs, which was nine times the statistically expected occurrence of 0.9. Unfortunately, the histological type of
the brain tumours was not reported. Eight families were also reported (0.9
expected) in which one child died of a brain tumour (3 glioblastomas, 2 gliomas,
1 medulloblastoma, 1 astrocytoma, and 1 sarcoma) while another died of cancer
of the bone or muscle. The author suggests that concordance of brain tumours
presumably occurs on a genetic basis as in heritable neurocutaneous syndromes,
and that a subclinical form of these syndromes may account for the excessive
occurrence of tumours of the brain and musculoskeletal system in the same sibship. One sibling did demonstrate tuberous sclerosis. Representation of a form
of (SBLA) familial cancer syndrome may be another possible explanation of this
association.

Li et al. (145) studied 38 families demonstrating cancer in two or more children aged 0 to 19 years. Three sibling pairs had brain tumours, in one family
synchronic with haematological malignancy. One of these pairs had a family
history of neurofibromatosis and brain tumours. In six families one child had
a brain tumour. The associated malignancies in the other siblings were
leukaemia (two families), bone cancer (two families), non-Hodgkin lymphoma
(one family), and soft tissue sarcoma (one family).

III. FAMILIAL OCCURRENCE IN OTHER GENERATIONS AND DISTANT RELATIVES

Case reports

1. Concordant cases

The first case of histologically verified gliomas in two generations
was noted by Ostertag in 1948 and reported as a personal communication by
Koch in 1949 (VII.C.1.1). He refers to a mother and daughter dying of glioblastomatosis of the parieto-occipital region. The report is of further
interest as the daughter was a premature, still-born child. The glioblastomatosis must have developed during intra-uterine life. Congenital examples
of gliomas in isolated cases have also been reported; 36 cases were collected from the literature by Ohta et al. (190) in 1977 (see associated
congenital conditions). Twenty-two other reports of histologically verified
glioma occurrence in more than one generation have been made. The relevant
data on these reports are summarized in the case reports and table 5.

Twenty-one reports of the occurrence of gliomas in two generations and two
reports in three generations are summarized. Two other reports dealing with
glioma occurrence in cousins (VII.C.1.12 and VII.C.1.22) have also been
registered here as a matter of choice. In 19 reports two relatives were
affected, in four reports three relatives, in one report six relatives
(five cases of which were histologically verified), and in one case seven
relatives (three cases of which were also histologically verified).

Two reports of familial occurence of (possible) gliomas were not registered
as a result of insufficient data: Bing and Haymaeker (307) report the
occurrence of cerebral neoplasms in three members of a family; Munslow and
Hill (182) cite a personal communication from Klemme who had identified
gliomas in two members of a family. No further information is available
concerning these cases.

Relationship:

The following relationships were encountered in the reports:

mother - son	4 cases
mother - daughter	3 cases
mother - daughter and son	2 cases
father - son	4 cases
father - daughter	3 cases
father - daughter and son	1 case
uncle - nephew	3 cases
uncle - niece	2 cases
aunt - nephew	1 case

The report by Thuwe et al. (VII.C.1.25) concerning seven relatives with
brain tumours in three generations is of special interest. Unfortunately,
the histological nature of the brain tumours could only be verified in
three cases. The macroscopic appearance of the brain tumour at autopsy in
two other cases was indicative of glioma.

A second report of the occurrence of brain tumours in three generations is
that of Blickenstorfer (VII.C.2.3). He reported a brother with a glioblastoma and a sister with a meningioma. A grandmother and an aunt of these
siblings also died of brain tumours but no information on histological
examination is given. This family has been registered among the discordant
CNS tumours.

Mention has been made of a significant maternal predominance (mother-child
as compared to father-child relationships) in cases of parent-child glioma
reports (3), but the present finding of nine mother-child and eight father-
child occurrences does not clearly support this conclusion.

Histological diagnosis:

  A. Astrocytic tumours: 20 cases
- Astrocytoma   8
- Astrocytoma grade I   4
- Astrocytoma grade II   5
- Astrocytoma grade III   3

  B. Oligodendroglial tumours: 2 cases
- Malignant oligodendroglioma 2

  C. Ependymal tumours: 2 cases
- Ependymoma   1
- Ependymoblastoma   1

  D. Poorly differentiated tumours: 27 cases
- Glioblastoma   22
- Gliomatosis   3
- Spongioblastoma   2

  E. Unspecified glioma: 5 cases

For the specified tumours a predominance of glioblastomas and astrocytomas is found, namely: poorly differentiated tumours (glioblastomas) 53%, astrocytic tumours 39.2%, oligodendroglial tumours 3.9% and ependymal tumours 3.9%.

In the affected families the histological diagnosis of the tumour was the same in 11 reports, different in 10 reports and of uncertain similarity in four. Interesting in this respect is the family reported by Kjellin et al. (VII.C.1.7) in which all three affected persons (father, daughter and son) had histologically identical gliomas, astrocytoma grade II.

Location of the tumour:

  A. Astrocytic tumours: 20 cases
- frontal   2
- temporal   3
- temporo-parietal   1
- occipital   1
- occipito-temporal   1
- corpus callosum   2
- thalamus   1
- third ventricle   1
- brain stem   3
- cerebellum   4
- unknown   1

  B. Glioblastoma group: 27 cases
- frontal   9
- temporal   3
- fronto-parietal   1
- fronto-temporal   3
- parietal   2
- temporo-parietal   1
- parieto-occipital   2
- occipital   1
- corpus callosum   1
- paraventricular   1
- unknown   3

All gliomas: 56 cases
- frontal   13
- temporal   8
- fronto-temporal   3
- parietal   2
- temporo-parietal   2
- fronto-parietal   1
- occipital   2
- parieto-occipital   3
- occipito-temporal   1
- corpus callosum   3
- thalamus   1
- third ventricle   2
- brain stem   3
- paraventricular   1
- cerebellar   4
- spinal   1
- unknown   6

The tumours occurred predominantly in the frontal and temporal regions, corresponding to the predeliction of familial gliomas in siblings for these areas. Parietal and occipital lobe occurrences were relatively infrequent. The tumours were usually located deep within the brain. The location was approximately the same in 12 of the reported cases, and clearly different in 11 others. The left hemisphere was affected more often than the right: 23 as compared to 13 cases. There was no multiple tumour occurrence.

Age of occurrence:

For this parameter reports of a parent and one or more children with gliomas were examined. There was considerable difference in the age of manifestation between the parent and the children groups. The mean age at tumour manifestation was 47.4 years for the parents and 27.1 years for the children. The mean age of 27.1 years for the affected children is also rather low compared to the usual age of occurrence of gliomas in non-familial cases. The occurrence of glioblastomatosis in a premature, still-born child has been mentioned earlier in this chapter.

Associated physical or mental conditions:

Some of the affected persons had *congenital abnormalities*. One of the patients (daughter) described by Koch (VII.C.1.2) had pigmented naevi and an abnormal configuration of the skull, possibly suggesting a relationship with the phacomatoses. Another patient had a naevus pigmentosus vinosus (VII.C.1.4).

Other incidentally associated diseases were: typhoid fever, a possible case of muscular dystrophy, and eclampsia. Two instances of *head injury* were noted.

Blood-groups were recorded in nine cases, seven patients having blood-group

A Rhesus positive, one patient AB Rhesus positive, and one patient B Rhesus
positive. For affected family members the blood-group was reported identical
in two instances and different in two others.
In three affected persons appendectomy was performed.
Associated *mental conditions* were: depressions (two patients), alcoholism
(one), and one patient committed suicide.
Family:

   In the family described by Koch (VII.C.1.2) concerning a mother and son
with gliomas, two other children died, one in the first year of life and
another at the age of 14 years, both of unknown cause. Some form of
dysplasia with blastomatous features in this family was suspected by the
author.
Four siblings *dying at an early age of unknown cause* were also reported in
the family with seven affected members studied by Thuwe et al. (VII.C.1.25).
In the report of Schianchi and Kraus-Ruppert (VII.C.1.23) on a father and
son with brain stem astrocytomas, two nephews of the father died of unspecified cause at ages 18 months and 8 days. In this family the occurrence of
multiple sclerosis and *Cockayne syndrome,* a rare autosomal recessive disorder, was also noted.
Four affected relatives reported by Lynch et al. (VII.C.1.18) are part of a
family with the remarkable cancer aggregation of sarcoma, brain tumours,
breast cancer, leukaemia, and adrenal cortical carcinoma, together called
the *SBLA cancer syndrome* (see associated diseases).
A *brain tumour* of unknown nature was discovered in a distant relative in
one report (VII.C.1.22).
Other *cancer occurrences* among the families were a lung tumour, cancer of
the bowel, carcinoma of the stomach (2 cases) and two relatives with unspecified cancer.

2. Discordant cases

   Thirteen reports of familial tumour occurrence in more than one generation or in more distantly related family members, one family member having
a glioma, have appeared in the literature. Eight reports concerned brain
tumours in two generations, two reports three generations, two reports
concerned cousins, and in one report a grandfather and granddaughter were
involved.
Some authors include a publication by Pittrich (203) among familial glioma
reports. In this report a daughter had a glioblastoma and her father

epileptic seizures with mental disturbances of unknown origin. The
presence of a brain tumour, however, was not confirmed in this case.
The histological glioma type in the 13 reports were: glioblastoma in
seven cases, unspecified glioma in four cases, one oligodendroglioma, one
neuroblastoma, and one case of astrocytoma.
The histological nature of the 'other' tumours was unspecified in 16
cases; in two cases meningiomas, in one a neurinoma, in one a medulloblastoma, and in one case bilateral neuroepitheliomas (retinoblastomas) were
diagnosed.

Associated physical or mental conditions:

A son with a neuroblastoma reported by Meyer (VII.C.2.6) also had a
naevus on the face. His brother died at 8 weeks of 'Krämpfen'; a nephew
died at 25 years of age while in a state of depression, and a niece had
epilepsy. Another brother in this report died of a sarcoma of the kidney.
In the family described by Van der Wiel (VII.C.2.13) one member (son of
the grandfather, father of the granddaughter) had a spina bifida occulta,
and a cousin died shortly after birth of anencephaly.
Rados (VII.C.2.1) reported the occurrence of a brain stem astrocytoma and
bilateral *retinoblastomas* in two maternally related cousins. This occurrence is possibly relevant considering the hereditary aspect of retinoblastomas.
In the family reported by Kemper (VII.C.2.11) consanguinity between the
grandparents existed; also two examples of *multiple sclerosis* and a few
relatives with mental disturbances were noted.
The report by Blickenstorfer (VII.C.2.3) of brain tumour occurrence in
three generations has been discussed previously.
Walker et al. (VII.C.2.12) reported a familial occurrence of two brain
tumours in each of three generations. In one generation it concerned two
brothers with malignant gliomas. Many other malignancies were demonstrated
among relatives in five generations, such as leukaemia, carcinomas of the
stomach, bowel, and breast, carcinoma of the adrenal glands, and sarcoma.
This family manifests the *SBLA family cancer syndrome* (see associated
inherited conditions).

As in the case of sibling studies, reports on glioma occurrence in
generations and distant relatives were insufficiently documented for
examination of other parameters.

Relative studies

A number of studies on relatives of glioma patients have been published. Pass (197) examined the close relatives of 30 patients with a brain tumour and found only one case of familial occurrence: two half-sisters with gliomas (VII.B.1.6). A remarkably large number of other tumours, however, was discovered in the examined relatives, and several cases of Von Recklinghausen's disease were also found.

Wanner (277) studied mental disturbances in 114 patients having brain tumours, and their relatives. Among 878 examined relatives only one case of brain tumour could be discovered, no further details of which are supplied.

In order to study mental symptoms Blickenstorfer (30) investigated seven patients operated upon because of occipital brain tumours and 463 of their relatives. For one family brain tumour occurrence in four relatives from three generations was noted (VII.C.2.3).

A series of 350 female brain tumour patients (including 15 spinal tumours) from the clinic of Münster were examined by Koch (127). Six (1.7%) familial occurrences of brain tumour were diagnosed, four of which were histologically verified. These occurrences were mainly of gliomas (including one glioblastoma) and neurinomas.

Meyer (172), examining a series of 459 cases of male brain tumour patients in the same clinic in Münster, 305 of which were histologically verified (glioma, glioblastoma, astrocytoma, meningioma, and hypophysis tumours), found seven cases of familial brain tumour occurrence (1.4%). The histologically verified familial cases were mainly gliomas-glioblastomas located deeply within the brain.

Hauge and Harvald (89, 91, 92) concluded hereditary factors to be of little significance in the etiology of brain tumours. They investigated 1813 relatives of 179 glioblastoma patients, and 2020 relatives of 174 astrocytoma patients. They found, respectively, 5 and 8 intracranial tumours among those relatives, whereas 5.7 and 4.3 would have been expected on the basis of calculations of occurrence of cerebral tumour among relatives in a control group population. In their discussion, however, the authors state that *the only group in which the material does not permit the exclusion of hereditary etiological factors is the group of astrocytomata in which the number of tumours observed among relatives is somewhat higher than the anticipated figure although this difference is not significant.*

In a series of 163 verified cases of glioblastoma multiforme in which family histories were recorded only three positive for familial brain tumour occurrence were found by Frankel and German (73), the type of tumours in the family members not being specified.

Examining the role of status dysraphicus in the etiology of gliomas, Van der Wiel (286) examined the relatives of 100 randomly selected patients with pathologically confirmed glioma of the brain. Of the 1290 deaths occurring in 5262 relatives of these patients seven were found to be the result of a verified glioma and five others of a probable but unverified glioma. In a control group of 2228 individuals not a single case died of glioma. Compared with the entire population of The Netherlands the glioma mortality of the tumour group was four times higher than statistically expected. As for dysraphic features the difference between the tumour and control groups was statistically significant and demonstrated status dysraphicus to constitute a predisposition for glioma occurrence. Difference in frequency of café-au-lait spot occurrence between the tumour and the control group was also highly significant. The author concluded gliomas to be a manifestation of an endogenous blastomatosis, more resembling the phacomatoses than carcinoma.

Metzel (171) studied 393 cases of glioma (including medulloblastoma and neurinoma) and found three histologically verified familial cases and two instances of clinically suspected familial brain tumour. As statistical analysis showed this frequency to be more than ten times that of a random occurrence, Metzel concluded hereditary influences to be probably involved in the etiology of at least certain glioma types.

In a study of 453 brain tumour patients, 385 of which were histologically verified (glioblastoma, astrocytoma, meningioma, hypophysis tumours, metastases), Kemper (117) found four histologically verified and two clinically diagnosed occurrences of familial brain tumour, a frequency of 1.32%. In the familial cases mainly gliomas (glioblastomas) and neurinomas were encountered. The study by Kemper (117) was conducted in the clinic of Münster, as were the studies of Koch (127) and Meyer (172). These authors concluded the familial cases of brain tumours to chiefly concern gliomatoses-glioblastomatoses and neurinomas. The possibility of a special disease entity within the group of dysplasias with blastomatous features (phacomatoses) is suggested by them.

Choi et al. (45) performed a retrospective study based on interviews with family members of 77 patients with histologically verified tumours of the glioma group (35 astrocytomas, 23 glioblastomas, 7 ependymomas, 6 medulloblastomas, and 6 unclassified and mixed gliomas). Eight brain tumours were found among the 1243 relatives of these patients as compared to one brain tumour among 1382 relatives of an equivalent size control group. The

difference in tumour occurrence rate for the two groups was statistically
significant. Statistical analysis of subgroup (i.c., astrocytoma, glioblastoma,
ependymoma) occurrence was not performed because of the small number of involved cases. Unfortunately no further confirmation of the histological diagnoses of the brain tumours occurring in the relatives was attempted. The
authors concluded their findings to be highly suggestive of familial aggregation of brain tumours, particularly for the glioma group.

Author	year	number of patients	tumour type	number of relatives examined	number of familial brain tumours	percentage
Pass	1938	30	brain tumours	?	1	3.3
Wanner	1950	114	brain tumours	878	1	0.9
Blickenstorfer	1951	7	gliomas	463	3 (1 family)	14.3
Koch	1954	350	brain tumours	-	6	1.7
Meyer	1956	459	brain tumours	-	7	1.5
Frankel	1958	163	glioblastomas	-	3	1.8
Van der Wiel	1959	100	gliomas	5262	12	12
Metzel	1964	393	gliomas	-	3 (5?)	0.8 (or 1.3)
Kemper	1964	453	brain tumours	-	6	1.3
Choi	1970	77	gliomas	1243	8	10.4

Reviewing the studies on the families of glioma - or brain tumour - patients
(see table), the percentages of familial occurrence ranged from 0.8 to 14.3%,
occurrence differences probably reflecting the varying number of relatives investigated in the individual studies. In the glioma group percentages varying
from approximately 1 to 14.3% are found with a mean of 7.86%. This is higher
than might be expected on a coincidental basis, the incidence of occurrence as
cited in several countries being approximately 4 per 100,000 population per
year. This appears to indicate a familial basis for glioma occurrence.

In an attempt to review the familial cases of brain tumour occurrence in The
Netherlands we requested the 20 largest neurological and neurosurgical clinics
in this country to refer their reports to us. Replies were received from 10 of
the clinics. Six families with familial brain tumour occurrence were reported
(VII.B.1.34 and 35, VII.C.1.20, 21, and 22, VII.C.2.13). The reported cases
were all based upon the memory of the clinicians involved, the majority of the
clinics not routinely including familial aspects within their filing system

records. The result of these inquiries, however, indicates that more of these
cases do in fact occur.

IV. ASSOCIATED HEREDITARY OR CONGENITAL CONDITIONS

A number of inherited or congenital conditions exist in which gliomas more
or less frequently occur.

A. *Autosomal dominant diseases*

Neurofibromatosis

Neurofibromatosis or Von Reckoinghausen's disease is a phacomatosis
characterized by cuteneous pigmentations (café-au-lait spots) and multiple
tumours arising from elements of the peripheral and central nervous system.
These manifestations result from developmental disturbances of neuroectodermal tissue. Two forms of the disease are distinguished: the peripheral
or classical form as described by Von Recklinghausen in 1882, characterized
by peripheral nerve and skin lesions, and a central form marked by bilateral
acoustic neurinomas and only few peripheral stigmata (4, 106, 113, 216). The
most common other CNS tumours accompanying neurofibromatosis are optic
gliomas, astrocytomas, spongioblastomas, ependymomas, gliomatosis, and
meningiomas (40, 103, 147, 211, 224). They predominantly occur in the central form.
The association of brain stem spongioblastoma with Von Recklinghausen's
disease in monozygotic male twins has been reported by Brady (308).
The reported percentages of intracranial neoplasms occurring in neurofibromatosis vary from 4 to 17% (103, 216). In a large review of reported cases
gliomatous tumours of the central nervous system have been observed in as
many as 45% of all affected individuals with the central form of neurofibromatosis (222). The wide range of occurrence estimates is mainly due to a
lack of uniform distinction between the central and peripheral forms of the
disease.
Neurofibromatosis is a not uncommon disorder with an incidence of about 1
in 3,000 (103, 216). The mode of inheritance is by autosomal dominant trait
in both forms. Penetrance is high, but expression is markedly variable (113,
128, 216). Sporadic cases can also occur resulting from new mutation of the
neurofibromatous gene (113, 216).

Tuberous sclerosis

Tuberous sclerosis or Bourneville's disease is one of the phacomatoses.
The disease entity is characterized by the triad of sebaceous adenomas,

mental deficiency, and epilepsy. The most common CNS lesions in this disease are cortical tubers, clusters of heterotopic cells in white matter,
and nodules in the walls of the cerebral ventricles (59).
Cerebral tumours have been noted in 1 to 5% of cases of this disease (106,
211) and have been thought to originate from the subependymal nodules
('candle cutterings') (227). The histological diagnosis of these tumours
is most frequently a giant cell astrocytoma, but glioblastoma, ependymoma,
and meningioma have been rarely reported (59, 246). The mode of inheritance
is by dominant transmission with great variability in gene manifestation
(128, 258). Many isolated cases also have been reported, probably caused by
fresh mutations (128, 140).
The incidence of this disease varies from 1 : 30,000 to 1 : 150,000 in
different studies (128).

Other phacomatoses

Gliomas are very rarely encountered in the other phacomatoses. One case
of a cerebellar ependymoma has been reported in Von-Hippel-Lindau's disease
(52). In the multiple nevoid basal cell carcinoma syndrome (NBCC) or
Gorlin's syndrome medulloblastomas can occur, usually appearing in the first
two years of life (84, 93, 185, see also familial aspects of medulloblastoma).

Status dysraphicus

Status dysraphicus is a constitutional anomaly characterized by the principal symptoms: spina bifida, kyphoscoliosis, anomalies of the spinal column,
funnel chest, hollow feet and club feet, acrocyanosis, areflexia, and enuresis, and other accessory symptoms such as lumbosacral hypertrichosis, palate
disorders, malformations of the urogenital tract, anisomastia and mental
deficiency (53, 146, 286). In order to study the relationship between the
dysraphic state and the genesis of gliomas Van der Wiel examined 100 histologically verified glioma patients and their relatives. Dysraphic features
were more common among the patients and their relatives than within a control
group. Especially signs of 'lethal dysraphism' - spina bifida aperta,
meningocele, and anencephaly - were more frequent among the relatives of the
brain tumour patients. He concluded that status dysraphicus constitutes a
predisposition for glioma development. The pattern of inheritance of this
constitutional disorder suggests an irregular dominant transmission (146,
286). It is uncertain, however, whether the concept of status dysraphicus
can be regarded as a distinct genetic entity (56, 255).

SBLA or family cancer syndrome

Brain tumours frequently occur in the SBLA syndrome, a rare familial

cancer syndrome characterized by the aggregation of S, sarcoma, B, breast
cancer and brain tumours, L, leukaemia, laryngeal carcinoma and lung cancer,
and A, adrenal cortical carcinoma.
Families with this tumour complex have been reported by Li and Fraumeni
(142, 143), Bottomley et al. (33), Walker et al. (276), Lynch et al. (151),
and Blattner et al. (29).
Histologically the most frequent brain tumours found in this syndrome are
glioblastomas, astrocytomas, and medulloblastomas. These brain tumours
predominantly manifest at an early age, the majority in the first decade.
Genetic analysis of the families showed that the predisposition to develop
malignancies is inherited by a completely (150, 151) or incompletely (29)
penetrant autosomal dominant gene with pleiotropic effects. Chromosomal
studies on the peripheral blood from family members showed that *increased
numbers of abnormal chromosomes were not consistently seen, although some
members seemed to have more aneuploidy than would be expected* (33).
Histological examination of the tumours by bright field microscopy revealed
*variable occurrences of intranuclear cytoplasmic invaginations, intranuclear
bodies, and acidophilic intracytoplasmic inclusions* (151). Genetic analysis
together with morphological findings suggests that the dominantly inherited
cancer-prone factor interacts with environmental factors (29, 149, 150, 151).
Gamma irradiation studies of cultured fibroblasts of members of a cancer
family demonstrated radioresistance to cell killing. This could be a manifestation of a basic cellular defect predisposing to a variety of tumours
(17) (see also case reports VII.B.2.14, VII.C.1.18, VII.C.2.12).

In general no stigmata of phacomatoses disorders are present in families
with a SBLA syndrome. However, families with characteristics of both the
phacomatosis complex and the SBLA cancer syndrome have been reported
VII.B.1.30, VII.B.2.12, VII.B.2.14).
Chen et al. (42) described a family with brain tumours, leukaemia, hepatomas,
laryngeal cancer and features of the phacomatoses such as café-au-lait spots,
black naevi, haemangiomas and hypoplasia of the corpus callosum.
Li et al. (144) studied a sibship with gliomas associated with leukaemia,
congenital malformations of heart and CNS, and hamartomatous skin lesions.
Chromosome analysis of the peripheral blood of the parents revealed isolated
abnormalities: fragments, breaks and aneuploidy. Elevated nerve-growth-
stimulating activity was found in the mother but she had no clinical signs
of neurofibromatosis. Other laboratory studies could not identify markers
of susceptibility to familial neoplasia.

Apart from the unique aggregation of malignancies in the SBLA cancer syndrome, brain tumours also have been found in association with isolated cancer types belonging to the syndrome complex.

Regelson et al. (212) reported one incidental finding of a cerebellar neuro-astrocytoma among 59 autopsied children with acute lymphoblastic leukaemia. In one series of 62 children with adrenocortical neoplasms Fraumeni and Miller (74) found two cases with associated astrocytomas. One of the children involved also had undescended testes and multiple small pigmented naevi, the other a bifid tip of the tongue and a short frenulum. Two other children had congenital or developmental anomalies of the brain, and two others spina bifida occulta.

Epstein et al. (65) presented a family in which 6 of 15 members over three generations developed 7 malignancies: osteogenic sarcoma appeared in three cases over two generations; in one family member a spongioblastoma multiforme occurred; other associated tumours were: adrenal and colon adenocarcinoma, and a squamous cell carcinoma of the forehead.

B. *Autosomal recessive diseases*

Ataxia telangiectasia

Ataxia telangiectasia or Louis Bar syndrome is a neurological disease of childhood characterized by slowly progressive cerebellar ataxia, chorea-athetosis and telangiectasias of the skin and conjunctivae (240). It is considered to be a phacomatosis as well as an immunodeficiency disease. The immunological defects in this syndrome are deficient cellular immunity, abnormal or absent thymic and lymphoid tissues, and reduced or absent levels of serum IgA (78, 120, 240). There is a marked tendency for development of malignancies, especially lymphoreticular diseases and leukaemias (78, 120, 240). Primary brain tumours are rarely associated with this syndrome, but a medulloblastoma and a cystic glioma have been reported (120, 245, 292). The pattern of inheritance is autosomal recessive (128). Chromosomal breaks and other karyotypic abnormalities are fairly common in lymphocyte cultures of these patients (79).

Glioma-polyposis or Turcot syndrome

In 1959 Turcot described a boy with polyposis of the distal colon and adenocarcinoma of the sygmoid and rectum who died of a medulloblastoma of the spinal cord at the age of 17 years. His sister, who had polyposis of the colon since the age of 13 years, died of a glioblastoma of the left frontal lobe when she was 21 years old. The family history of these siblings did not reveal reports of a similar disease (VII.B.2.6).

This association of polyposis of the colon and gliomas, especially glioblastomas and medulloblastomas, has since then been known as the glioma-
polyposis or Turcot syndrome.

Subsequently two other families with this syndrome were reported by Baughman
et al. (18) and Todd et al. (263). These families are extensively described
in the case reports VII.B.1.24 and VII.B.1.36. In one family four siblings
were affected, in the other three siblings. The histological diagnosis of
the brain tumour was glioblastoma multiforme in six cases, and in one case
an astrocytoma grade III. The medical history of the family reported by
Baughman et al. revealed one additional case of a brain tumour, a posterior
fossa ependymoma in a 3-year-old maternal second-cousin.

Individual cases with this syndrome also have been reported (135, 223).

In all patients affected with this syndrome the gliomas manifest at an
early age, mainly between the ages of 10 and 20 years. As the disease entity
of polyposis of the colon has an autosomal dominant inheritance, the exact
genetic pattern of this rare syndrome remains open to question, but an autosomal recessive mode of inheritance seems probable. The possibility of
environmental effects has not been excluded.

C. *Sex-linked inherited conditions*

Sporadic cases of glioma occurrence have been reported in association
with sex-linked inherited disease.

One case of a cerebellar astrocytoma has been reported in association with
the Wiskott-Aldrich syndrome (5), a primary immunodeficiency disease occurring in childhood in which reticuloendothelial malignancies are frequently
found. It is inherited in a sex-linked recessive pattern.

Blaauw and Schenk (VII.B.1.25) described two haemophiliac brothers, each
dying of a cervical subependymoma. In one case the subependymoma was also
associated with a syringomyelic cavity.

Haemophilia, a haemorrhagic disease due to deficiency of the globulin factor
VIII necessary for thromboplastin formation, is inherited in an X-linked
recessive fashion. The gene has been located on the long arm of the
X-chromosome (183).

D. *Congenital, possibly hereditary, conditions*

A relationship between syringomyelia and tumours of the central nervous
system has been reported by several authors.

Poser (204) reviewed 245 autopsied cases of syringomyelia from the literature and found 40 cases (16.4%) with intramedullary tumours. A review of
209 autopsied cases with intramedullary tumours showed 65 cases (31%)
associated with syringomyelia. He also collected 234 autopsy cases with
both syringomyelia and tumours of the central nervous system. In 32 of
these 234 cases (13.7%) either Von Recklinghausen's disease or Von Hippel-
Lindau's disease was also present.

Sloof et al. (247) studied a series of 33 autopsied cases with intramedullary tumours and found 19 cases with an associated cavity. Among 38 cases
with the clinical diagnosis of syringomyelia 29 cases with an associated
medullary neoplasm were found by Ferry et al. (69). These authors also noted
a relationship between syringomyelia and hereditary tumour-forming syndromes
such as neurofibromatosis and Von Hippel-Lindau's disease. Barnett and
Rewcastle (15) made a secondary diagnosis of syringomyelia in 5 out of 17
cases with intramedullary spinal cord tumours. Among 12 cases with the
primary diagnosis of syringomyelia one had a spinal cord tumour.

The most frequently associated CNS tumours in these studies are ependymomas,
astrocytomas and glioblastomas. They are mainly located in the spinal cord,
but can also occur in other parts of the central nervous system.

The authors of these studies suggest that both syringomyelia and the CNS
tumours result from a single process of developmental disturbance and that
some relationship with the pathogenesis of the phacomatoses must exist.
Familial occurrence of syringomyelia has also been reported, but the inheritance of this disease has not been proven.

De Weerdt and Schut (283) studied the relationship between the occurrence
of brain tumours and spina bifida, a distinct congenital anomaly, and the
relationship between brain tumour occurrence and mongoloid idiocy, but no
correlation was demonstrated between these conditions. The possibility of a
high frequency of CNS tumour occurrence in association with Down's syndrome
has been postulated (173), but not confirmed in later studies (295).

Gold et al. (315), studying risk factors for brain tumour occurrence in
children, reported a significantly increased frequency of epilepsy in
siblings of children with brain tumours as compared to siblings of normal
children. In several cases epilepsy or strokes occurring at relatively
early age were also encountered in the maternal parents of these children.

Congenital glioma occurrence also has been reported. Ohta et al. (190)
collected 36 cases from the literature, nine examples being found in still-
births. The sex distribution of these congenital gliomas was approximately

equal. The commonest types of gliomas were astrocytomas, glioblastomas, and spongioblastomas. The astrocytomas were most frequently located in the cerebellum and brain stem, the glioblastomas principally in the supratentorial space. Among familial cases of gliomas one case of glioblastomatosis occurred in a still-born child; his mother also died of glioblastomatosis at the age of 23 years (VII.C.1.1).

Incidental cases of glioma have also been reported in other inherited conditions such as the Rubinstein-Taybi syndrome, Gaucher's disease, Paget's disease, Fanconi's anaemia, and some others (180).

V. CYTOGENETIC ASPECTS

While chromosome analysis of different neoplastic cell types has been performed, relatively little information concerning gliomas is available in the literature.

Spriggs et al. (253) examined chromosomes in dividing cells from human tumours including one primary malignant glioma of the brain. The histogram showed the majority of cells having hypertriploid or near tetraploid numbers of chromosomes. Lubs and Salmon (148) analysed an oligodendroglioma and a glioblastoma. The cells of the oligodendroglioma demonstrated a tetraploid karyotype; the glioblastoma contained two distinct lines of cells, one line with chromosome numbers in the diploid range and the other in the tetraploid range. Identical acrocentric marker chromosomes were present in both lines, and many instances of breakage and structural rearrangement were found. The glioblastoma, however, had been irradiated 14 months prior to examination.

Bicknell (24) studied 21 human brain tumours but *satisfactory cells* were seen in only three cases. Cells from an ependymoma had chromosome numbers varying from 56 to 90. Many extra chromosomes were seen in group C, and less frequently in the smaller groups D through G. Infrequent excess or deficiencies of chromosomes in groups A or B, and occasionally abnormal chromosomes or fragments were seen. The chromosome numbers of a glioblastoma multiforme clustered mainly just above and below normal. The third tumour was an astrocytoma grade III. Chromosome numbers in this neoplasm fell into several clusters, one near the normal value, one near twice normal, and a few near 4 to 6 times normal. Extra chromosomes were most often present in the C group (6 - 12). All three patients were exposed to diagnostic irradiation before tissue samples were obtained. From a review of the literature the author concluded that in every reported case of central nervous system neoplasm chromosomal abnormalities have been found, but that no specific number of chromosomes, pattern of chromosome excess or deficiency, or abnormal extra chromosomes common to the tumour type have been demonstrated. He stressed further that clinical artifacts and effects of exposure to radiation must be kept in mind in evaluating studies of tumour chromosomes.

Wilson et al. (288) studied 11 glioblastomas. Satisfactory cells for chromosome analysis were obtained from three as fresh tumour tissue, and from the other eight after short periods in cell culture. The predominant pattern was a near-diploid karyotype with most frequent deviations occurring in group 6 - 12. Comparing previous reports with their results the authors concluded that: 1. glioblastomas often contain cells with diploid and hypodiploid karyotypes, some tumours also containing additional clusters of near-tetraploid cells; 2. chromosomes in group 6 - 12 (C group) are most likely to deviate from the normal diploid karyotype; 3. glioblastomas may contain marker chromosomes that are usually large submetacentrics or acrocentrics.

In a case of glioblastoma evaluated by Manuelidis (322), the majority of cells showed a range of 70 - 90 chromosomes per cell. Cytogenetic investigations of tissue cultures from human glioblastomas transplanted to the eye and brain of guinea-pigs were also undertaken. The histological characteristics of the tumours in both transplantation sites were identical, but chromosomal counts showed different patterns: culture lines arising from the brain had a peak around the hypertriploid range while those from the eye revealed two distinct cellular populations, one in the triploid and the other in the hexaploid range. An analysis of the chromosomal representation of seven astrocytic glioma cell lines in four studies by Mark et al. (160, 161, 162, 163) revealed an increased proportion of chromosomes nrs 7 and 19, and a reduction of chromosomes nrs 4 and 22 and most likely also nrs 10 and 12. Three different types of markers were observed: 12q-, 13q- and 14q-. The numeral and structural observations in the glioma cell lines were interpreted as indicating the existence of several different karyotypic patterns in this type of neoplasm. The similarities between different cell lines were assumed to be related to their origin from the same tissue type rather than to other factors, as for example oncogenic agents.

The genotypic and phenotypic characteristics of these cell lines, completed with a number of new permanent cell lines derived from human gliomas, were studied by Bigner et al. (26). They found that while many common properties of the different lines were present, each line had a unique profile for the evaluated parameters. This genotypic and phenotypic diversity and individuality of the cell lines was their most striking finding. According to the authors *this heterogeneity most likely reflects the individuality of the tumors of origin and individual genotypes and capacity for a range of phenotypic expression of the cells.*

Karyotypic analysis of a human malignant glioma cell line performed by Diserens et al. (57) showed a chromosome number ranging from 70 to 80 with a modal number of 78 XXYY, and the constant finding of three marker chromosomes; one large acrocentric chromosome of unspecified origin, and two 9p- markers.

The chromosomal pattern in one case of familial glioma has been examined by Koch and Waldbaur (132). They reported a father and son with astrocytomas; the son had a normal karyotype of 46 XY, but the cell line was not reported.

It seems from the literature that a diversity of chromosomal abnormalities may be found in glioma cells. Some authors report glioma cells to contain a number of chromosomes near the diploid range, others near the hypertriploid-tetraploid range and still others near both. The deviations in number are most often found in the C group of chromosomes, nrs 6 to 12. Abnormal (marker) chromosomes may be present in glioma cells and are reported in various degrees and numbers.

A major problem lies in the interpretation of these chromosomal abnormalities. It is uncertain whether these chromosomal disorders are the cause or the result of tumour growth (see also familial aspects of medulloblastoma).

S U M M A R Y

I. TWIN STUDIES

1. Four reports on monozygotic twins with concordant glioma are available in the literature.
2. Dizygotic twins with concordant glioma have not been reported.
3. The histological type of glioma and age at manifestation are similar in the separate twin-pairs.
4. Studies on twin population indicate that genetic factors have little influence on the genesis of gliomas in twins.

II. FAMILIAL OCCURRENCE IN SIBLINGS

5. Thirty-two reports on two siblings with histologically verified glioma, three (possibly six) reports on three affected siblings and one report on four affected siblings are available.
6. The risk of occurrence of gliomas in two siblings on the basis of chance alone varies from 0.8×10^{-5} in a sibship of two to 36×10^{-5} in a sibship of ten; the chance of occurrence in three out of three siblings being 0.0048×10^{-5} and for three out of ten siblings 0.57×10^{-5}.
7. The ratio of reported cases on occurrence in three siblings as compared to occurrence in two siblings is approximately 9 times greater than expected on a chance basis.
8. Males are more often affected than females: 63.75 to 36.25%.
9. The gender of affected siblings within a family was the same in 71.4% of the reports on two siblings.
10. The distribution of histological types of glioma is approximately the same in familial cases as in isolated cases, glioblastomas and (high grade) astrocytomas occurring in 83.6% of the cases.
11. The histological nature of the gliomas occurring in affected siblings within one family was identical in 85.7% of the cases.
12. The most frequent locations of gliomas in familial cases were the temporal and frontal regions, and less frequently the parieto-occipital region.
13. The tumours were most frequently situated deeply within the brain.
14. The mean age at symptom occurrence in siblings is approximately the same as in isolated cases.
15. Studies of siblings show an increased number of familial occurrences of glioma than would be expected on a chance basis.

16. The association of glioma with other malignancies, especially leukaemia, and cancer of the bone and muscle, is higher than expected.

III. FAMILIAL OCCURRENCE IN GENERATIONS

17. Twenty-one reports of verified gliomas in two generations, and two reports in three generations are available.
18. Two relatives were affected in 17 reports, in four reports three relatives were affected, in one report six relatives (five cases verified), and in one report seven relatives (five cases verified).
19. Mother-child(ren) and father-child(ren) glioma occurrence were approximately equal in number.
20. Glioblastomas and (high grade) astrocytomas were the most frequently encountered glioma types: 92.2%.
21. The tumours occur predominantly in the frontal and temporal regions and are frequently located deeply within the brain.
22. The mean age at occurrence in children (second generation) was lower than in the parent group: 27.1 years as compared to 47.4 years.
23. The mean age of familial glioma occurrence in the second generation is lower than that found in isolated cases.
24. One familial occurrence of glioblastoma is reported in a premature, still-born child.
25. Blood-group A Rhesus positive was the most frequently encountered blood-type in the examined cases.
26. Cancer of the stomach was the most frequent malignancy noted among members of the reported families with glioma occurrence in siblings and different generations (12 occurrences).
27. Sixteen occurrences of deaths of unknown cause occurring at an early age were noted among the close relatives of the reported familial cases of glioma in siblings and other generations.
28. In studies of relatives of glioma patients familial occurrence of glioma is reported in 1 to 14.3% of cases in different series, with a mean of 7.9%. This occurrence is more frequent than would be expected on a chance basis.

IV. ASSOCIATED INHERITED CONDITIONS

29. Gliomas frequently occur in neurofibromatosis and tuberous sclerosis, both phacomatoses and autosomal dominantly inherited diseases.

30. A positive correlation has been found between the presence of dysraphic features and glioma occurrence.
31. Gliomas occur in the SBLA cancer syndrome, a family cancer syndrome with a dominant pattern of inheritance.
32. Families with characteristics of both the SBLA cancer syndrome and the phacomatoses have been reported.
33. Glioblastomas occur in association with polyposis of the colon, the glioma-polyposis or Turcot syndrome, a disease with a probably autosomal recessive pattern of inheritance.
34. Glioblastomas in the Turcot syndrome manifest at an early age, mainly in the second life decade.
35. The association of glioma and syringomyelia has been demonstrated.
36. An increased frequency of epilepsy in siblings of children with brain tumours has been found.
37. Congenital glioma occurrence has been reported, the commonest types being astrocytomas, glioblastomas, and spongioblastomas.

V. CYTOGENETIC STUDIES

38. A variety of chromosomal abnormalities have been reported in glioma cells.
39. Deviation of chromosomal numbers are especially found in the C group (nrs 6 - 12).
40. Various degrees and numbers of marker chromosomes may be present in glioma cells.

Schimke (232) states that *present information would suggest that not more than 5 percent of CNS tumours are genetic but when inherited, may well be transmitted as an autosomal dominant trait, although again polygenic inheritance cannot be excluded.* Our data indeed suggest that genetic factors have an influence on the genesis of certain types of gliomas. This influence finds its expression in the group of glioblastomas and (high grade) astrocytomas, with a preferential site of occurrence in the frontal and temporal regions. Familial glioma occurrence also appears associated with a number of known inherited conditions.
In order to better determine the role of genetic factors in glioma development the collection of case material is needed. Examination and description of cases and the study of family members is essential to the search for possibly associated disorders. Studies on cytogenetic aspects of familial occurrences are urgently required.

REFERENCES

1. ACKER REH van   1977
    Gliomas: New ways of treatment?
    Clin Neurol Neurosurg 80:112-115
2. AIRD RB   1963
    Treatment of brain tumors.
    Med Clin North Am 47:1675-1689
3. AITA JA   1967
    In: Lynch HT (ed) Hereditary factors in carcinoma.
    Recent Results Cancer Res 12:86-95
4. AITA JA   1968
    Genetic aspects of tumors of the nervous system.
    Nebraska Med J 53:121-124
5. AMIET A von   1963
    Aldrich's syndrome: a report of two cases.
    Ann Paediat 201:315
6. ANDERSON M, HUGHES B, JEFFERSON M, SMITH WT, WATERHOUSE JAH   1980
    Gliomatous transformation and demyelinating disease.
    Brain 103:603-622
7. ANNEGERS JF, SCHOENBERG BS, OKAZAKI H, KURLAND LT   1981
    Epidemiologic study of primary intracranial neoplasms.
    Arch Neurol 38:217-219
8. APUZZO ML, MITCHELL MS   1981
    Immunological aspects of intrinsic glial tumors. Review article.
    J Neurosurg 55:1-18
9. ARENDT A   1975
    Ependymomas.
    In: Vinken PJ, Bruyn GW (eds) Handbook of Clinical Neurology.
    North-Holland Publ Co, Amsterdam vol 18:105-150
10. ARMSTRONG RM, HANSON CW   1969
    Familial gliomas 1969
    Neurology 19:1061-1063
11. BAILEY P   1924
    A study of tumors arising from ependymal cells.
    Arch Neurol 11:1-27
12. BAILEY P, BUCY PC   1929
    Oligodendrogliomas of the brain.
    J Pathol Bacteriol 32:735-751
13. BAILEY P, CUSHING H   1926
    A classification of the tumors of the glioma group on a histogenetic
    basis with a correlated study of prognosis.
    Lippincott, Philadelphia.
14. BARNARD RO   1968
    The development of malignancy in oligodendrogliomas.
    J Pathol Bacteriol 96:113-123

446

15. BARNETT HJM, REWCASTLE NB 1973
    In: Barnett HJM, Foster JB, Hudgson P (eds)
    Syringomyelia.
    WB Saunders Co, London p 261-301
16. BARONE BM, ELVIDGE AR 1970
    Ependymomas. A clinical survey.
    J Neurosurg 33:428-438
17. BATZDORF U, MALAMUD N 1963
    The problem of multicentric gliomas.
    J Neurosurg 20:122-136
18. BAUGHMAN Jr FA, LIST CF, WILLIAMS JR, MULDOON JP, SEGARRA JM,
    VOLKEL JS 1969
    The glioma-polyposis syndrome.
    N Engl J Med 281:1345-1346
19. BECH-HANSEN NT, BLATTNER WA, SELL BM, McKEEN EA, LAMPKIN BC,
    FRAUMENI Jr JF, PATERSON MC 1981
    Transmission of in-vitro radioresistance in a cancer-prone family.
    Lancet I:1335-1337
20. BEHREND RC 1974
    Epidemiology of brain tumours.
    In: Vinken PJ, Bruyn GW (eds) Handbook of Clinical Neurology.
    North-Holland Publ Co, Amsterdam vol 16:56-88
21. BENDER W, PANSE F 1932
    Familiäres Gliom. (Zur Genetik der Gliome).
    Monatsschr Psychiatr Neurol 83:253-285
22. BESOLD G 1896
    Ueber zwei Fälle von Gehirntumor (Hämangiosarkom oder sogenanntes
    Peritheliom in der Gegend des dritten Ventrikels) bei zwei
    Geschwistern.
    Dtsch Z Nervenheilk 8:49-74
23. BEST PV 1963
    Intracranial oligodendrogliomatosis.
    J Neurol Neurosurg Psychiatry 26:249-256
24. BICKNELL JM 1967
    Chromosome studies of human brain tumors.
    Neurology 17:485-490
25. BIELSCHOWSKY M 1919
    Entwurf eines Systems der Heredodegerationen des Zentralnerven-
    systems einschliesslich der zugehörigen Striatumerkrankungen.
    J Psychol Neurol (Lpz) 24:48
26. BIGNER DD, BIGNER SH, PONTÉN J, WESTERMARK B, MAHALEY MS, RUOSLAHTI E,
    HERSCHMAN H, ENG LF, WIKSTRAND CJ 1981
    Heterogeneity of genotypic and phenotypic characteristics of fifteen
    permament cell lines derived from human gliomas.
    J Neuropathol Exp Neurol 40:201-229
27. BLAAUW G, SCHENK VWD 1971
    Cervical cord tumor in two haemophilic brothers.
    J Neurol Sci 14:409-416
28. BLAIN JG, GUAY JP, DEROME G 1980
    L'astrocytome malin: évaluation.
    Union Med Can 109:97-102
29. BLATTNER WA, McGUIRE DB, MULVIHILL JJ, LAMPKIN BC, HANANIAN J,
    FRAUMENI Jr JF 1979
    Genealogy of cancer in a family.
    JAMA 241:259-261

30. BLICKENSTORFER E 1951
Sieben Fälle operierter Okzipitalhirntumoren unter besonderer
Berücksichtigung der psychischen Symptomatologie und deren Zusam-
menhänge mit der Familienkonstitution.
Wien Z Nervenheilk 4:94-119

31. BLOOM HJG, PECKHAM MJ, RICHARDSON AE 1973
Glioblastoma multiforme. A controlled trial to assess the value of
specific active immunotherapy and radiotherapy.
Br J Cancer 27:253-267

32. BÖHMIG KH 1918
Gehirntumor bei zwei Geschwistern.
Arch Psychiat Nervenkr 59:527-533

33. BOTTOMLEY RH, TRAINER AL, CONDIT PT 1971
Chromosome studies in a "cancer family".
Cancer 28:519-528

34. BROMOWICZ J, ARASZKIEWICZ H, KINDERMAN B 1971
Familial occurrence of neoplasms of the central nervous system.
Neurol Neurochir Pol 5:721-725

35. BROOKS WH 1972
Geographic clustering of brain tumors in Kentucky.
Cancer 30:923-926

36. BROOKS WH, CALDWELL HD, MORTARA RH 1974
Immune responses in patients with gliomas.
Surg Neurol 2:419-423

37. BROOKS WH, LATTA RB, MAHALEY MS, ROSZMAN TL, DUDKA L, SKAGGS C 1981
Immunobiology of primary intracranial tumors. Part 5: Correlation of
a lymphocyte index and clinical status.
J Neurosurg 54:331-337

38. BROOKS WH, NETSKY MG, NORMANSELL DE, HORWITZ DA 1972
Depressed cell-mediated immunity in patients with primary intracranial tumors. Characterization of a humoral immuno-suppressive factor.
J Exp Med 136:1631-1647

39. BROOKS WH, ROSZMAN TL, MAHALEY MS, WOOSLEY RE 1977
Immunobiology of primary intracranial tumours. II: Analysis of
lymphocyte subpopulations in patients with primary brain tumours.
Clin Exp Immunol 29:61-66

40. CANALE DJ, BEBIN J 1972
Von Recklinghausen disease of the nervous system.
In: Vinken PJ, Bruyn GW (eds) Handbook of Clinical Neurology.
North-Holland Publ Co, Amsterdam vol 14:132-162

41. CASENTINI L, GULLOTTA F, MÖHRER U 1981
Clinical and morphological investigations on ependymomas and their
tissue cultures.
Neurochirurgia 24:51-56

42. CHEN KM, BRODY JA, KURLAND LT, ELIZAN TS 1970
Clinical and genetic patterns of neurological diseases other than
amyotrophic lateral sclerosis on Guam.
Neurology 20:954-964

43. CHIN HW, HAZEL JJ, KIM TH, WEBSTER JH 1980
Oligodendrogliomas. I: A clinical study of cerebral oligo-
dendrogliomas.
Cancer 45:1458-1466

44. CHOI NW, SCHUMAN LM, GULLEN WH 1968
    Epidemiology of central nervous system neoplasms: a case-control study.
    Neurology 18:306
45. CHOI NW, SCHUMAN LM, GULLEN WH 1970
    Epidemiology of primary central nervous system neoplasms. II: Case-control study.
    Am J Epidemiol 91:467-485
46. CLARENBACH P, KLEIHUES P, METZEL E, DICHGANS J 1979
    Simultaneous clinical manifestation of subependymoma of the fourth ventricle in identical twins.
    J Neurosurg 50:655-659
47. CLIFTON MD, AMROMIN GD, PERRY MC, ABADIR R, WATTS C, LEVY N 1980
    Spinal cord glioma following irradiation for Hodgkin's disease.
    Cancer 45:2051-2055
48. COHEN MS, KUSHNER MJ, DELL S 1981
    Frontal lobe astrocytoma following radiotherapy for medulloblastoma.
    Neurology 31:616-619
49. COHNHEIM J 1878
    Vorlesungen über allgemeine Pathologie.
    Berlin (cited by Zülch 1956 and 1974, and Kemper 1964)
50. COLAFRANCESCHI M, MENNONNA P 1970
    Gliomi ad insorgenza familiare. Osservazione in due fratelli.
    Arch de Vecchi Anat Patol 56:568-579
51. COURVILLE CB 1936
    Multiple primary tumours of the brain. Review of the literature and report of twenty-one cases.
    Am J Cancer 26:703-731
52. CRAIG WMck, WAGENER HP, KERNOHAN JW 1941
    Lindau-von Hippel disease: a report of four cases.
    Arch Neurol Psychiat 46:36-58
53. CURTIUS F 1957
    Altes und Neues zum Status dysraphicus.
    Nervenarzt 28:185-188
54. CUSHING H 1932
    Intracranial tumours.
    Charles C Thomas, Springfield, Ill
55. DASTUR DK, LALITHA VS 1969
    Pathological analysis of intracranial space-occupying lesions in 1000 cases including children.
    Part 2: Incidence, types and unusual cases of glioma.
    J Neurol Sci 8:143-170
56. DEGENHARDT KH 1964
    Missbildungen des Rückenmarks.
    In: Becker PE (ed) Humangenetik
    Thieme, Stuttgart vol 2:533
57. DISERENS AC, TRIBOLET N de, MARTIN-ACHARD A, GAIDE AC, SCHNEGG JF, CARREL S 1981
    Characterization of an established human malignant glioma cell line: LN-18.
    Acta Neuropathol (Berl) 53:21-28
58. DOHRMANN GJ, FARWELL JR, FLANNERY JR 1976
    Ependymomas and ependymoblastomas in children.
    J Neurosurg 45:273-283

59. DONEGANI G, GRATTAROLA FR, WILDI E 1972
    Tuberous sclerosis.
    In: Vinken PJ, Bruyn GW (eds) Handbook of Clinical Neurology.
    North-Holland Publ Co, Amsterdam vol 14:340-390
60. DRUCKREY H, IVANKOVIC S, PREUSSMANN R 1965
    Selektive Erzeugung maligner Tumoren im Gehirn und Rückenmark von
    Ratten durch N-Methyl-N-nitrosoharnstoff.
    Z Krebsforsch 66:389-408
61. DRUCKREY H, PREUSSMANN R, IVANKOVIĆ S, SCHMÄHL D 1967
    unter Mitarbeit von AFKHAM J, BLUM G, MENNEL HD, MÜLLER M,
    PETROPOULOS P, SCHNEIDER H
    Organotrope carcinogene Wirkungen bei 65 verschiedenen N-Nitroso-
    Verbindungen an BD-Ratten.
    Z Krebforsch 69:103-201
62. DUFFELL D, HINZ R, NELSON E 1964
    Neoplasms in hamsters induced by Simian virus 40.
    Am J Pathol 45:59-73
63. DUINEN MTA van 1976
    The ependymoma of the cauda equina.
    Thesis, Utrecht, The Netherlands
64. EARNEST III F, KERNOHAN JW, CRAIG WM 1950
    Oligodendrogliomas. A review of two hundred cases.
    Arch Neurol Psychiatry 63:964-976
65. EPSTEIN LI, BIXLER D, BENNETT JE 1970
    An incident of familial cancer. Including 3 cases of osteogenic
    sarcoma.
    Cancer 25:889-891
66. FAIRBURN B, URICH H 1971
    Malignant gliomas occurring in identical twins.
    J Neurol Neurosurg Psychiatry 34:718-722
67. FARWELL JR, DOHRMANN GJ, MARRETT LD, MEIGS JW 1979
    Effect of SV40 virus-contaminated polio vaccine on the incidence and
    type of CNS neoplasma in children: A population-based study.
    Trans Am Neurol Assoc 104:261-264
68. FEIRING EH, DAVIDOFF LM 1947
    Two tumors, meningioma and glioblastoma multiforme, in one patient.
    J Neurosurg 4:282-289
69. FERRY DJ, HARDMAN HM, EARLE KM 1969
    Syringomyelia and intramedullary neoplasms.
    Med Ann D C 38:363-365
70. FINKEMEYER H, PFINGST E, ZÜLCH KJ 1975
    The astrocytomas of the cerebral hemispheres.
    In: Vinken PJ, Bruyn GW (eds) Handbook of Clinical Neurology.
    North-Holland Publ Co, Amsterdam vol 18:1-49
71. FISCHER-WASELS B 1938
    Die Erblichkeit in der Geschwülstentwicklung.
    Fortschr Erbpathol 2:221-261
72. FOKES Jr EC, EARLE KM 1969
    Ependymomas: clinical and pathological aspects.
    J Neurosurg 30:585-594
73. FRANKEL SA, GERMAN WJ 1958
    Glioblastoma multiforme. Review of 219 cases with regard to natural
    history, pathology, diagnostic methods and treatment.
    J Neurosurg 15:489-503

74. FRAUMENI Jr JF, MILLER RW 1967
    Adrenocortical neoplasms with hemihypertrophy, brain tumors, and
    other disorders.
    J Pediatr 70:129-138
75. GARCIA JH, OKAZAKI H, ARONSON SM 1963
    Blood-group frequencies and astrocytomata.
    J Neurosurg 20:397-399
76. GARSON JA, QUINDLEN EA, KORNBLITH PL 1981
    Complement fixation by ig M and ig G autoantibodies on cultured
    human glial cells.
    J Neurosurg 35:19-26
77. GASS H, WAGENEN WP van 1950
    Meningioma and oligodendroglioma adjacent in the brain.
    J Neurosurg 7:440-443
78. GATTI RA, GOOD RA 1971
    Occurrence of malignancy in immunodeficiency diseases. A literature
    review.
    Cancer 28:89-98
79. GERMAN J 1972
    Genes which increase chromosomal instability in somatic cells and
    predispose to cancer.
    Prog Med Genet 8:61-101
80. GEROSA M, RAUMER R, AMADORI G, SEMENZATO G, GASPAROTTO G, CARTERI A,
    1979
    Immunobiology of primary neoplasms of the CNS. Preliminary results.
    J Neurosurg Sci 23:165-175
81. GEYER H, PEDERSEN O 1939
    Zur Erblichkeit der Neubildungen des Zentralnervensystems und seiner
    Hüllen.
    Z ges Neurol Psychiatr 165:284-294
82. GLASAUER FE, YUAN RHP 1963
    Intracranial tumors with extracranial metastases.
    J Neurosurg 20:474-493
83. GLAUBERMAN LM 1936
    Neurologia i genetika 1:361 (cited by Manuelidis 1972)
84. GORLIN RJ, SEDANO HO 1972
    Multiple nevoid basal cell carcinoma syndrome.
    In: Vinken PJ, Bruyn GW (eds) Handbook of Clinical Neurology.
    North-Holland Publ Co, Amsterdam vol 14:455-473
85. GROSS SW, COHEN R, PANICHAVANTANA S 1969
    Cerebellar glioblastomas.
    J Mt Sinai Hosp NY 36:123-129
86. GROSZ K, PLASCHKES SJ 1960
    The occurrence of cerebral tumors in a brother and sister.
    Isr Med J 19:302-305
87. HALLERVORDEN J 1936
    Erbliche Hirntumoren.
    Nervenarzt 9:1-8
88. HALPERN L 1943
    Harefuah 25(3):43 (cited by Peyser and Beller 1951 and Manuelidis
    1972)
89. HARVALD B, HAUGE M 1956
    On the heredity of glioblastoma.
    J Natl Cancer Inst 17:289-296

90. HASS WK 1966
    Soluble tissue antigens in human brain tumor and cerebrospinal
    fluid.
    Arch Neurol 14:443-447
91. HAUGE M, HARVALD B 1957
    Genetics in intracranial tumours.
    Acta Genet 7: 573-591
92. HAUGE M, HARVALD B 1960
    Studies in the etiology of intracranial tumours.
    Acta Psychiatr Neurol Scand 35:163-170
93. HAWKINS III JC, HOFFMAN HJ, BECKER LE 1979
    Multiple nevoid basal-cell carcinoma syndrome (Gorlin's syndrome):
    Possible confusion with metastatic medulloblastoma. Case report.
    J Neurosurg 50:100-102
94. HAYMAKER W, RUBINSTEIN LJ, MIQUEL J 1972
    Brain tumors in irradiated monkeys.
    Acta Neuropathol (Berl) 20:267-277
95. HEINONEN OP, SHAPIRO S, MOUSON RR, HARTZ SC, ROSENBERG L, SLONE D 1973
    Immunization during pregnancy against poliomyelitis and influenza in
    relation to childhood malignancy.
    Int J Epidemiol 2:229-235
96. HENSCHEN F 1955
    Tumoren des Zentralnervensysteems und seiner Hüllen.
    In: Lubarsch, Henke, Rössle (eds) Handbuch der speziellen patholo-
    gischen Anatomie und Histologie. Bd 13 Nervensyst 3 Teil.
    Springer, Berlin p 413 (cited by Kemper 1964)
97. HESHMAT MY, KOVI J, SIMPSON C, KENNEDY J, FAN KJ 1976
    Neoplasms of the central nervous system. Incidence and population
    selectivity in the Washington DC, Metropolitan area.
    Cancer 38:2135-2142
98. HOCHBERG FH, LINGGOOD R, WOLFSON L, BAKER WH, KORNBLITH P 1979
    Quality and duration of survival in glioblastoma multiforme. Com-
    bined surgical, radiation, and lomustine therapy.
    JAMA 241:1016-1018
99. HOCHBERG FH, PRUITT A 1980
    Assumptions in the radiotherapy of glioblastoma.
    Neurology 30:907-911
100. HOEVE J van der 1923
    Eye diseases in tuberous sclerosis of the brain and in
    Recklinghausen disease.
    Trans Ophthalmol Soc U K 43:534-540
101. HOEVE J van der 1933
    Les phacomatoses de Bourneville, de Recklinghausen et de von
    Hippel-Lindau.
    J Belge Neurol Psychiat 33:752-762
102. HOFFMANN H 1919
    Gehirntumoren bei zwei Geschwistern. Ein Beitrag zur Vererbung der
    Geschwülste.
    Z Ges Neurol Psychiatr 51:113-123
103. HOPE DG, MULVIHILL JJ 1981
    Malignancy in neurofibromatosis.
    Adv Neurol 29:33-56

104. HOPPE HJ 1952
    Diskordantes Auftreten von Hirntumoren bei erbgleichen Zwillingen.
    Zentralbl Neurochir 12:34-36
105. HORRAX G, WU WQ 1951
    Postoperative survival of patients with intracranial oligo-
    dendroglioma with special reference to radical tumor removal. A
    study of 26 patients.
    J Neurosurg 8:473-479
106. HORTON WA 1976
    Genetics of central nervous system tumors.
    Birth Defects XII:91-97
107. HOSHINO T, TOWNSEND JJ, MURAOKA I, WILSON CB 1980
    An autoradiographic study of human gliomas: growth kinetics of
    anaplastic astrocytoma and glioblastoma multiforme.
    Brain 103:967-984
108. HUTCHISON GB 1976
    Late neoplastic changes following medical irradiation.
    Cancer 37:1102-1107
109. ISAMAT F, MIRANDA AM, BARTUMEUS F, PRAT J 1974
    Genetic implications of familial brain tumors.
    J Neurosurg 41:573-575
110. JANISCH W, SCHREIBER D 1975
    Experimental brain tumours.
    In: Vinken PJ, Bruyn GW (eds) Handbook of Clinical Neurology
    North-Holland Publ Co, Amsterdam vol 18:1-41
111. JELLINGER K 1978
    Glioblastoma multiforme: morphology and biology.
    Acta Neurochir 42:5-32
112. JOUGHIN JL 1928
    Coincident tumor of the brain in twins.
    Arch Neurol Psychiatry 19:948-950
113. KANTER WR, ELDRIDGE R, FABRICANT R, ALLEN JC, KOERBER T 1980
    Central neurofibromatosis with bilateral acoustic neuroma. Genetic,
    clinical and biochemical distinctions from peripheral neurofibroma-
    tosis.
    Neurology 30:851-859
114. KAPP J 1975
    Brain tumours with tuberous sclerosis.
    In: Vinken PJ, Bruyn GW (eds) Handbook of Clinical Neurology.
    North-Holland Publ Co, Amsterdam vol 18:299-303
115. KATSURA S, SUZUKI J, WADA T 1959
    A statistical study of brain tumours in the neurosurgical clinics of
    Japan.
    J Neurosurg 16:570-580
116. KAUFMAN HH, BRISMAN R 1972
    Familial gliomas. Report of four cases.
    J Neurosurg 37:110-112
117. KEMPER K 1964
    Vorkommen von Hirntumoren bei Zwillingen und in Familien.
    Thesis, Münster, Germany
118. KERNOHAN JW, MABON RF, SVIEN HJ, ADSON AW 1949
    A simplified classification of the gliomas.
    Proc Mayo Clin 24:71-75

119. KERNOHAN JW, SAYRE GP 1952
     Tumors of the central nervous system.
     In: Atlas of Tumor Pathology, Fasc 35.
     Armed Forces Inst of Pathol, Washington DC
120. KERSEY JH, SPECTOR BD, GOOD RA 1973
     Primary immunodeficiency diseases and cancer: the immunodeficiency-
     cancer registry.
     Int J Cancer 12:333-347
121. KEUTER EJW 1960
     Predisposition to postvaccinal encephalitis.
     Thesis, Elsevier, Amsterdam
122. KING AB, EISINGER G 1966
     May glioma multiforme be hereditary?
     Guthrie Clin Bull 35:169-175
123. KJELLIN K, MÜLLER R, ASTRÖM KE 1960
     The occurrence of brain tumors in several members of a family.
     J Neuropathol Exp Neurol 19:528-537
124. KO L, KNOESTER A, WECHSLER W 1980
     Morphological characterization of nitrosurea-induced glioma cell
     lines and clones.
     Acta Neuropathol (Berl) 51:23-31
125. KOBAYASHI N, ALLEN N, CLENDENON NR, KO LW 1980
     An improved rat brain-tumor model.
     J Neurosurg 53:808-815
126. KOCH G 1949
     Erbliche Hirngeschwülste.
     Z menschl Vererb Konstitutionslehre 29:400-423
127. KOCH G 1954
     Beitrag zur Erblichkeit der Hirngeschwülste (vorläufige Mitteilung).
     Acta Genet Med Gemellol 3:170-191
128. KOCH G 1972
     Genetic aspects of the phakomatoses.
     In: Vinken PJ, Bruyn GW (eds) Handbook of Clinical Neurology.
     North-Holland Publ Co, Amsterdam vol 14:488-561
129. KOCH G 1981
     Results of the 40-year, longitudinal study of a series of twins of
     Berlin (450 monozygotic and dizygotic twin pairs).
     In: Advances in twin research, Vol III. Proceedings Third Inter-
     national Congress on Twin Studies, Jerusalem 16-20 June 1980
     Alan R Liss Inc New York
130. KOCH G, KRISCHEK J, TIWISINA T 1957
     Beitrag zur Klinik, Pathogenese und Erbpathologie dysontogenetischer
     (dysraphischer) Störungen des Zentralnervensystems (Septum
     pellucidum-Cysten, Hirntumor) bei eineiigen Zwillingen.
     Z menschl Vererb Konstitutionslehre 34:105-123
131. KOCH G, MIDDENDORF E 1960
     Vorkommen von Glioblastoma multiforme bei 3 Schwestern im Alter von
     50 bis 54 Jahren (neuere Betrachtungen zur Ätiologie dyson-
     togenetischer Geschwülste).
     Med Welt (Stuttg) II(48):2541-2544.
132. KOCH G, WALDBAUR H 1981
     Erbliche Hirngeschwülste. (Brain tumour family syndrome)
     Z Allg Med 57:1219-1224

133. KORNBLITH PL, DOHAN Jr C, WOOD WC, WHITMAN BO 1974
Human astrocytoma: serum-mediated immunologic response.
Cancer 33:1512-1519
134. KRETSCHMER H 1974
Die extrakranielle Metastasierung intrakranieller Geschwülste.
Zentralbl Neurochir 35:81-112
135. KROKOWICZ P 1979
The Turcot syndrome.
Acta Clin Scand 145:113-115
136. KRUEGER E, KRUPP G 1952
Oligodendroglioma arising from structures of the posterior fossa.
Neurology 2:461
137. KUHNEN B 1953
Beobachtungen an sieben Zwillingspaaren mit Hirntumoren.
Acta Genet Med Gemellol 2:407-430
138. KUMAR S, TAYLOR G 1973
Specific lymphocytotoxicity and blocking factors in tumors of the
central nervous system.
Br J Cancer 28:135-141
139. KURLAND LT, MYRIANTHOPOULOS NC, LESSELL S 1962
Epidemiologic and genetic considerations of intracranial neoplasms.
In: Field WS, Sharkey PC (eds) The biology and treatment of
intracranial tumors.
Charles C Thomas, Springfield, Ill p 5-48
140. LAGOS JC, GOMEZ MR 1967
Tuberous sclerosis: reappraisal of a clinical entity.
Proc Mayo Clin 42:26-49
141. LEVY HL, MAHALEY SM, DAY ED 1972
In vitro demonstration of cell-mediated immunity in human brain
tumors.
Cancer Res 32:477-482
142. LI FP, FRAUMENI Jr JF 1969
Rhabdomyosarcoma in children: epidemiologic study and identification
of a familial cancer syndrome.
J Natl Cancer Inst 43:1365-1373
143. LI FP, FRAUMENI Jr JF 1969
Soft-tissue sarcomas, breast cancer, and other neoplasms. A familial
syndrome?
Ann Intern Med 71:747-752
144. LI FP, McINTOSCH S, PENG-WHANG J 1977
Double primary cancers in 2 young sibs, leukemia in another, and
dextrocardia in a fourth.
Cancer 39:2633-2636
145. LI FP, TUCKER MA, FRAUMENI Jr JF 1976
Childhood cancer in sibs.
J Pediatr 88:419-423
146. LIEBALDT GP, LEIBER B 1972
Cutaneous dysplasias associated with neurological disorders.
In: Vinken PJ, Bruyn GW (eds) Handbook of Clinical Neurology
North-Holland Publ Co, Amsterdam vol 14:110-111
147. LOTT IT, RICHARDSON EP 1981
Neuropathological findings and the biology of neurofibromatosis.
Adv Neurol 29:23-32

148. LUBS Jr HA, SALMON JH 1965
     The chromosomal complement of human solid tumors. II. Karyotypes of
     glial tumors.
     J Neurol 22:160-168
149. LYNCH HT 1981
     SBLA syndrome.
     In: Vinken PJ, BRUYN GE (eds) Handbook of Clinical Neurology.
     North-Holland Publ Co, Amsterdam vol 42:769-771
150. LYNCH HT, GUIRGIS HA, LYNCH PM, LYNCH JF, HARRIS RE 1977
     Familial cancer syndromes. A survey.
     Cancer 39:1867-1881
151. LYNCH HT, MULCAHY GM, HARRIS RE, GUIRGIS HA, LYNCH JF 1978
     Genetic and pathologic findings in a kindred with hereditary sarcoma
     breast cancer, brain tumors, leukemia, lung, laryngeal, and adrenal
     cortical carcinoma.
     Cancer 41:2055-2064
152. MACCABE JJ 1975
     Glioblastoma.
     In: Vinken PJ, Bruyn GW (eds) Handbook of Clinical Neurology.
     North-Holland Publ Co, Amsterdam vol 18:49-72
153. MacKAY MCJ 1952
     Tumor cerebri en ontwikkelingsstoornissen. Onderzoekingen en medede-
     lingen
     Inst Praev Geneesk Leiden
154. MacPHERSON 1976
     Association between previous tuberculous infection and glioma.
     Br Med J 2:1112
155. MAHALEY Jr MS, BROOKS WH, ROSZMAN TL, BIGNER DD, DUDKA L, RICHARDSON S
     1977
     Immunobiology of primary intracranial tumors. Part 1: Studies of the
     cellular and humoral general immune competence of brain-tumor patients.
     J Neurosurg 46:467-476
156. MAHALEY MS, STEINBOK P, ARONIN P, DUDKA L, ZINN D 1981
     Immunobiology of primary intracranial tumors. Part 4: Levamisole as
     an immune stimulant in patients and in the ASV glioma model.
     J Neurosurg 54:220-227
157. MANCUSO TF 1963
     Tumors of the central nervous system. Industrial considerations.
     Acta Unio Int Contra Cancer 19:488-489
158. MANSUY L, ALLÈGRE G, COURJON J, TOMMASI M, THIERRY A 1967
     Analyse d'une série opératoire de 49 oligodendrogliomes. Avec 3
     localisations infratentorielles.
     Neurochirurgie 13:679-700
159. MANSUY L, THIERRY A, TOMMASI M 1975
     Oligodendrogliomas.
     In: Vinken PJ, Bruyn GW (eds) Handbook of Clinical Neurology.
     North-Holland Publ Co, Amsterdam vol 18:81-103
160. MARK J, PONTÉN J, WESTERMARK B 1974a
     A G-band analysis of an established cell line of a human malignant
     glioma.
     Humangenetik 22:323-326
161. MARK J, PONTÉN J, WESTERMARK B 1974b
     Origin of the marker chromosomes in an established hypotriploid
     glioma cell line studied with G-band technique.
     Acta Neuropathol 29:223-228

162. MARK J, PONTÉN J, WESTERMARK B 1974c
     Cytogenetical studies with G-band technique of established cell
     lines of human malignant gliomas.
     Hereditas 78:304-308
163. MARK J, WESTERMARK B, PONTÉN J, HUGOSSON R 1977
     Banding patterns in human glioma cell lines.
     Hereditas 87:243-260
164. MAYO CM, BARRAN KD 1966
     Concurrent glioma and primary intracranial sarcoma.
     Neurology 16:662-672
165. MAYR E, DIAMOND LK, LEVINE RP, MAYR M 1956
     Suspected correlation between bloodgroup frequency and pituitary
     adenomas.
     Science 124:932-934
166. McFARLAND J, MEADE TS 1932
     The genetic origin of tumors supported by their simultaneous and
     symmetrical occurrence in homologous twins.
     Am J Med Sci 184:66-80
167. MEINKE W, GOLDSTEIN DA, SMITH RA 1979
     Simian virus 40-related DNA sequences in a brain tumor.
     Neurology 29:1590-1594
168. MENNEL HD, ZÜLCH KJ 1972
     Formale Pathogenese experimenteller Hirntumoren.
     Acta Neuropathol (Berl) 21:140-153
169. MENZIES CB, THOMAS DGT, BEHAN PO 1980
     Impaired thymus-derived lymphocytic function in patients with
     malignant brain tumour.
     Clin Neurol Neurosurg 82:157-168
170. METZEL E 1963
     Uber die familiär gehäuften Gliome.
     Arch Psychiat Nervenkr 204:537-555
171. METZEL E 1964
     Betrachtungen zur Genetik der familiären Gliome.
     Acta Genet Med Gemellol 13:124-132
172. MEYER R 1956
     Vorkommen von Hirntumoren bei Zwillingen und in Familien
     (statistische Erhebungen in einer unausgelesenen Serie von 459
     männlichen Hirntumorträgern).
     Thesis, Münster, Germany
173. MILLER RW 1966
     Relation between cancer and congenitaL defects in man.
     N Engl J Med 275:87-93
174. MILLER RW 1968
     Deaths from childhood cancer in sibs.
     N Engl J Med 279:122-126
175. MILLER RW 1971
     Deaths from childhood leukemia and solid tumors among twins and
     other sibs in the United States, 1960-67.
     J Natl Cancer Inst 46:203-209
176. MODAN B, BAIDATZ D, MART H, STEINITZ R, LEVIN SG 1974
     Radiation induced head and neck tumors.
     Lancet 1:277-279

177. MOERLOOSE Ph de, JEANNET M, MARTIN-ACHARD A, TRIBOLET N de, SEILER R, GUANELLA N 1978
HLA and glioma.
Tissue Antigens 12:146-148
178. MOERTEL CG 1966
Multiple primary malignant neoplasms. Their incidence and significance.
Springer, New York p 103
179. MORANTZ RA, SHAIN W 1978
Trauma and Brain Tumors: An Experimental Study.
Neurosurgery 3:181-186
180. MULCAHY GM, HARLAN WL 1976
Occurrences of central nervous system tumors, with special reference to relative genetic factors.
In: Lynch HT (ed) Cancer Genetics.
Charles C Thomas, Springfield, Ill p 263-325
181. MUNK J, PEYSER E, GRUSKIEWICA J 1969
Radiation-induced intracranial meningiomas.
Clin Radiol 20:90-94
182. MUNSLOW RA, HILL AH 1955
Multiple occurrences of gliomas in a family.
J Neurosurg 12:646-650
183. MYRIANTHOPOULOS NC 1981
Hemophilia A (classic hemophilia).
In: Vinken PJ, Bruyn GW (eds) Handbook of Clinical Neurology.
North-Holland Publ Co, Amsterdam vol 42:739-740
184. NAGASHIMA C, NAKASHIO K, FUJINO T 1963
Meningioma and astrocytoma adjacent in the brain.
J Neurosurg 20:995-999
185. NEBLETT CR, WALTZ TA, ANDERSON DE 1971
Neurological involvement in the nevoid basal cell carcinoma syndrome.
J Neurosurg 35:577-584
186. NOETZEL H 1959
Gliome bei zwei Geschwisterpaaren.
Zentralbl Neurochir 19:169-173
187. NOETZLI M, MALAMUD N 1962
Postirradiation fibrosarcoma of the brain.
Cancer 15:617-622
188. NORRIS FD, JACKSON EW 1970
Childhood cancer deaths in California-borns twins. A further report on types of cancer found.
Cancer 25:212-218
189. OEHLER F 1936
Über die Erblichkeit der ekto-mesodermalen Blastomatosen unter besonderer Berücksichtigung der familiären Hirntumoren.
Arch Psychiatr Nervenkr 1054:324-357
190. OHTA T, KAJIKAWA H, TAKEUCHI J 1977
Congenital tumours of the brain.
In: Vinken PJ, Bruyn GW (eds) Handbook of Clinical Neurology.
North-Holland Publ Co, Amsterdam vol 31:35-74
191. OMMAYA AK 1976
Immunotherapy of gliomas: A review.
Adv Neurol 15:337-357

458

192. OSTERTAG B   1936
    Einteilung und Charakteristik der Hirngewächse.
    Gustav Fischer, Jena
193. PADMALATHA C, HARRUFF RC, GANICK D, HAFEZ GR   1980
    Glioblastoma multiforme with tuberous sclerosis. Report of a case.
    Arch Pathol Lab Med 104:649-650
194. PAILLAS JE, COMBALBERT A, BERARD-BADIER M, BILLE J, FRANK R   1964
    Etude sur l'évolution des oligodendrogliomes de l'encéphale. A pro-
    pos d'une série opératoire de 34 cas.
    Acta Neurol Belg 64:537-551
195. PARKINSON D, HALL CW   1962
    Oligodendrogliomas. Simultaneous appearance in frontal lobes of
    siblings. Case reports.
    J Neurosurg 19:424-426
196. PASQUIER B, PASQUIER D, N'GOLET A, PANH MH, COUDERC P   1980
    Extraneural metastases of astrocytomas and glioblastomas. Clinico-
    pathological study of two cases and review of literature.
    Cancer 45:112-125
197. PASS KE   1938
    Erbpathologische Untersuchungen in Familien von Hirntumorkranken.
    Z ges Neurol Psychiatr 161:204-211
198. PATTERSON RH, CAMPBELL WG, PARSONS H   1961
    Ependymoma of the cauda equina with multiple visceral metastases.
    J Neurosurg 18:145-150
199. PEDERSEN O, GEYER H   1938
    Diskordantes Auftreten von Hirntumoren bei erbgleichen Zwillingen.
    Zentralbl Neurochir 2:53-63
200. PELGROM von MOTZ I, BOTS GTAM, ENDTZ LJ   1977
    Astrocytoma in three sisters.
    Neurology 27:1038-1041
201. PERCY AK, ELVEBACK LR, OKAZAKI H, KURLAND LT   1972
    Neoplasms of the central nervous system. Epidemiologic con-
    siderations.
    Neurology 22:40-48
202. PEYSER E, BELLER AJ   1951
    Brain tumors in two brothers.
    Acta Med Orient (Tel-Aviv) 10:229-232
203. PITTRICH H   1941
    Stirnhirngeschwülste.
    Archiv für Psychiatrie 113:1-60
204. POSER CM   1956
    The relationship between syringomyelia and neoplasm.
    Charles C Thomas, Springfield, Ill
205. POUILLART P, PALANGHIE T, POISSON M, BUGE A, HUGUENIN P, MORIN P,
    GAUTIER H   1979
    Treatment of adult malignant gliomas.
    Recent Results Cancer Res 68:399-407
206. RABOTTI GF, GOGUSEV J, TEUTSCH B, MONGIAT, LARDEMER F, HAGUENAU F
    1978
    Transformation in vitro of glial hamster cells by Rous sarcoma
    virus.
    J Natl Cancer Inst 60:113-124

207. RABOTTI GF, GROVE AS, SELLERS RL, ANDERSON WR 1966b
     Induction of multiple brain tumours (gliomata and leptomeningeal
     sarcomata) in dogs by Rous sarcoma virus.
     Nature 209:884-886
208. RABOTTI GF, RAINE WA 1964
     Brain tumours induced in hamsters inoculated intracerebrally at
     birth with Rous sarcoma virus.
     Nature 209:524-525
209. RABOTTI GF, SELLERS RL, ANDERSON WR 1966a
     Leptomeningeal sarcomata and gliomata induced in rabbits by Rous
     sarcoma virus.
     Nature 209:524-525
210. RASMUSSEN TB, KERNOHAN JW, ADSON AW 1940
     Pathologic classification with surgical consideration of intra-
     spinal tumors.
     Ann Surg III:513-530
211. RECONDO J de, HAGUENAU M 1972
     Neuropathologic survey of the phakomatoses and other disorders.
     In: Vinken PJ, Bruyn GW (eds) Handbook of Clinical Neurology.
     North-Holland Publ Co, Amsterdam vol 14:19-101
212. REGELSON W, BROSS IDJ, HANANIAN J, NIGOGOSYAN G 1965
     Incidence of second primary tumors in children with cancer and
     leukemia. A seven-year survey of 150 consecutive autopsied cases.
     Cancer 18:58-72
213. REGGIANI R, SOLIMÉ F, DEL VIVO RE, NIZZOLI V 1971
     Intracerebral oligodendroglioma with metastatic involvement of the
     spinal cord. Case report.
     J Neurosurg 35:610-613
214. RENKAWEK K, KROH H, KRÁSNICKA Z 1972
     Experimental gliomas cultured in vitro. Morphological and histoche-
     mical study.
     Z Krebforsch 77:247-256
215. RIBBERT H 1904
     Geschwulstlehre.
     Cohen, Bonn (cited by Zülch 1956 and 1974)
216. RICCARDI VM 1981
     Von Recklinghausen neurofibromatosis.
     N Engl J Med 305:1617-1627
217. RIDLEY A, CAVANAGH JB 1971
     Lymphocytic infiltration in gliomas: evidence of possible host
     resistance.
     Brain 94:117-124
218. RIESE W, MEREDITH JM, ZFASS IS 1944
     Cerebral glioma in siblings.
     South Med J 37:424-428
219. RINGERTZ N, REYMOND A 1949
     Ependymomas and choroid plexus papillomas.
     J Neuropathol Exp Neurol 8:355-380
220. RINGKJOB R 1968
     Treatment of intracranial gliomas and metastatic carcinomas by local
     application of cytostatic agents.
     Acta Neurol Scand 441:318-322

460

221. RODA JE, HEREDERO JJ, VILLAREJO FJ, RODA JM   1980
     Tumoural antigens on experimental and human glioblastoma.
     Acta Neurochir (Wien) 53:187-204
222. RODRIGUEZ HA, BERTHRONG M   1966
     Multiple primary intracranial tumors in von Recklinghausens's neuro-
     fibromatosis.
     Arch Neurol 14:467-475
223. ROTHMAN D, KENDALL AB   1975
     Dilemma in a case of Turcot's (glioma-polyposis) syndrome: report of
     a case.
     Dis Colon Rectum 18:514-515
224. RUBENSTEIN AE, MYTILINEAU C, YAHR MD, REVOLTELLA RP   1981
     Neurological aspects of neurofibromatosis.
     Adv Neurol 29:11-21
225. RUBINSTEIN LJ   1972
     Tumors of the central nervous system.
     In: Atlas of tumor pathology, 2nd series, Fasc 6.
     Armed Forces Inst of Pathol, Washington DC p 1-126
226. RUBINSTEIN LJ, LOGAN WJ   1970
     Extraneural metastases in ependymoma of the cauda equina.
     J Neurol Neurosurg Psychiatry 33:763-770
227. RUSSEL DS, RUBINSTEIN LJ   1977
     Pathology of the Tumours of the nervous system, 4th ed.
     Edward Arnold, London p 146-283
228. SAHAR A, STREIFLER M   1966
     Multiple intracranial tumours of diverse origin.
     Neurochirurgia 9:18-27
229. SALEMAN M   1980
     Survival in glioblastoma: historical perspective.
     Neurosurgery 7:435-439
230. SCHARRER E, BRUNNGRABER CV   1973
     Gliome bei Vater und Sohn.
     Z Neurol 205:287-205
231. SCHERER HJ   1940
     Cerebral astrocytomas and their derivatives.
     Am J Cancer 40:159-198
232. SCHIMKE RN   1978
     Genetics and cancer in man.
     Churchill Livingstone, Edinburgh p 95-103
233. SCHNECK SA, PENN I   1971
     De-novo brain tumours in renal-transplant recipients.
     Lancet I:983-086
234. SCHOENBERG BS, CHRISTINE BW, WHISNANT J   1976
     The descriptive epidemiology of primary intracranial neoplasms: the
     Connecticut experience.
     Am J Epidemiol 104:499-510
235. SCHREIBER D, WARZOK R, GÜTHERT H, SCHNEIDER J   1980
     Tumoren des Zentralnervensystems im Biopsie- und Autopsiegut.
     4. Mitteilung: Glioblastome.
     Zentralbl Allg Pathol 124:416-423
236. SCHREIBER D, WARZOK R, GÜTHERT H   1981
     Tumors of the CNS in biopsy and autopsy material.
     5th communication: oligodendrogliomas.
     Zentralbl Allg Pathol 125:12-18

237. SCHREIER HA, SHERRY N, SHAUGHNESSY E 1977
     Lead poisoning and brain tumors in children: a report of 2 cases.
     Ann Neurol 1:599-600
238. SCHRÖDER R, MÜLLER W, BONIS G, VORREITH M 1970
     Statistische Beiträge zum Grading der Gliome. III. Astrozytome und
     Oligodendrogliome.
     Acta Neurochir 23:1-29
239. SCHUMAN LM, CHOI NW, GULLEN WH 1967
     Relationship of central nervous system neoplasms to toxoplasma gon-
     dii infection.
     Am J Public Health 57:848-856
240. SEDGWICK RP, BODER E 1972
     Ataxia telangiectasia.
     In: Vinken PJ, Bruyn GW (eds) Handbook of Clinical Neurology
     North-Holland Publ Co, Amsterdam vol 14:267-339
241. SELVERSTONE B, COOPER DR 1961
     Astrocytomas and ABO blood groups.
     J Neurosurg 18:602-604
242. SHAPIRO WR, YOUNG DF 1976
     Treatment of malignant glioma. A controlled study of chemotherapy
     and irradiation.
     Arch Neurol 33:494-500
243. SHEIKH KMA, APUZZO MLJ, WEIRS MH 1979
     Specific cellular immune responses in patients with malignant glioma.
     Cancer Res 39:1729-1734
244. SHELINE GE 1977
     Radiation therapy of brain tumors.
     Cancer 39:873-881
245. SHUSTER J, HARTZ Z, STIMSON CW, BROUGH AJ, POULIK MD 1966
     Ataxia telangiectasia with cerebellar tumor.
     Pediatrics 37:776-786
246. SIMA AAF, ROBERTSON DM 1979
     Subependymal giant-cell astrocytoma.
     J Neurosurg 50:240-245
247. SLOOFF JL, KERNOHAN JW, MACCARTY CS 1964
     Primary intramedullary tumors of the spinal cord and filum ter-
     minale.
     WB Saunders Co, Philadelphia p 43-61
248. SLOWIK F, BALOGH I 1980
     Extracranial spreading of glioblastoma multiforme.
     Zentralbl Neurochir 41:57-68
249. SMITH DR, HARDMAN JM, EARLE KM 1969
     Metastasizing neuroectodermal tumours of the central nervous system.
     J Neurosurg 31:50-58
250. SMITH KO, NEWMAN JT, STORY JL, WISSINGER JD 1974
     Viruses and brain tumors.
     Clin Neurosurg 21:362-382
251. SOGG RL, DONALDSON SS, YORKE CH 1978
     Malignant astrocytoma following radiotherapoy of a cranio-
     pharyngioma. Case report.
     J Neurosurg 48:622-627
252. SOLOMON A, PERRET GE, McGORMICK WF 1969
     Multicentric gliomas of the cerebral and cerebellar hemispheres.
     J Neurosurg 31:87-93

253. SPRIGGS AI, BODDINGTON MM, CLARKE CM 1962
     Chromosomes of human cancer cells.
     Br Med J 2:1431-1435
254. STARZL TE, PENN I, PUTNAM CW, GROTH CG, HALGRIMSON CG 1971
     Iatrogenic alterations of immunologic surveillance in man and their
     influence on malignancy.
     Transplant Rev 7:112-145
255. STERTZ G, GEYER H 1937
     Zur Erbpathologie der spinalen Ataxie unter besonderer
     Berücksichtigung der "Status dysraphicus".
     Z Ges Neurol Psychiatr 157:795-806
256. STRONG AJ, SYMON L, MACGREGOR BJL, O'NEILL BP 1976
     Coincidental meningioma and glioma. Report of two cases.
     J Neurosurg 45:455-458
257. SULLA J, FAGULA J, STOPEKOVÁ, KUNDRÁT, VÝROSTKO J 1979
     Astrocytóm mozgu u dvoch súrodencov (astrocytoma of the brain in two
     siblings)
     Rozhl Chir 58:331-333
258. SYBERT VP, HALL JG 1979
     Inheritance of tuberous sclerosis.
     Lancet 7:783
259. SYMONDS C 1960
     Disease of mind and disorder of brain.
     Br Med J 2:1-5
260. TANGHETTI B, GATTA G, GIUNTA F, MARINI G 1980
     Multiple gliomas of the brain. Report of three cases.
     J Neurosurg Sci 24:155-159
261. THUMS K 1939
     Die Brauchbarkeit der Zwillingsmethode für die Erblichkeitsfor-
     schung bei Gehirntumoren.
     III Cong Neurol Intern Kopenhagen
262. THUWE I, LUNDSTRÖM B, WALINDER J 1979
     Familial brain tumour.
     Lancet 1:504
263. TODD DW, CHRISTOFERSON LA, LEECH RW, RUDOLF L 1981
     A family affected with intestinal polyposis and gliomas.
     Ann Neurol 10:390-392
264. TORRE E de la, ALEXANDER Jr E, DAVIS Jr CH, CRANDELL L 1963
     Tumors of the lateral ventricles of the brain. Report of eight
     cases, with suggestions for clinical management.
     J Neurosurg 20:461-470
265. TRIBOLET N de, DERUAZ JP, ZANDER E 1979
     Familial gliomas.
     Neurochirurgia 22:225-228
266. TROUILLAS P, LAPRAS C 1970
     Immunothérapie active des tumeurs cerebrales. A propos de 20 cas.
     Neurochirurgie 16:143-170
267. TURCOT J, DESPRÉS JP, StPIERRE F 1959
     Malignant tumors of the central nervous system associated with
     familial polyposis of the colon: report of two cases.
     Dis Colon Rectum 2:465-468
268. TUROWSKI K 1978
     Familial gliomas.
     Neurol Neurochir Pol 1:85-86

269. UNIO INTERNATIONALIS CONTRA CANCRUM 1959
     Histologische Nomenklatur menschlicher Tumoren.
     Z Krebforsch 63:75-98
270. UNIO INTERNATIONALIS CONTRA CANCRUM 1965
     Illustrated tumor nomenclature.
     Springer, Berlin
271. UNIO INTERNATIONALIS CONTRA CANCRUM 1969
     Illustrated tumor nomenclature. Second reviewed edition.
     Springer, Berlin
272. VERSLUYS JJ 1934
     Zwillingspathologischer Beitrag zur Ätiologie der Tumoren.
     Z Krebforsch 41:239-259
273. VOIGT K, MARQUARDT B 1979
     Angiographischer Nachweis infratentorieller Tumoren mit Konkordanter
     Manifestation, Lokalisation und Histologie bei eineiigen Zwillingen.
     Fortsch Röntgenstr 130:89-94
274. VOGT U 1972
     Neurologische Diagnose und Verlauf des Glioblastoms.
     Dtsch Med Wochenschr 97:717-722
275. WAGA S, HANDA H 1976
     Radiation-induced meningioma with review of literature.
     Surg Neurol 5:215-219
276. WALKER MD, RUMACK BH, ROSENBLUM ML 1971
     Malignant central nervous system tumour and other neoplasms in a
     large family.
     Neurology 21:440-441
277. WANNER O 1950
     Genealogische Überprüfung des Wesens der Geistesstörungen bei Hirn-
     tumor.
     Nervenarzt 21:252-254
278. WARD DW, MATTISON ML, FINN R 1973
     Association between previous tuberculous infection and cerebral
     glioma.
     Br Med J 1:83-84
279. WARZOK R, GÜTHERT H 1978
     Die Tumoren des Zentralnervensystems im Biopsie- und Autopsiegut.
     I. Mitteilung: Häufigkeit, Alters- und Geschlechtsverteilung.
     Zentralbl Allg Pathol 122:462-474
280. WARZOK R, GÜTHERT H, SCHREIBER D 1979
     Tumoren des Zentralnervensystems im Biopsie- und Autopsiegut.
     3. Mitteilung: Astrozytome.
     Zentralbl Allg Pathol 123:553-561
281. WATTS C 1976
     Meningioma following irradiation.
     Cancer 38:1939-1940
282. WECHSLER W, KLEIHUES P, MATSUMOTO S, ZÜLCH KJ, IVANKOVIC S,
     PREUSSMANN R, DRUCKREY H 1969
     Pathology of experimental neurogenic tumors chemically induced
     during prenatal and postnatal life.
     Ann NY Acad Sci 159:360-408
283. WEERDT de CJ, SCHUT T 1972
     Some aspects of heredity of brain tumours.
     Psychiatr Neurol Neurochir (Amst) 75:293-298

284. WEIR B 1973
     The relative significance of factors affecting postoperative sur-
     vival in astrocytomas, grades 3 and 4.
     J Neurosurg 38:448-452
285. WEIR B, BAND P, URTASUN R, BLAIN G, McLEAN D, WILSON F, MIELKE B,
     GRACE M 1976
     Radiotherapy and CCNU in the treatment of high-grade supratentorial
     astrocytomas.
     J Neurosurg 45:129-134
286. WIEL HJ van der 1959
     Inheritance of glioma.
     Thesis, Elsevier, Amsterdam
287. WILKINS RH, ODAN GL 1965
     Attempted induction of gliomas utilizing Simian virus 40.
     Arch Neurol 13:149-154
288. WILSON CB, KAUFMANN L, BARKER M 1970
     Chromosome analysis of glioblastoma multiforme.
     Neurology 20:821-828
289. YAMADA K, TAKAGI N, SANDBERG AA 1966
     Chromosomes and causation of human solid tumors.
     Cancer 19:1879-1890
290. YATES PO, PEARCE KM 1960
     Recent change in bloodgroup distribution of astrocytomas.
     Lancet 1:194-195
291. YOSHIDA J, CRAVIOTO H 1978
     Nitrosurea-induced brain tumours: An in vivo and in vitro tumor
     model system.
     J Natl Cancer Inst 61:365-374
292. YOUNG RR, AUSTEN KF, MOSER HW 1964
     Abnormalities of serum gamma I A globulin and ataxia telangiec-
     tasia.
     Medicine (Baltimore) 43:423-433
293. YUNG WA, HORTEN BC, SHAPIRO WR 1980
     Meningeal gliomatosis: A review of 12 cases.
     Ann Neurol 8:605-608
294. ZAWORSKI RE, OYASU R 1973
     Lead Concentration in Human Brain Tissue. An Autopsy Study.
     Arch Environ Health 27:383-386
295. ZELLWEGER H 1977
     Down syndrome.
     In: Vinken PJ, Bruyn GW (eds) Handbook of Clinical Neurology.
     North-Holland Publ Co, Amsterdam vol 31:367-470
296. ZIMMERMAN HM, ARNOLD H 1943
     Experimental brain tumors. II.Tumors produced with benzpyrene.
     Am J Pathol 19:939-955
297. ZÜLCH KJ 1951
     Die Hirngeschwülste.
     Johann Ambrosius Barth, Leipzig (cited by Koch 1954)
298. ZÜLCH KJ 1951
     Vorzugssitz, Erkrankungsalter und Geschlechtsbevorzugung bei
     Hirngeschwülsten als bisher ungeklärte Formen der Pathoklise.
     Dtsch Z Nervenheilk 166:91-102

299. ZÜLCH KJ 1956
     Biologie und Pathologie der Hirngeschwülste.
     In: Olivecrona H, Tönnis W (eds) Handbuch der Neurochirurgie, Bd III
     Springer, Berlin
300. ZÜLCH KJ 1965
     Brain tumours. Their biology and pathology. 2nd ed.
     Springer, Berlin
301. ZÜLCH KJ 1969
     Biology and morphology of glioblastoma multiforme.
     Acta Radiol Ther Phys Biol 8:65-77
302. ZÜLCH KJ 1980
     Principles of the new World Health Organization (WHO) classification
     of brain tumors.
     Neuroradiology 19:59-66
303. ZÜLCH KJ, MENNEL HGD 1971
     Gehirntumor und Trauma.
     Hefte Unfallheilkd 107:33-44
304. ZÜLCH KJ, MENNEL HD 1974
     The biology of brain tumours.
     In: Vinken PJ, Bruyn GW (eds) Handbook of Clinical Neurology
     North-Holland Publ Co, Amsterdam vol 16:1-55

Additional references

305. ADELOYE A 1979
     Neoplasms of the brain in the African.
     Surg Neurol 11:247-255
306. ANNEGERS JF, KURLAND LT, HAUSER WA 1979
     Brain tumors in children exposed to barbiturates (letter to the
     editor).
     J Natl Cancer Inst 63:3
307. BING R, HAYMAEKER W 1939
     Textbook of nervous diseases.
     CV Mosby Co, St. Louis
308. BRADY WJ 1962
     Brain stem gliomas causing hydrocephalus in twins with von
     Recklinghausen's disease.
     J Neuropathol Exp Neurol 21:555-565
309. CLEMMESEN J, HJALGRIM-JENSEN S 1978
     Is phenobarbital carcinogenic? A follow-up of 8,078 epileptics.
     Ecotoxocol Environ Safety 1:457-470
310. CLEMMESEN J, HJALGRIM-JENSEN S 1981
     Brain tumors in children exposed to barbiturates (letter to the
     editor).
     J Natl Cancer Inst 66:215
311. GILLESPIE R, MAHALEY Jr MS 1981
     Brain tumors: gliomas, pituitary tumors, pineal region tumors, and
     metastatic tumors.
     In: Appel SH (ed) Current Neurology
     John Wiley and Sons, New York vol 3:420-453
312. GOLD EB, GORDIS L 1979
     Patterns of incidence of brain tumours in children.
     Ann Neurol 5:565-568

313. GOLD E, GORDIS L, TONASCIA J, SZKLO M 1978
     Increased risk of brain tumors in children exposed to barbiturates.
     J Natl Cancer Inst 61:1031-1034
314. GOLD EB, GORDIS L, TONASCIA JA, SZKLO M 1979
     Brain tumors in children exposed to barbiturates (letter to the
     editor).
     J Natl Cancer Inst 63:3-4
315. GOLD E, GORDIS L, TONASCIA J, SZKLO M 1979
     Risk factors for brain tumors in children.
     Am J Epidemiol 109:309-319
316. GORLIN RJ, SEDANO HO 1977
     Syndromes of skeletal anomalies with CNS malformations.
     In: Vinken PJ, Bruyn GW (eds) Handbook of Clinical Neurology.
     North-Holland Publ Co, Amsterdam vol 31:236-238
317. JANISCH W, ROTH FW, FELECETTI D 1979
     Pathogenetic factors in the induction of brain tumors by nitro-
     soureas. In: Paoletti P, Walker MD, Butti G, Knerich R (eds) Multi-
     disciplinary aspects of brain tumor therapy.
     North-Holland Publ Co, Amsterdam p 9-14
318. KAISER J, GULLOTTA F 1980
     Kupferbestimmung in Astrozytomen und Glioblastomen mit Cuproin.
     Neurochirurgia 23:20-23
319. LAMPERTH-SEILER E 1974
     Harnweg- und Hirntumoren bei Gummiarbeitern.
     Schweiz Med Wochenschr 104:1655-1659
320. LONDON WT, HOUFF SA, MADDEN DL, FUCCILLO DA, GRAVELL M, WALLEN WC,
     PALMER AE, SEVER JL 1978
     Brain tumors in Owl Monkeys inoculated with a human polyomavirus
     (JC-virus).
     Science 201:1246-1249
321. LYNCH HT, KRUSH AJ, THOMAS RJ, LYNCH J 1976
     Cancer family syndrome. In: Lynch HT (ed) Cancer genetics.
     Charles C Thomas, Springfield, Ill p 355-388
322. MANUELIDIS EE 1972
     Genetics of glioblastomas. In: Minckler J (ed) Pathology of the ner-
     vous system.
     McGraw-Hill, New York vol 3:2917-2926
323. PENN J 1976
     Second malignant neoplasms associated with immunosuppressive medica-
     tions.
     Cancer 37:1024-1032
324. RADOS A 1946
     Occurrence of glioma of retina and brain in collateral lines in same
     family.
     Arch Ophthalmol 35:1-12
325. REAGAN TJ, FREIMAN IS 1973
     Multiple cerebral gliomas in multiple sclerosis.
     J Neurol Neurosurg Psychiatry 36:523-528
326. SCHIANCHI P, KRAUS-RUPPERT R 1980
     Familial brain tumors: rhombencephalon-astrocytoma grade I in father
     and son.
     Acta Neuropathol (Berl) 52:153-155

327. SCHOENBERG BS, GLISTA GG, REAGAN TJ   1975
      The familial occurrence of glioma.
      Surg Neurol 3:139-145
328. SIMS WL, MARX MB, BROOKS WH   1979
      A follow-up study of the geographic distribution of selected
      malignancies among Kentucky residents, 1969-1976.
      J Natl Med Ass 71:685
329. TUROWSKI K, CZOCHRA M   1979
      ABO bloodgroups in glioblastoma multiforme.
      Neurol Neurochir Pol XIII:173-176
330. WENT LN   1981
      Retinoblastoma.
      In: Vinken PJ, Bruyn GW (eds) Handbook of Clinical Neurology.
      North-Holland Publ Co, Amsterdam vol 42:768-769
331. WILKINS RH   1972
      Genetic factors related to the induction and hereditary transmission
      of primary intracranial neoplasms.
      In: Kirsch WM, Grossi-Paoletti E, Paoletti P (eds) The experimental
      biology of brain tumors.
      Charles C Thomas, Springfield, Ill p 551-560

468

STANDARD REQUEST FORM

Dear Colleague,

We are compiling a "Commented Register of Familial Brain Tumours" to be published in 1981 or 1982 by Martinus Nijhoff Publishers.
        0   Reference will be made in this publication to your report which appeared in:

        0   We have been informed that one or more patients with familial brain tumour have been under your care. According to this information:

If possible we would like to receive additional information in regard to the categories marked below:
- relationship of family members
- race or nationality of patient
- age of symptom occurrence
- if performed, operation procedure and result
- age at operation
- age at death
- diagnosis
- method of diagnosis establishment (biopsy, autopsy, histology)
- neoplasm location
- clinical course
- associated physical or mental conditions
- number of unaffected siblings
- complete description of case
- familial data

For your convenience a reply-form is provided with this letter.
        We thank you for your kind cooperation.

        Sincerely yours,

L.J. Endtz, M.D.   M.R. Halprin, M.D.   C.C. Tijssen, M.D.

REPLY-FORM

Please return this form to:

                  C.C. Tijssen, M.D.
                  Department of Neurology
                  Municipal Hospital Leyenburg
                  Leyweg 275
                  THE HAGUE, The Netherlands

Additional information concerning

          0   cases published in:

          0   unpublished cases

relationship of
family members

race or nationality

age of symptom occurrence

operation procedure

age at operation

age at death

diagnosis

biopsy

autopsy

histology

neoplasm location

clinical course

associated physical or
mental conditions

number of unaffected siblings

familial data

        0   I give permission to use the information
mentioned above in a "Commented Register on Familial Brain Tumours"
edited by C.C. Tijssen, M.R. Halprin and L.J. Endtz, the reference to
be quoted as "personal communication".
        0   I give permission to reproduce diagram/
  photo/table/figure: of our publication which appeared in:
                     in the "Commented Register" mentioned above.

                Signed,

INTERNATIONAL REGISTER OF FAMILIAL BRAIN TUMOURS (IRFBT)

Comprehensive Cancer Centre
Vondellaan 47
2332 AA Leyden, The Netherlands

Cases of familial brain tumours published until 1982 have
been assembled in 'Familial Brain Tumours, a Commented
Register' (Martinus Nijhoff Publishers, The Hague, 1982).
The IRFBT is engaged in the active search for new cases
of familial brain tumours and would like to invite clinicians worldwide to submit reports, either published or
unpublished, to this register. Care will be taken to update the register at appropriate times.

The IRFBT would appreciate receiving information concerning new reports of
familial brain tumours in regard to the following categories:
- gender
- relationship of family members
- race or nationality
- age of symptom occurrence
- operation procedure
- age at operation
- age at death
- diagnosis
- biopsy
- autopsy
- histology
- neoplasm location
- clinical course
- associated physical or mental conditions
- number of unaffected siblings
- familial data
- genetic studies
- other epidemiological factors

Please enclose permission for use or reproduction of your material with
your communication.

On behalf of the IRFBT:

C.C. Tijssen, M.D.

M.R. Halprin, M.D.

L.J. Endtz, M.D.